ELECTROCONVULSIVE THERAPY

ELECTROCONVULSIVE THERAPY

Third Edition

Richard Abrams, M.D.

UNIVERSITY OF HEALTH SCIENCES

THE CHICAGO MEDICAL SCHOOL

New York   Oxford

OXFORD UNIVERSITY PRESS

1997

Oxford University Press

Oxford   New York
Athens   Auckland   Bangkok   Bogota   Bombay   Buenos Aires
Calcutta   Cape Town   Dar es Salaam   Delhi   Florence   Hong Kong
Istanbul   Karachi   Kuala Lumpur   Madras   Madrid   Melbourne
Mexico City   Nairobi   Paris   Singapore   Taipei   Tokyo   Toronto

and associated companies in
Berlin   Ibadan

Copyright © 1988, 1992, 1997 by Richard Abrams, M.D.

Published by Oxford University Press, Inc.
198 Madison Avenue, New York, New York 10016

Oxford is a registered trademark of Oxford University Press

Library of Congress Cataloging-in-Publication Data
Abrams, Richard, 1937–
Electroconvulsive therapy / Richard Abrams.—3rd ed.
p.   cm.   Includes bibliographical references and index.
ISBN 0-19-510944-9
1. Electroconvulsive therapy.   I. Title.
[DNLM: 1. Electroconvulsive Therapy.
WM 412 A161e   1997]   RC485.A27   1997
616.89'122—dc21   DNLM/DLC   for Library of Congress   96-36879

2   4   6   8   9   7   5   3

Printed in the United States of America
on acid-free paper

*For Karen, Deirdre,
Jessina, Erin, Kemo,
and Matilda*

Preface

Of the more than 500 articles on ECT I reviewed since the second edition of this book—more than enough to justify a third edition—the present revision references about a quarter, requiring more than 20,000 new words to integrate and present the information they contain. Reading these articles, one is struck by how many address those technical and medical aspects of treatment that have emerged as central to the primary aim of most clinical ECT research for the last several decades: improving efficacy while reducing side-effects.

Now clinicians desiring to optimize the therapeutic ratio of their treatment must, in selecting electrical stimulus parameters and monitoring electroencephalographic response patterns, exercise a sophistication heretofore unknown, and certainly untaught even today in most residency training programs.

The inherent safety of ECT, augmented by routine oximetry and electrocardiographic monitoring, enables appropriately trained clinicians to administer it successfully to patients traditionally believed to be too old or infirm to withstand the rigors of induced convulsions—the "high-risk" geriatric-cardiac patient who is rapidly becoming the modal candidate for ECT in university hospitals everywhere.

Clearly, the time is long past when clinicians giving ECT could just "push the button" and hope for the best. Indeed, the degree of technical and medical sophistication now required for proper administration of this therapy may be daunting to some older practitioners, however experienced, who have not kept up. It is for them, as well as the younger graduates whose residency training programs have failed to instruct them adequately, or at all, in this most medical of psychiatric therapies, that this book is intended.

Chicago, IL   R.A.
February 12, 1997

Contents

ELECTROCONVULSIVE THERAPY

1

History of Electroconvulsive Therapy

The traditional litany on the history of the medical uses of electricity, beginning with the Roman use of electric fish to treat headaches (Harms, 1956; Sandford, 1966; Brandon, 1981), is simply beside the point; electroconvulsive therapy (ECT) evolved solely as a result of Ladislaus von Meduna's original investigations on the effects of camphor-induced convulsions in schizophrenic patients. It is the chronology of the medical (and specifically, psychiatric) uses of convulsions that provides the appropriate historical perspective to his work.

This chapter draws extensively and often without specific attribution from the excellent historical reviews of the subject by Mowbray (1959), Sandford (1966), Fink (1979, 1984), Brandon (1981), Kalinowsky (1982, 1986), Endler (1988), and Endler and Persad (1988); from Cerletti's (1950) personal recollections; from the English translations of the autobiography of Meduna (1985); from Accornero's (1990) eyewitness account of the discovery of ECT; and from my own numerous conversations over 25 years, and my published interview with, Lothar Kalinowsky (Abrams, 1988).

According to Mowbray (1959), Paracelsus, the sixteenth-century Swiss physician and alchemist, "... gave camphor by mouth to produce convulsions and to cure lunacy." The first published citation, however, is generally attributed to Leopold von Auenbrugger, the originator of the percussion method of examining the heart and lungs, who, in 1764, treated "mania vivorum" with camphor every 2 hours to the point of convulsions (Mowbray, 1959; Sandford, 1966). The next publication (and the first in English) was by one Dr. Oliver, whose case report in 1785 in the *London Medical Journal* described the successful use of camphor in a patient who had been "seized with mania with few intervals of reason" (Kalinowsky, 1982). Fifteen minutes after a

3

single dose of camphor, the patient had a grand mal seizure and awakened in a rational state. The case was later cited by Burrows in his 1828 textbook, *Commentaries on Insanity*:

> In a case of insanity, where two scruples [of camphor] were exhibited, it produced a fit and a perfect cure followed. When given to the same gentleman two years afterwards, upon a relapse, i.e., a recurrence, it had the same effect, even to an alarming degree; but the patient did not, as before, progressively recover from a single dose, for it was repeated afterwards in smaller doses of ten grains.

Next came Weickhardt, a councilor of the Russian Imperial College, who reported in a Viennese textbook in 1798 that he had obtained cures in 8 out of 10 cases of mania with camphor-induced seizures (Mowbray, 1959; Sandford, 1966; Meduna, 1985). The last citation given before the method fell into obscurity for almost a century is from an unpublished 1851 manuscript in Hungarian by a Dr. Szekeres, who described the technique for treating mania recommended by a Dr. Pauliczky, who gave

> ... camphor, beginning with a dose of 10 grains and increasing the dosage by five grains daily up to 60 grains a day. After this the patient will have dizziness and epileptic attacks. When he awakes from these, his reasoning will return (Sandford, 1966).

An English translation of Meduna's autobiography (1985) reveals that none of this work was known to Meduna until a year after he had published his first report on induced seizure therapy in schizophrenia, at which time a Hungarian psychiatrist accused him of plagiarizing Weickhardt's eighteenth-century ideas. Stung by the unfairness of the accusation, which was subsequently published in a Hungarian medical journal, Meduna says

> ... I began to read old manuscripts and found that the convulsive method had been used 20 years before Weickhardt by Auenbrugger ... I found other reports: Simmon, whose nationality I could not ascertain, used camphor to produce epileptic attacks to cure insanity; as did Pauliczky, a Polish scientist of the 18th century, and a Dr. Laroze of Paris, probably at the beginning of the 19th century.

Meduna's decision to treat schizophrenic patients by inducing epileptic seizures stemmed directly from the results of neuropathologic studies (Meduna, 1932) in which he observed an "overwhelming and almost crushing growth of the glial cells" in the brains of epileptic patients compared with an equally evident lack of glial-cell growth in the brains of schizophrenic patients. He thought these observations to be evidence of a "biological antagonism" and decided to pursue this line of inquiry further. He was encouraged in this approach by a friend and colleague, Dr. Julius Nyirö, who had observed that epileptic patients had a much better prognosis if they were also diagnosed as having schizophrenia; Dr. Nyirö actually had attempted (unsuccessfully) to treat epileptic patients with injections of blood from schizophrenic patients (Nyirö and Jablonszky, 1929). Not mentioned by Meduna in his autobiography or in Fink's (1984) historical review is Mowbray's (1959) assertion that these earlier authors also had reported using pentylenetetrazol to produce convulsions in their schizophrenic patients.

After unsatisfactory animal trials of strychnine, thebaine, nikethamide, caffeine, brucine, and absinthe (!), Meduna learned from the International League Against Epilepsy that one of its officers had written a monograph about producing artificial convulsions with camphor monobromide. Choosing the less toxic simple camphor, Meduna successfully produced experimental epilepsy in guinea pigs (Meduna, 1934). Two months later, on January 23, 1934, Meduna injected camphor in oil into a schizophrenic patient who had been in a catatonic stupor for 4 years, never moving, never eating, being incontinent, and requiring tube-feeding.

> After 45 minutes of anxious and fearful waiting the patient suddenly had a classical epileptic attack that lasted 60 seconds. During the period of observation I was able to maintain my composure and to make the necessary examinations with apparent calm and detached manner. I examined his reflexes, the pupils of his eyes, and was able to dictate my observations to the doctors and nurses around me; but when the attack was over and the patient recovered his consciousness, my legs suddenly gave out. My body began to tremble, a profuse sweat drenched me, and, as I later heard, my face was ashen gray.

Thus, convulsive therapy was born. The patient went on to full recovery after a short series of seizures, as did the next five patients treated; by the end of a year, Meduna had collected results, which he then published, from a sample of 26 schizophrenic patients: 10 who recovered, 3 who enjoyed good results, and 13 who did not change

(Fink, 1984). Meduna soon replaced camphor with the chemically related pentylenetetrazol (Cardiazol, Metrazol), which he preferred because of its solubility and rapid onset of action.

Pentylenetetrazol convulsive therapy spread rapidly throughout
Europe; however, the extremely unpleasant sensations induced in cons-
cious patients during the preictal (or myoclonic) phase of the treatment
soon led investigators in Rome to seek alternative methods of induction
(Cerletti, 1956). Von Fritsch and Hitzig had already demonstrated that
epileptic seizures could be produced in dogs by electrical stimulation
of the exposed brain, and von Schilf had suggested the feasibility of
producing convulsions in humans with extracerebral electrodes (Mowbray, 1959; Sandford, 1966).

In 1934, Chiauzzi, working in Cerletti's laboratory, produced seizures in animals by passing a 50-Hz, 220-V stimulus for 0.25 seconds
across electrodes placed in the mouth and rectum; in May of 1937, Bini,
another of Cerletti's assistants (and himself a fine clinician who later
wrote a leading Italian textbook on psychiatry), reported similar animal
studies at an international meeting in Münsingen, Switzerland, on new
therapies for schizophrenia. About 50% of the dogs thus stimulated died,
and, according to Kalinowsky (1986), it was Bini who first realized the
danger of passing current through the heart with oral-rectal electrodes
and who demonstrated the safety of applying both electrodes to the
temples of the dogs he was studying. Bini confirmed this during a visit
with another of Cerletti's assistants, Fernando Accornero, to the Rome
slaughterhouse where, they had been told, pigs were killed by electricity.
In actuality, the pigs were first convulsed by an electrical stimulus to
the head and then dispatched while they were comatose. The fact that
such transcerebral electrical stimulation did not actually kill the pigs
provided encouragement for continued attempts by Cerletti and Bini to
define the electrical stimulus parameters that might be safe and effective
for application to humans (Cerletti, 1950; Accornero, 1988).

This goal was soon accomplished, and the first patient to receive
electroconvulsive therapy was a 39-year-old unidentified man found
wandering about the train station without a ticket. He was delusional,
hallucinating, and gesticulating, and alternated between periods of mutism and incomprehensible, neologistic speech (Cerletti, 1940, 1956).
After he was observed for several weeks, he was diagnosed as having
schizophrenia; he received his first treatment on 11 April 1938. Present
were Cerletti, Bini, and only one or two others. An initial stimulus of
80 V for 0.25 seconds was subconvulsive. Two subsequent stimuli of
the same voltage, but with durations of 0.5 and 0.75 seconds
each, were administered several minutes apart (Bini, 1938), despite the

statement of the patient that he did not want a third stimulus. No effect was observed on the patient, and no further attempts to induce a seizure were made that day. A few days later, a second attempt was made, this time with the entire research team in attendance. Again the initial stimulus was unintentionally subconvulsive (80 V for 0.2 seconds): The patient exhibited a brief myoclonic reaction without loss of consciousness and began to sing loudly. He lapsed into silence while those in attendance discussed what to do next, and then solemnly intoned clearly and without jargon, ''Not again, it's murderous!'' Despite this ominous warning, which understandably caused some apprehension among those present, the patient was restimulated at 110 V for 0.2 seconds and a grand mal seizure ensued. After awakening,

> The patient sat up of his own accord, looked about him calmly with a vague smile, as though asking what was expected of him. I asked him: ''What has been happening to you?'' He answered, with no more gibberish: ''I don't know; perhaps I have been asleep.''

The patient's eventual full recovery with a course of 11 ECTs was dramatic, but not the important contribution made by the Italian investigators—the striking effectiveness of induced convulsions had already been shown many times since 1934—rather, it was the demonstration that such convulsions could safely, reliably, and inexpensively be induced by electrical means, that constituted the technical advance for which Cerletti and Bini justly achieved fame, and that stimulated the rapid spread of this uniquely effective therapeutic modality.

Cerletti and Bini (1938) published their results a few months later in an Italian journal, but Bini (1938) enjoyed the first English-language publication on the topic when his paper on ''experimental researches on epileptic seizures induced by the electric current'' was published in a supplement to the *American Journal of Psychiatry*. (The topic was his research in dogs, but he alluded to the first use of ECT in man in the cryptic sentence: ''These experiments have so far been conducted almost exclusively in animals.'')

Introduction of Electroconvulsive Therapy to the United States

Present during the second ECT administered several days after the first was Lothar B. Kalinowsky, a young German psychiatrist who had left Berlin for Rome in 1933, when Hitler came to power. Along with Bini,

Accornero, and several other associates, Kalinowsky was a member of a research team that investigated the multiform effects of ECT on the organism and eventually published its results in a special issue of an Italian journal of experimental psychiatry (Cerletti, 1940). Kalinowsky left Rome with his wife in 1939—one jump ahead of the Nazis—and traveled extensively in Switzerland, France, Holland, and England before emigrating to the United States in 1940, where he received an appointment at the New York State Psychiatric Institute. While in England, he and Dr. J. Sanderson McGregor treated some patients at the Netherne Hospital at Coulsdon with a device constructed according to plans Kalinowsky brought with him from Rome; the results of this work provided the basis for the first English-language publications on the clinical use of ECT (Kalinowsky, 1939; Shepley and McGregor, 1939).

Kalinowsky was not the first to give ECT in the United States as all of the possessions that he had shipped, including his ECT device, were delayed for 10 years by the war. That honor belongs to Drs. Renato Almansi and David Impastato, who administered the first treatment at Columbus Hospital in New York City in early 1940, with a device Almansi had obtained in Rome (Almansi and Impastato, 1940). A few months later, Dr. Douglas Goldman—who subsequently invented nondominant unilateral ECT—demonstrated ECT at the annual meeting of the American Psychiatric Association (Fink, 1987). Later that same year, Kalinowsky—who by then had had another device built—started giving ECT at the Psychiatric Institute, which, because of its academic reputation as a research center, soon became a focal point for the spread of the new treatment method in this country.

As Fink (1979) pointed out, convulsive therapy burst on the scene during an era of unprecedented therapeutic optimism in psychiatry, following hard on the heels of Wagner-Jauregg's malarial fever therapy for general paresis of the insane (1917) and Klaesi's prolonged sleep therapy (1922), and virtually coeval with Sakel's insulin coma therapy (1933) and Moniz' psychosurgery (1935). One by one, the other treatments flourished briefly and then fell into desuetude, to be replaced by less complex and more definitive methods. Only ECT flourished and remains widely used to this day, doubtless because of its demonstrable efficacy, safety, and relative ease of administration, all due, in large measure, to the advances in technique (e.g., succinylcholine muscle relaxation, barbiturate anesthesia, oxygenation, unilateral electrode application, brief-pulse stimulation) that have been introduced over the years.

An analysis of National Institutes of Mental Health national survey data for the years 1975, 1980, and 1986 showed that the declining use of ECT ended in the 1980s (Thompson et al., 1994). In 1986, 36,558 patients received ECT, which represented a decrease from the 58,667 who received ECT in 1975, but an increase over 1980, when 31,514 patients were so treated. Strikingly, recipients of ECT were primarily older white patients in private institutions. The figures presented are doubtless underestimates of the true usage, primarily because of sampling error such as chance omission from the sample of a few large-volume ECT centers. The authors estimated that the 36,558 patients treated in 1986 received approximately 300,000 ECTs—equivalent to the number of procedures performed for coronary bypass, tonsillectomy, inguinal hernia, or appendectomy—thus making ECT one of the most common procedures carried out in patients given general anesthesia.

Analyzing data from the American Psychiatric Association Professional Activities survey of 1988–1989, Hermann et al. (1995) found that 1,102 psychiatrists reported treating 4,398 patients during the previous month. Extrapolating from these results, the authors estimated that 4.9 patients per 10,000 population received ECT annually—a modest increase over the 1978 American Psychiatric Association estimate of 4.4 per 10,000 population—yielding an estimate of 100,000 patients treated in the United States during the year studied.

Because ECT is given in virtually every other country of the world—and not infrequently at much higher rates of usage than in the United States—it is likely that between 1 and 2 million patients per year receive ECT worldwide.

Will ECT also be replaced by a less intrusive, pharmacologic, therapy that alters brain function in the desired direction (e.g., via a hypothalamic neuropeptide) but without the auxiliary convulsion and its attendant risks and drama? Perhaps, but, I think, not soon. The rate of accumulation of new techniques and discoveries in the application of neurotransmitter pharmacodynamics to the treatment of mentally ill patients (and depressives, in particular) has slowed considerably, and despite manufacturers' claims, no significant progress in the pharmacological treatment of major depression has occurred since the introduction of imipramine in 1958.

Moreover, incremental advances in the technique of ECT have refined the treatment to the point that, with high- or maximum-dose brief-pulse right unilateral ECT, many patients can now enjoy the full therapeutic benefit of ECT without the usual cognitive side effects that were so prominent with sine-wave bilateral ECT. Most importantly, those patients requiring bilateral ECT (as well as unilateral ECT) can now receive it in a more physiological form than before, using the smaller pulse widths, lower frequencies, and longer stimulus trains that are more consistent with the parameters of neuronal depolarization and recovery (Abrams, 1996), and therefore less likely to be neurotoxic.

It is more likely that in the foreseeable future, the application of increasingly sophisticated research methods will augment our understanding of the mechanisms inherent in the therapeutic action of ECT and promote continued refinement of its technique of administration. One such refinement already under consideration uses magnetic fields to induce electrical currents, and thereby seizures, in the brain (George and Wasserman, 1994; Sackeim, 1994c). Because the skull and its associated extra- and intracranial tissues are transparent to the magnetic field, rapid-rate transcranial magnetic stimulation can generate electrical stimuli directly in the brain without considerations of impedance or seizure threshold—most patients should require a similar dosage for seizure induction—and more physiologic stimulus parameters can be used. Because electrical currents are not passed directly through the temporal lobes, memory dysfunction should be reduced; because the magnetic coils permit more accurate focusing of the electrical fields generated in the brain, stimuli can be applied more accurately than is presently achievable via placement of external electrical treatment electrodes (e.g., as for bilateral or unilateral ECT).

2

Efficacy of Electroconvulsive Therapy

Experimental Data

It is axiomatic that rigorous experimental methods are required to demonstrate the efficacy of a medical treatment. Whether the comparison is with placebo (sham treatment) or with an alternative active therapy, a prospective design with random assignment of consecutive patients to treatment groups and blind assessment of outcome using objective measures are absolute requirements. Both the diagnostic criteria and the precise treatment parameters must be specified, and appropriate statistical analyses must be employed (or the data presented in sufficient detail for readers to perform their own calculations). Scrupulous adherence to these rules is especially crucial when studying an emotionally charged and physiologically active treatment such as ECT, for it is often used for illnesses (depression, mania) with a high spontaneous remission rate.

The first part of this chapter assesses the efficacy of ECT by reviewing the evidence from controlled trials in the three disorders for which such data are available: depression, schizophrenia, and mania. The results of uncontrolled or otherwise methodologically weak studies, anecdotal reports, and case history studies are referred to in the second part.

Depressive Illness

SHAM ELECTROCONVULSIVE THERAPY STUDIES

The studies of genuine versus sham ECT published through 1966 and reviewed by Barton (1977), Fink (1979), and Taylor (1982) generally support the efficacy of ECT in treating severe depression, although

11

each suffers from inadequate methods of varying degree (Crow and Johnstone, 1986). The following review concentrates on the random assignment studies published since then, each of which satisfies the methodological requirements outlined earlier.

Freeman, Basson, and Crighton (1978) treated 40 primary depressives with either 2 genuine (bilateral, partial sine-wave) or 2 simulated ECTs during their first week of treatment, after which, for ethical reasons, all patients received genuine bilateral ECT for the remainder of the course. Anesthesia was identical for both groups and included atropine, barbiturate, and muscle relaxant. Mean scores on the Hamilton, the Wakefield, and the Visual Analogue depression scales after the first two treatments were significantly lower after genuine than after simulated ECT, and patients in the simulated ECT group ultimately received significantly more treatments prescribed by clinicians who were blind to group assignment. (The Beck self-rating depression scale did not reveal any significant between-group differences, perhaps because depressed patients, particularly those with retardation, have difficulty completing it.)

Lambourn and Gill (1978) assigned 32 patients with psychotic depression to receive either 6 brief-pulse, low-dose (10 joules, J), unilateral ECTs or an equal number of identical anesthesia inductions without the passage of electricity. Mean Hamilton rating-scale scores obtained 24 hours after the sixth treatment did not differ significantly for the two groups.

In the Northwick Park ECT trial, Johnstone et al. (1980) gave 70 endogenous depressives a 4-week course of 8 partial sine-wave bilateral ECTs or 8 anesthesia inductions without electrical stimulation. Mean Hamilton depression scale scores after 4 weeks were significantly lower in the genuine ECT group by about 26%, a difference that was no longer present at 1- and 6-month follow-up intervals, during which additional treatment (including ECT) had been given ad libitum. The advantage of genuine over sham ECT in this study was most marked in the subgroup of delusional depressives (Clinical Research Centre, 1984).

West (1981) treated 22 primary depressives with courses of 6 genuine or sham ECTs. The patients then completed the Beck self-rating scale for depression, were blindly rated on both doctors' and nurses' rating scales, and were then switched to the alternate treatment if indicated. There was a highly statistically significant and clinically important improvement in the genuine compared with the sham ECT group, and 10 out of 11 sham ECT patients (but no genuine ECT patients) were switched to the alternate method, from which they derived the expected degree of improvement.

In the Leicestershire trial, Brandon et al. (1984) studied 95 major depressives who were allocated to up to 8 genuine (bilateral, partial sine-wave) or sham ECT, administered twice weekly. A significantly greater improvement in Hamilton depression scale scores was seen in the genuine (compared with the sham) ECT group at 2 and 4 weeks, but not at 12 and 28 weeks. As in the Northwick Park trial, the largest between-group differences occurred in the subgroup of delusional depressives.

In the Nottingham ECT study, Gregory et al. (1985) randomly assigned 60 depressives to partial sine-wave ECT with bilateral or unilateral placmcnt, or to sham ECT. Both genuine methods were superior to sham ECT after 2, 4, and 6 treatments, as measured by the Hamilton and the Montgomery and Asberg depression scales, which were administered blindly.

Thus, 5 out of 6 methodologically impeccable studies of simulated compared with real ECT in the treatment of depressive illness show both a statistically significant and clinically substantial advantage for the genuine article in reducing depression scale scores during and immediately following the treatment course. It is not surprising that evaluations done later in the maintenance phase of the treatment course or at follow-up generally fail to show such an advantage; during the intervening weeks patients typically received a variety of "doctor's choice" treatments, including both ECT and drugs, administered unsystematically.

The single study (Lambourn and Gill, 1978) that failed to show an advantage for real compared with sham ECT also differs from all the others in having used brief-pulse, low-dose (10 J) unilateral ECT as the active treatment. A similar low-dose technique using an even higher stimulus energy (mean = 18 J) was shown by Sackeim et al. (1987a) to be clinically ineffective for right unilateral ECT. Recent evidence demonstrates that this method must be administered with high stimulus dosing to maximize efficacy (Abrams, Swartz, and Vedak, 1991).

ELECTROCONVULSIVE THERAPY COMPARED WITH
ANTIDEPRESSANT DRUGS

The case for a therapeutic advantage of ECT over antidepressant drugs rests primarily on three studies: Greenblatt, Grosser, and Wechsler (1964), the Medical Research Council trial (MRC, 1965), and

Gangadhar et al. (1982). Although many studies have provided interesting and useful insights into special aspects of the relative efficacy of the two treatment methods, none has the scientific rigor necessary for an unequivocal demonstration of the superiority of ECT. Abrams (1982b) and Rifkin (1988) have detailed the methodological flaws of the published comparisons of ECT and antidepressant drugs in the treatment of depressive illness. Half of the studies have to be excluded from consideration because of retrospective design; nonblind evaluation and faulty data analyses account for most of the remainder. These are by no means trivial points. In a retrospective study, for example (they are all chart-reviews), patients have not been assigned randomly to treatments; there is no sure way to equate the groups for psychopathology or illness severity; the reasons why physicians or patients chose one or the other treatment constitute a major source of bias; there is no control over drug dosage or numbers of ECTs administered; and outcome assessment (even if done by "blinded" reviewers) is necessarily based on the nonsystematic observations recorded at the time by nonblind clinicians with unknown biases.

Even studies that apparently follow a rigorous method may fade into insubstantiality on closer scrutiny. A case in point is the previously mentioned study by Greenblatt, Grosser, and Wechsler (1964) that is widely cited as a demonstration of the therapeutic superiority of ECT over imipramine in the treatment of depressive illness. In this trial, 281 patients were randomly assigned to receive either ECT, a maximum obligatory dose of 200 mg/day of imipramine, phenelzine, isocarboxazid, or placebo and evaluated blindly. The authors indeed found ECT to be superior to imipramine across the total sample studied, but diagnoses were heterogeneous and included psychoneurotic depression, schizophrenia, and a large number categorized only as "other," in addition to the diagnostically relevant categories of manic-depressive, depressed, and involutional psychotic reaction. A combined analysis is clearly noninformative with such diagnostic heterogeneity. Although a table provides separate percentages for each diagnostic subgroup of patients who were markedly improved with each treatment, the actual numbers of patients receiving each method are not given, nor are chi-square values or significance levels provided. The authors nevertheless affirm that their analyses show ECT to be significantly more effective than imipramine for the treatment of involutional psychotic reaction (85% versus 42% markedly improved) but not for the depressed phase of manic-depressive illness (78% versus 59% markedly improved); these groups were not combined for analysis.

In the multihospital Medical Research Council trial (MRC, 1965), 269 patients with endogenous depression were randomly assigned to four different treatment groups, two of which comprised 4 to 8 ECTs (65 patients) and imipramine, 100 to 200 mg/day (mean = 193 mg/day; 63 patients). Fifty-eight patients in each group completed the first 4 weeks of treatment, at which time physicians' blind global assessments showed 71% of the ECT group to have no or slight symptoms, compared with 52% of the imipramine group (χ^2 = 8.75; p = 0.0005).

Gangadhar, Kapur, and Kalyanasundaram (1982) studied 24 primary endogenous depressives who were randomly assigned to receive a course of genuine bilateral or sham ECT given over a 12-week trial in conjunction with either placebo capsules or imipramine, 150 mg/day. The first 6 treatments were given over 2 weeks, followed by one treatment per week for 2 additional weeks and then one "maintenance" treatment at the 6th, 8th, and 12th weeks of the trial (total, 11 treatments). Genuine ECT plus placebo capsules was significantly superior to sham ECT plus imipramine in lowering Hamilton depression scale scores after 6 treatments; no significant between-group differences on this scale were observed at subsequent assessment intervals. Assuming that imipramine does not antagonize the antidepressant effects of ECT—Price et al. (1978) suggest that this may not be the case—this study also demonstrates the efficacy of genuine versus sham ECT. Although the sample size is small and the dose of imipramine used is low, this is the only study to employ the critical format of genuine ECT plus placebo compared with sham ECT plus active drug in conjunction with all of the other methodologic requirements.

All three studies, however, can be criticized for the low drug dosages employed. Although there is little doubt that imipramine, 100 to 200 mg/day, is an effective treatment for some patients, most psychopharmacologists today would peg the therapeutic range of this antidepressant at 200 to 300 mg/day and might also require plasma-level monitoring. The two-phase study of Wilson et al. (1963) addresses the question of dosage, albeit in a very small sample. In the initial phase, depressives were randomly assigned to four treatment groups, of which two (6 patients each) were ECT plus placebo and sham ECT plus imipramine at a dose of 150 to 220 mg/day (mean = 180 mg/day). Assessment on the Hamilton Scale after 5 weeks showed a large and highly significant advantage for ECT. In the second phase of the study, 14 new patients were treated—4 with ECT and 10 with imipramine alone—at a higher dosage: 215 to 270 mg/day. After 5 weeks on this regimen, the high-dose imipramine group showed significantly more improvement than the first- and second-phase ECT groups combined (although the authors erroneously describe the two methods as identical). The rating procedure, however, presents an important problem in this study: Different numbers of raters were used at different assessment periods; one of the raters was never blind; and one was not a psychiatrist. Moreover, the authors do not say which raters participated in the second-phase assessments or how the Hamilton scores were derived when more than one rater was used.

Another aspect of the imipramine dose-response relation was studied by Glassman et al. (1977), who treated 42 nondelusional psychotic depressives with a fixed milligram per kilogram dose of imipramine and examined the relation of plasma level to clinical outcome. The proportion of imipramine-responders increased directly with plasma levels: 29% for plasma levels of 150 ng/mL, 64% at 150 to 225 ng/mL, and 93% for levels of 225 ng/mL. The study is rendered meaningless, however, by the authors' failure to specify their criteria for defining treatment response.

Thus, although ECT is clearly more effective than moderate doses of imipramine in treating several subtypes of endogenous depression, it is less obvious that this difference would obtain under the optimal conditions of higher drug dosages, perhaps with plasma-level monitoring. To be sure, most practitioners neither administer high-dose antidepressant drugs nor routinely monitor plasma levels; in this sense, ECT can justifiably be considered superior to the mediocre antidepressant therapy that is generally prescribed.

In a different paradigm, Dinan and Barry (1989) randomly assigned 30 severely depressed patients who did not respond to treatment with tricyclics—of whom 23 met criteria for melancholia—to receive either 6 bilateral ECTs or the addition of lithium to the tricyclic. There was no difference between groups in blindly obtained, depression-scale score reductions at the end of 3 weeks, although patients receiving the lithium-tricyclic combination improved faster. This is the most favorable outcome obtained to date for drug therapy of depression when compared with ECT and supports the rapid antidepressant efficacy previously reported for the lithium-tricyclic combination (DeMontigny et al., 1983; Heninger et al., 1983).

ELECTROCONVULSIVE THERAPY VS. DRUGS IN DEPRESSIVE
ILLNESS: OTHER STUDIES OF INTEREST

The study of DeCarolis et al. (1964), as reviewed by Avery and Lubrano (1979), provides unique information on an important clinical question: What is the response to ECT in depressives who have failed high-dose antidepressant drug therapy? These authors intially treated a diagnostically heterogeneous sample of 437 depressives with imipramine, 200 to 350 mg/day. All patients who failed to improve after 30 days on this regimen were then given a course of 8 to 10 ECTs. Endogenous depressives constituted the largest diagnostic subgroup (*n* = 282), of which 172 (61%) responded to imipramine. Of the remaining 109 patients (one patient dropped out), 93 (85%) then responded to a course of ECT. In the subgroup of 181 delusional depressives, only 72 (40%) responded to imipramine, compared with 91 (83%) of the 109 imipramine nonresponders who went on to receive ECT. Although assessment of outcome was not blind in this study, this seems at least partially counterbalanced by the powerful bias against ECT response introduced by withholding this treatment until patients had first failed high-dose antidepressant drug therapy.

A paper by Coryell (1978) considers a different question: What is the response of patients who had received ECT and antidepressants during different depressive episodes? In this study, hospital charts were reviewed and blindly rated for all patients who received ECT for depression in the pre-antidepressant era (1920–1959) and who later received tricyclic antidepressants from 1961 to 1975 for a different episode. Complete recovery occurred in 94% of the episodes treated with ECT compared with 53% of those treated with antidepressants. Drug dosages were low by present standards, however, and no data are provided on the relative efficacy of the two methods within patients (e.g., how often the ECT response was superior to the tricyclic response).

ECT VS. ISOFLURANE

Because of a superficial analogy between ECT-induced postictal suppression and the total suppression of cerebral activity that can occur with deep isoflurane anesthesia, Langer et al. (1985) conducted an open clinical trial of this procedure in 11 treatment-resistant depressed patients who preferred not to undergo ECT, and claimed thereby to have achieved a very rapid antidepressant effect that was comparable to ECT. Stimulated by that article, Greenberg et al. (1987) conducted an open replication trial in 6 patients with recurrent depressive disorder, 5 of whom had recovered with ECT from prior episodes. No clinical antidepressant activity of deep isoflurane anesthesia was observed during the study, and 5 of the 6 patients went on to recover with ECT.

An open study of isoflurane anesthesia and ECT in depressed patients (Carl et al., 1988) is simply incomprehensible as insufficient methodology is provided to determine what was done to whom, or why, and what the results were. This same group published a subsequent open clinical trial (Engelhardt et al., 1993) in which 12 treatment-resistant depressed patients were first given 6 isoflurane inductions, and those who failed to respond—or improved only temporarily—were then given ECT. In a nonblind assessment, the authors rated 7 of the 12 patients as markedly improved after isoflurane anesthesia, but only 3 of them could be discharged from the hospital. The remaining 9 patients went on to receive ECT, but the authors unaccountably omit mention of whether any of them were subsequently discharged from the hospital. As the authors point out, however, isoflurane anesthesia is contraindicated in patients with coronary or cerebral vascular disease, a fact that would certainly prevent a substantial number of patients who receive ECT from ever becoming candidates for this procedure.

Most recently, Langer et al. (1995) reported an open, nonrandom, clinical comparison of ECT with isoflurane anesthesia in depression, purporting to find isoflurane anesthesia the more effective therapy. Remarkably, all patients continued to receive antidepressant drug therapy throughout the study period.

However, their study is invalidated by inadequate ECT technique. Using a Siemens Konvulsator partial sine wave device set to the intermittent stimulus mode, with peak current of 500 mA, these authors delivered a stimulus only 2 seconds long. (If they didn't induce a seizure, they immediately restimulated at 600 mA.) Langer et al. (1995) do not provide figures for the mean charge they used, but it is easy to calculate using the correction factor of 0.64 provided by the manufacturer of the Siemens device. Each second of stimulation in the intermittent mode provides 0.125 second (25 pulses per second of 0.005 second each) of current flow, so:

$$500 \text{ mA} \times 0.64 \times 0.125 \text{ sec.} \times 2 \text{ sec.} = 80 \text{ mC}$$

For the 600-mA setting, the dose would have been 96 mC. Such a low dosage range is doubtless responsible for the incredibly poor results these authors obtained with bilateral ECT: just 49% improvement in depression scores after 6 treatments.

In comparison, Lamy et al. (1994), who also used an old Siemens Konvulsator, delivered an 800-mA peak current for an average of 6 seconds' stimulation (range 4 to 10 seconds), yielding a mean stimulus charge of 384 mC and achieving recovery in most patients with bilateral ECT. Similarly, Abrams, Swartz and Vedak (1991) reported 79%

improvement with 6 bilateral ECTs, using a mean stimulus charge of 378 mC delivered via a brief-pulse instrument.

Efficacy in Mania

Only one prospective controlled trial of ECT in mania has been published at the time of this writing (Small et al., 1988): A sample of 34 newly admitted manic patients were diagnosed as bipolar I according to the Research Diagnostic Criteria and were randomly assigned to receive a course of brief-pulse ECT (n = 17) or lithium therapy (n = 17). The mean number of ECTs administered was 9.3, and lithium dosages were adjusted to yield serum lithium levels between 0.6 and 1.2 mmol/L. Concomitant neuroleptic drug therapy was permitted ad libitum. After completion of the ECT course, patients in this group were placed on maintenance lithium therapy.

Ratings by nonblind observers as well as blind evaluations of videotaped interviews were done at weekly intervals for the first 8 weeks, using a variety of rating instruments, including the Brief Psychiatric Rating Scale, Clinical Global Assessment scale, and Bech-Rafaelson Manic Rating Scale. At all rating intervals after the first week, and for each of the three previous measures, ECT induced greater improvement than lithium, a difference that reached statistical significance on most measures at weeks 6, 7, and 8. The results of the blind and nonblind ratings were in general agreement throughout the study. The mean daily dose of neuroleptic agents received during the trial was similar for both groups. It is notable that a significant advantage for ECT emerged in this study despite the fact that the first group of ECT patients treated initially received unilateral electrode placement, failed to respond (or got worse), and then responded to bilateral placement, thereby confirming an earlier retrospective study that demonstrated a therapeutic advantage for the latter method in manic patients (Small et al., 1985; Milstein et al., 1987). Had all ECT patients received bilateral ECT from the outset, the observed advantage over lithium might well have been larger.

Efficacy in Schizophrenia

Evaluating the efficacy of ECT in schizophrenia is more difficult than in depression because of the greater variability in the diagnostic criteria for the former disorder. Most investigators who were quite specific in their description of the signs and symptoms of endogenous depression were unaccountably satisfied with merely proclaiming their schizo-phrenic patients to be either chronic or acute, with an occasional sub-type thrown in. Moreover, no attempt was made until the 1980s to exclude schizophrenic patients who had prominent affective symptoms from ECT studies, raising the spectre of misdiagnosis because many patients with a mixture of affective and schizophrenic symptoms ac-tually suffer from affective disorder (Abrams and Taylor, 1976c, 1981; Pope and Lipinski, 1978; Pope et al., 1980).

Moreover, just as in the studies in depressive illness already re-viewed, most of the older ECT studies in schizophrenia are method-ologically defective. The few acceptable studies from this era are briefly reviewed here, followed by a more detailed examination of the few methodologically acceptable studies conducted in recent years.

Miller et al. (1953) assigned 30 chronic catatonic schizophrenics to genuine ECT or to pentothal anesthesia with or without the addition of nonconvulsive electrical stimulation. Partially blind assessment (two of the four interviewers were blind) after 3 to 4 weeks of treatment showed no differences among the three groups for reduction of psy-chotic symptoms or for improvement in social performance. Brill et al. (1959) compared 20 genuine ECTs with an equal number of thiopental or nitrous oxide anesthesia inductions in 67 male chronic schizophrenics and found no significant difference among the methods, as blindly assessed on three separate outcome measures 1 month after treatment. Heath et al. (1964) gave short courses of 4 or 8 genuine or sham (thiopental anesthesia) ECTs to 45 chronic schizophrenics and found no significant changes or intergroup differences 1 month after treatment on a blindly administered nurses' behavior rating scale.

Langsley, Enterline, and Hickerson (1959) randomly assigned 106 acutely schizophrenic or manic patients to a course of 12 to 20 ECTs or 200 to 2000 mg/day chlorpromazine (CPZ) (mean = 800 mg/day). Blind evaluation at 8 and 12 weeks revealed no between-group differ-ences on either a psychiatrist's or nurse's rating scale. King (1960) randomly assigned 84 newly admitted female schizophrenics to a course of 20 ECTs or 900 to 1200 mg/day CPZ for one month. Hospital discharge rates were the same for both groups, as were the subsequent relapse rates while on maintenance CPZ.

It is reasonable to conclude from these data that ECT is no better than sham ECT in the treatment of chronic schizophrenia and no better than neuroleptic agents in the treatment of nonchronic schizophrenia.

Modern Studies Including a Sham Electroconvulsive Therapy Group

Taylor and Fleminger (1980) studied 20 paranoid schizophrenic patients diagnosed according to the Present State Examination and referred for ECT after having failed at least 2 weeks of low-dose therapy with neuroleptic agents (e.g., 300 mg/day CPZ, 15 mg/day trifluoperazine). Chronically ill patients were excluded from this study, as were those who had a short (6 months) history of psychiatric problems. Patients were randomly assigned to a course of 8 to 12 genuine or sham ECTs (10 in each group), administered thrice-weekly, during which neuroleptic drugs were continued at the same low pre-ECT dosages in both groups. Blind ratings on the Comprehensive Psychiatric Rating Scale revealed lower scores for the genuine ECT group at 2 weeks, 4 weeks, and 8 weeks, but not 1 month after the treatment course ended. Half of the patients in each group had pretreatment Beck Depression Inventory scores of 20, indicative of clinical depression; although genuine ECT caused a greater reduction in these scores compared with sham ECT at 2, 4, and 8 weeks, the differences were not quite significant.

In a separately published part of the Leicester ECT trial described earlier (Brandon et al., 1984), Brandon et al. (1985) randomly assigned 17 patients who were diagnosed by the PSE-based Catego program as having schizophrenia to receive 8 genuine ($n = 9$) or sham ($n = 8$) ECTs administered over a 4-week course. Those patients already on stable doses of neuroleptic drugs were continued on them; there was no difference in mean dosage between the groups. Blind psychiatric evaluations on the Montgomery-Asberg Schizophrenia Scale at 2 and 4 weeks showed significantly greater improvement with genuine compared with sham ECT; this was no longer the case at the 12- and 28-week follow-up examinations. No effort was made in this trial to exclude patients with affective symptoms: Mean Hamilton Depression scale scores were 26 and 37 for the genuine and sham ECT groups, respectively, well within the range of most studies of ECT in major depressive disorders.

The small sample sizes and failure to exclude patients with prominent affective symptoms limits the conclusions that can be drawn from these two studies: They both clearly demonstrate a therapeutic effect of ECT in nonchronic schizophrenic patients receiving neuroleptic drugs and diagnosed according to modern British criteria.

Bagadia et al. (1983) randomly assigned 38 predominantly nonchronic schizophrenic patients diagnosed according to the Research

Diagnostic Criteria (RDC) to receive either 6 genuine bilateral ECTs plus placebo (n = 20) or 6 sham ECT plus 600 mg/day CPZ (n = 18). Blind evaluation on the Brief Psychiatric (BPRS) and Clinical Global Impressions rating scales after 7 and 20 days of treatment revealed no significant between-group differences. This study is notable for its larger sample size and for excluding patients who had exhibited depressive or manic symptoms sufficient for a diagnosis of schizoaffective or affective illness. Although the number of ECTs given was small by any standard, the study design demonstrates that a short course of ECT is no more or less effective a treatment for schizophrenia than an equally short course of moderate-dose neuroleptic treatment.

Studies Without a Sham Electroconvulsive Therapy Control Group

Janakiramaiah et al. (1982) randomly assigned groups of 15 schizophrenic patients each to receive 6 weeks of treatment with one of four methods: ECT plus 500 mg/day CPZ; ECT plus 300 mg/day CPZ; 500 mg/day CPZ; or 300 mg/day CPZ. Diagnoses were made according to the RDC. Eight to 15 bilateral sine-wave ECTs were administered three times per week. Blind ratings on the BPRS at weekly intervals were significantly different among the four methods by analysis of variance at the first through fifth weeks of treatment: the ECT plus 500 mg/day CPZ group was the most effective at the end of the first week, and the 300 mg/day CPZ group fared worse than any of the others at the 2- to 5-week assessments. In the main effects analysis, ECT always resulted in lower BPRS scores compared with no ECT (regardless of CPZ dose), but these differences only reached significance at the end of the second and third weeks of treatment. The interactive effect of CPZ and ECT, that is, the efficacy of combined treatment compared with either treatment given separately, was significant at the end of the third through fifth treatment weeks. (The study is marred by the fact that 5 patients in the group receiving ECT plus 300 mg/day CPZ revealed to the "blind" examiner that they were receiving ECT.) In sum, this study shows that although at different times during the treatment course ECT was better than no ECT, and ECT plus CPZ was better than either treatment given alone, by the end of 6 weeks, schizophrenic patients fared equally well with or without ECT. Essentially, ECT served to accelerate the treatment response to low-dose CPZ.

The literature is best summarized by the following statements:

1. ECT is no better than sham ECT in the treatment of chronic schizophrenia.
2. ECT is better than sham ECT in the treatment of nonchronic schizophrenic patients who have many affective symptoms.

Efficacy in Other Disorders

No data exist from controlled trials to support the use of ECT in disorders other than those described earlier; such usage belongs to the art rather than to the science of psychiatry. Of course, such art has an important place: Ill patients must be treated, emergencies responded to, and families assured that no reasonable treatment alternatives have been overlooked. In truth, most suffering patients are primarily interested in seeking out a physician with great experience and reputed success in the treatment of their illness, correctly believing that if the physician is also honest, and learned, he will choose the most effective method of cure. How much does it really matter to the patient or doctor that data from controlled trials do not exist to support the use of ECT in the particular disorder under consideration? If a clinician has successfully used ECT under similar clinical circumstances in the past, he has ample justification for yet another therapeutic trial, especially when other treatments have already failed.

Clinical Considerations

This section is a personal interpretation and elaboration of the anecdotal clinical lore that has evolved during more than a half-century of ECT practice. Such uncontrolled observations are useful for the following reasons:

1. Controlled trials of ECT do not exist for all diagnoses. Some psychiatric syndromes for which ECT is often prescribed (e.g., mania) have not yet been been the subject of flawless controlled trials, and others (e.g., catatonic stupor, depressive pseudodementia) occur infrequently enough to make it doubtful that they ever will be. Yet the universal clinical experience has been that manics, catatonics, and depressive pseudodements respond to ECT at least as well as to other treatments, even when they have failed to respond to intensive pharmacotherapy, and occasionally achieve dramatic remissions that surprise even ardent foes of ECT.

2. The results of controlled trials may be conflicting: For example, the carefully controlled and sharply contradictory study of Wilson and Gottlieb (1967), which clearly demonstrates that right-unilateral ECT causes more verbal impairment than bilateral ECT, or Lambourn and Gill's (1978) methodologically impeccable demonstration that sham ECT is just as effective in relieving depressions as the genuine article. After attempting in vain to incorporate these and other similarly contradictory studies into a comprehensive view of the ECT process, most writers have simply chosen to ignore them, albeit without scientific grounds for doing so. The point is that practicing clinicians, as well as their more rigorously scientific colleagues, pick and choose daily from among the available data those results that best support their personal biases and experience and reject those that do not.

3. Controlled trials do not have a monopoly on truth. This sentiment may seem strange in view of the opening sentence of the preceding chapter, but only because truth is here being considered at a different level of discourse. Double-blind, random-assignment methodology was not required to demonstrate the efficacy of penicillin in meningococcal meningitis and will not be needed to prove the efficacy of the first drug that cures a few patients with acquired immune deficiency syndrome. When a drowned boy is restored to life through phased warming and the intravenous administration of complexly balanced electrolyte solutions, no one suggests the need for a placebo-controlled study to confirm the results. Likewise, the dramatic response of a mute, stuporous, rigid, incontinent, and drooling catatonic patient to one or two induced seizures also partakes of the truth, a truth that has generally been more difficult to accept with regard to ECT than with most other treatments.

4. Data from controlled trials may be incomplete. Some psychiatric disorders (e.g., melancholia), although subjected to controlled study for responsiveness to ECT, have protean manifestations that have not always been examined with enough thoroughness to draw definitive conclusions. The presence of depressive delusions, for example, long considered by clinicians to define an extremely ECT-sensitive subpopulation (e.g., Crow and Johnstone, 1986), has never been used to stratify a sample of melancholics in a prospective, random-assignment study of the efficacy of ECT.

Finally, although much of this volume is devoted to a critical review of the supporting research data for each topic covered, it is nevertheless intended as a clinical guide to ECT, and clinicians can never allow themselves to be bound solely by the narrow confines of data from controlled trials. This is simply because many, if not most, psychiatric patients present with syndromes that do not fit the nicely defined categories of research studies that have the luxury of specifying inclusion and exclusion criteria and minimal scores on standardized rating scales. For these patients, there simply are no definitive research data to guide the clinician's choice of treatment, yet treat he must. As is true for anyone who publishes frequently on the topic of ECT, I receive numerous queries from clinicians requesting advice on the management of a particularly difficult patient. The question is never "what objective data from controlled trials are there to support the use of ECT in my patient," but always "in your clinical experience, how should my patient be treated?" The present chapter addresses the latter class of questions, relying not only on an extensive clinical case-report literature but also on the cumulative wisdom of teachers and colleagues, all filtered through the residue of personal clinical experience.

Choice and Timing of Electroconvulsive Therapy

It is no secret that patients with affective disorder, unipolar or bipolar types, are prime candidates for ECT; however, despite the chastening lessons of the cross-national study (Kendell et al., 1971) and several articles documenting the pitfalls of misdiagnosing affective disorder as schizophrenia (Lipkin et al., 1970; Carlson and Goodwin, 1973; Taylor and Abrams, 1975; Abrams and Taylor, 1974, 1976c, 1981; Pope and Lipinsky, 1978; Pope et al., 1980), many affectively disordered patients who might otherwise have fully recovered or substantially benefited from ECT (or lithium, for that matter) still receive neuroleptic drugs in the mistaken belief that their psychotic symptoms indicate a diagnosis of schizophrenia. Melancholia often presents with a stereotypic syndrome that is easy to recognize: Agitation or retardation, weight loss, early waking, self-reproach, anhedonia, impaired concentration, low self-esteem, and ruminations of guilt, worthlessness, hopelessness, or suicide present an unmistakable clinical picture that augurs well for full remission with ECT. The presence of such psychotic features as delusions (e.g., of guilt, sin, poverty) or hallucinations (e.g., a rotting odor, a voice counseling suicide), far from suggesting a diagnosis of schizophrenia, only further cements the diagnosis of melancholia. If a delusional mood is also present or the patient appears dazed, perplexed, or clouded, the effects of ECT can be dramatic, with the patient awakening from the first or second treatment as from a dream, thoroughly astounded to learn of his whereabouts and recent strange behaviors. Although 6 to 8 ECTs (mean = 6.5) constitute the modal range for a treatment course in melancholia (Fink, 1979), an occasional patient may require considerably more. I remember well one woman in her early 70s whose severe unipolar depression did not respond at all to the first 10 ECTs. Treatment was continued despite these disappointing results because of her classical presentation and a history of an excellent response of similar symptoms to ECT 30 years earlier. Improvement became evident by the 12th ECT and was complete after the 15th, illustrating the general rule that as long as the clinical syndrome is prognostically favorable, ECT should be continued until the expected degree of improvement is obtained. Although there is probably a maximum number of ECTs that should not be exceeded in a single treatment course, I know of no way to determine it. (I have seen only one patient with classic melancholia who did not respond to ECT, a late-onset unipolar depressive whose presentation was so typical and whose symptoms so severe that he received 22 ECTs without significant improvement before the treatment was finally declared a failure.)

Conversely, there is no reason to adhere slavishly to a minimum number of treatments. I can think of several instances, especially in older patients, where marked improvement occurred after the third or fourth ECT, only to fade and then disappear with additional treatments. Whether this course of events represents a dose-response curve analagous to that reported for the tricyclic antidepressant nortriptyline or simply the deleterious effects of developing cognitive dysfunction, the advisable course of action when a patient has shown marked improvement early in the treatment course is to withhold further ECT pending the return of symptoms. The rationale for the common clinical practice of giving two additional ECTs to prevent relapse after full recovery has been achieved was not confirmed in a controlled follow-up study by Barton et al. (1973). Finally, some depressed patients who do not respond to the usual rate of administration of 3 times a week may nonetheless recover if double ECTs are given each session (Swartz and Mehta, 1986).

Of all the possible behavioral responses to ECT, the euphoric-hypomanic pattern (Fink and Kahn, 1961) is best. In my view, it always indicates that enough ECT has been given. Its occurrence after right-unilateral ECT as well as after bilateral ECT suggests that it represents not merely a nonspecific organic frontal lobe response, but rather a focused limbic effect of ECT (a direct hit), producing an affective overshoot with gradual return to euthymia several days after treatment has stopped. The relation of this syndrome to mania is discussed elsewhere in this volume (p. 201).

Antidepressants should be discontinued during ECT. No additive or synergistic effect of combining ECT and antidepressants has been demonstrated (Abrams, 1975; Siris, Glassman and Stetner, 1982), and Price et al. (1978) actually found a statistically significant reduction in affective improvement in patients in their ECT sample who had received concomitant tricyclic antidepressants compared with those who had not. Lithium, as noted in Chapter 6, should not be coadministered with ECT because it may cause severe organic confusional states and prolong the apnea induced by succinylcholine.

Two clinical variants of melancholia are exquisitely responsive to ECT: catatonic stupor and depressive pseudodementia.

1. *Catatonic stupor*: Known in the older literature as melancholia attonita, this syndrome of stupor, mutism, negativism, catalepsy, and incontinence of saliva, urine, and feces may linger for weeks or months until abruptly dissolved by a few (sometimes, just one) induced seizures. Again, a diagnosis of schizophrenia is not inherent to this syndrome, which is diagnostically nonspecific and occurs most frequently in patients who satisfy research criteria for affective disorders (Abrams and Taylor, 1976c). Other individual catatonic features (e.g., echolalia, echopraxia, mannerisms, stereotypies) are not associated with a particularly good response to ECT, perhaps because they are more often seen in patients with chronic schizophrenia. A positive, albeit transient, response of catatonic stupor to intravenous sodium amobarbital (the "amytal interview") often predicts a favorable outcome with ECT. Indeed, while awaiting completion of the pretreatment workup before starting ECT in a catatonic patient, 250 mg of sodium amytal given intramuscularly 30 minutes before meals will often enable him to eat and drink. Parenteral benzodiazepines—e.g., lorazepam—are also effective for this purpose.

2. *Depressive pseudodementia* (*dementia syndrome of depression*): If this syndrome of disorientation and impaired memory accompanying depressive symptoms in an older person is misdiagnosed as

senile dementia and the luckless patient is placed in a nursing home, he may not have long to live. A few ECTs, however, can rapidly restore such an apparently deteriorated individual to rosy health, an occurrence rendered all the more remarkable by the family's frequent comment that "_____ hasn't looked this well in years." One of the most striking examples of this phenomenon, dubbed "the Rip Van Winkle syndrome," occurred in a 72-year-old man (Fisman, 1988), who recovered fully from a "presenile dementia" with a course of ECTs given 14 years after the diagnosis was made and the patient interred in a nursing home. In their literature review, Price and McAllister (1989) found 10 reports describing a total of 22 cases of depressive pseudodementia treated with ECT (mean age = 64.2 years), all of whom improved, with only 23% showing significant ECT-induced cognitive impairment.

There is little risk in inadvertently treating a patient whose depressive symptoms are only an early manifestation of Alzheimer's dementia. ECT has been used successfully under such circumstances without worsening the cognitive symptoms or accelerating the progression of the underlying disorder (see Chapter 5), so there is nothing to be lost in questionable cases by a therapeutic trial.

A melancholic patient should receive ECT in preference to any other treatment under circumstances of increased clinical urgency or intolerance to psychotropic drugs:

1. *The presence of delusions or hallucinations*: Psychotic depression is notoriously resistant to antidepressant drugs but very responsive to ECT (Hordern et al, 1963; Glassman et al., 1975; Davidson et al., 1978; Crow and Johnstone, 1986). Although tricyclic-neuroleptic combinations are reported to be more effective in delusional depression than tricyclics alone (Spiker et al., 1986), it seems unwarranted to expose a depressed patient to the risk of tardive dyskinesia when the safe and rapidly effective alternative of ECT is available.
2. *The presence of stupor*: Neither full-blown catatonic stupor nor the more severe degrees of psychomotor retardation respond well to antidepressant drugs, yet both are rapidly responsive to ECT. Moreover, there is often some urgency involved, because such patients do not eat well, or at all, and have often lost significant body mass by the time they are first seen.

3. *The presence of suicidal ruminations or behavior*: Completed suicide presents the single greatest risk in melancholia, yet it rarely occurs once ECT has been initiated. No similar experience has been accumulated for antidepressant drugs, which are believed to increase the risk of completed suicide early in the treatment course if psychomotor retardation is relieved before despondency.

4. *Coexisting severe medical disease*: The pronounced cardiovascular effects of some tricyclic antidepressants have been reported to increase the risk of sudden death in cardiac patients (Coull et al., 1970; Moir et al., 1972), making ECT often seem to be the more conservative treatment choice. Hepatic and renal disease also increase the risks of drug therapy, due to impaired metabolism and excretion, but not the risk with ECT.

5. *Depressive pseudodementia*: Antidepressants seem only to aggravate this syndrome, presumably because of their anticholinergic effects.

6. *Old age*: Elderly melancholics also seem particularly intolerant to the anticholinergic effects of many tricyclics, which often cause severe constipation or even precipitate anticholinergic delirium. If anything, the response to ECT improves with the age of the patient, and fewer treatments are generally required to achieve remission.

7. *Pregnancy*: All psychotropic drugs, including lithium, cross the placental barrier and exert unknown, but doubtless protean and unfavorable effects on the fetus both during and after development, continuing into the postnatal period if the mother nurses. ECT is not known to exert any such adverse fetal effects (Chapter 5) and should be used in preference to drugs in pregnant women and during the nursing period.

8. *Drug therapy failure*: Any patient who has failed a course of adequate antidepressant therapy should be offered ECT in preference to another trial with a different compound. In practice, this covers many depressives who are admitted to the hospital after failing to respond to outpatient pharmacotherapy. Of course, any patient with a history of previous unresponsiveness to antidepressants should receive ECT as the initial treatment.

9. *Patient preference*: The 1990 APA Task Force on ECT report (American Psychiatric Association, 1990) also thoughtfully includes patient preference among the indications for the primary use of ECT, something psychiatrists have paid surprisingly little attention to when administering biologic treatments.

Mania

Mania, the obverse of melancholia, responds so well to ECT that it is difficult to account for the absence until recently of any prospective controlled trials of induced seizures in this disorder. Perhaps the rapidly spreading use (and remarkable efficacy) of lithium therapy at a time when the importance of controlled trials of ECT was also being recognized had an inhibiting effect; probably the general disinclination of manics to cooperate with any form of treatment, let alone random assignment to ECT or drugs, also played a role. At the time of this writing, the study of Small et al. (1988) cited earlier remains the only published controlled trial of ECT in mania.

Several retrospective studies shed light on the efficacy of ECT in mania. In a chart-review study, McCabe (1976) compared a sample of manic patients who received ECT in the predrug era (1945–1949) with an age- and sex-matched control sample of manics who were hospitalized at the Iowa Psychopathic Hospital before ECT had been introduced (1935–1941). All subjects were selected on the basis of the same research criteria, and the resultant groups were remarkably similar on most of 27 clinical psychopathologic variables studied. On all outcome measures (duration of hospitalization, condition at discharge, percent discharged home, degree of social recovery), the ECT-treated group fared substantially and significantly better than the untreated control sample, with the most striking difference being that 96% of the ECT patients were discharged to their homes, compared with only 44% of the untreated patients.

A second chart-review study from the same hospital (McCabe and Norris, 1977) examined the question from a different vantage point, comparing the outcome in the same two groups already described with that obtained in a third age- and sex-matched sample of manics who received CPZ therapy from 1958 to 1964. Not surprisingly, ECT and CPZ were both superior to no treatment and were about equal overall in their beneficial effects in mania; however, 10 patients who did not respond well to CPZ therapy went on to recover with ECT. In another retrospective chart-review study (Thomas and Reddy, 1982), ECT, CPZ, and lithium were reported to be equally effective; however, the three groups were not as well matched compared with groups in the studies from Iowa, and the sample sizes (10 in each group) were much smaller.

Black et al. (1987) reviewed the charts of 438 patients hospitalized for mania over a 12-year period and found that a significantly greater percentage who received ECT could be classed as having "marked improvement" compared with those who received adequate or inadequate lithium therapy or no therapy at all. Unilateral and bilateral ECT were equally effective.

In a review of all patients receiving ECT at McLean Hospital from 1973 to 1986, Alexander et al. (1988) found that 10 of 18 manic patients (56%) were significantly improved (n = 9) or recovered (n = 1) with ECT. A similar review at Aarhus Hospital in 1984 (Strömgren, 1988) revealed a far more salutary response: ECT induced a moderate (n = 6) or satisfactory (n = 10) effect in mania in 16 out of 17 series administered, virtually all with right unilateral ECT.

Most manic patients come to ECT only after treatment with lithium or neuroleptic drugs has failed and the patient, who has typically been in a state of relentless excitement for several days, is on the verge of exhaustion. Even under these unfavorable circumstances, ECT works. Other than psychomotor excitement, a particularly favorable feature that is usually present in patients with acute mania, no individual manic symptom or symptom-cluster is especially predictive of a good response to ECT. Conversely, the presence of psychotic symptoms, however outlandish or bizarre, in no way reduces the likelihood of recovery as long as the full manic syndrome is also present (Taylor and Abrams, 1975).

It has long been standard clinical practice to administer double bilateral ECTs on consecutive treatment days during the first session or two of a manic patient's treatment course, perhaps reflecting the clinical urgency often felt by the time such patients are finally referred for ECT. Recent evidence (Small et al., 1988), however, suggests that manics are responsive to conventional single bilateral ECTs when administered at the usual rate (albeit with concurrent neuroleptic therapy).

Schizophrenia

There is little doubt that many patients diagnosed as having acute or schizoaffective schizophrenia respond remarkably well to ECT; there is also little doubt that most of these patients are misdiagnosed manics (Abrams and Taylor 1974, 1976c, 1981; Taylor and Abrams, 1975). When the diagnosis of schizophrenia is made by first excluding patients with prominent affective syndromes (Taylor and Abrams, 1978), most of the ECT-responsive clinical variance is thereby also excluded.

This should not be taken to mean that patients with an early, insidious onset of emotional blunting, avolition, first-rank symptoms, and formal thought disorder should never be offered ECT. On the contrary, every such patient deserves one full trial of ECT (preferably earlier rather than later in their illness course) to insure that no treatment will be overlooked that has a chance, however slim, of halting the otherwise relentless progression of this devastating illness (Abrams, 1987). Two uncontrolled studies (Friedel, 1986; Gujavarty, Greenberg, and Fink, 1987) suggest that such a trial, in conjunction with neuroleptic drug therapy, may yield unexpectedly favorable results. Controlled studies, with and without coadministration of neuroleptic drugs, should now be undertaken to demonstrate the efficacy of such treatment.

In those rare instances when the catatonic syndrome of negativistic stupor is a manifestation of schizophrenia, ECT works just as well to remove the stupor as it does in patients with affective disorder, but often reveals a core schizophrenic syndrome that is resistant to further ECT.

Symptomatic Psychoses

Numerous individual case reports over the last half-century testify to the effectiveness of ECT in psychotic states secondary to a wide variety of toxic, metabolic, infectious, traumatic, neoplastic, epileptic, and endocrine disorders (Taylor, 1982). Particularly striking are the results that are often achieved with ECT in drug-induced states, especially amphetamine psychosis, and in the acute epileptiform psychoses. A favorable response is less likely in cases in which the underlying disorder has been chronically in place or remains uncorrected at the time of treatment. In general, it is reasonable to reserve ECT for those patients with symptomatic psychoses that have neither responded to medical treatment of the underlying condition nor to a week's trial of neuroleptic drugs.

Neuroses and Personality Disorders

Regardless of the current terminology used to classify these disorders, they are rarely responsive to (and often aggravated by) ECT. This is particularly true for anxiety-related syndromes such as panic disorder.

Use of Electroconvulsive Therapy in Children and Adolescents

Neither the first APA ECT Task Force Report (American Psychiatric Association, 1978) nor the Consensus Conference on ECT (Consensus Conference, 1985) address the indications for ECT in children or adolescents, and the second APA ECT Task Force Report (American Psychiatric Association, 1990) asserts only that they "are similar to those for adults." Excluding fully postpubertal adolescents (e.g., age 16 years and above) from consideration as not different from adults in any medically relevant way leaves an extremely sparse literature remaining on the subject. Further excluding the older literature on the use of induced seizures in autism, childhood schizophrenia, and other childhood encephalopathic disorders leaves but a handful of cases—only three of which were prepubertal—to provide guidance.

Warnecke (1975) reported the successful use of ECT to treat a severe depression that emerged in a 14-year-old boy after he had an acute manic episode that had responded well to neuroleptic drugs.

Carr et al. (1983) used right unilateral ECT to treat a 12-year-old prepubertal girl who met criteria for bipolar affective disorder, manic type. Seven ECTs induced full remission of her pronounced and chronic manic psychosis, despite a recent history of asymmetric, left-sided EEG slowing and enlargement of the frontal horns and bodies of the lateral ventricles on computed tomographic (CT) scan.

Black and colleagues (1985) described an excellent response to unilateral ECT in an 11-year-old prepubertal boy with major depression, and Powell, Silveira, and Lindsay (1988) obtained similarly favorable results with unilateral ECT during three separate episodes of recurrent familial depressive stupor in a 13-year-old prepubertal boy who remained well over a 4-year follow-up interval. Bertagnoli and Borchardt (1990) also successfully used unilateral ECT to treat a 15-year-old adolescent girl suffering from bipolar affective disorder; she remained symptom-free on maintenance lithium therapy during a 9-month follow-up interval.

Guttmacher and Cretella's (1988) survey of 10 years of experience with ECT at Strong Memorial Hospital is puzzling, both for the generally unfavorable outcome and the astoundingly high incidence (75%) of prolonged seizures recorded in the 4 patients, aged 12 to 15 years, who received ECT during that time. The 3 patients who failed to respond were hardly prime candidates for ECT: One had flattened affect and poverty of speech; another was socially isolated, emotionally blunted, and unresponsive to therapeutic levels of desipramine; and the third had a history of delayed language onset, a facial seizure, incontinence and echolalia, made guttural noises, had failed to respond to successive trials of imipramine, haloperidol, clonidine, clonazepam, and monoamine oxidase inhibitors, and was considered a candidate for psychosurgery. Even the sole designated responder had his ECT discontinued after 16 treatments because "the treatment team felt it to be ineffective" (improvement only began 7 days after his last treatment). Two of the prolonged seizures occurred in patients who were also receiving medications known to lower the seizure threshold: desipramine and trifluoperazine; the third was observed in the brain-damaged patient with epilepsy.

The survey methodology may have elicited this unusual outcome by asking physicians "if they had ever treated a patient aged 15 years or younger and if they had ever had a patient who experienced a seizure lasting more than 4 minutes," thus potentially biasing respondents to recall selectively those children and adolescents with prolonged seizures, in whom pre-existing brain pathologic conditions may have been responsible both for treatment resistance and prolonged seizures.

One of the most striking cases was reported by Cizlado and Wheaton (1995), who administered a course of 19 ECTs (15 bilateral, 4 unilateral) to an 8.5-year-old girl who developed a severe syndrome of catatonic stupor while undergoing antidepressant drug therapy for major depression. Clinical improvement was not observed until the 8th treatment, following which a neuroleptic was added to the treatment regimen (without any apparent medical basis). After the 11th ECT, dramatic improvement was observed with each additional seizure through the 16th, when full recovery was obtained. At 6-month follow-up, she remained well on maintenance fluoxetine therapy.

From the available data, then, it is apparent that when the clinical indications are straightforward and the prognosis favorable—as in unipolar or bipolar affective disorder—the response to ECT in children and adolescents is no different from that obtained in adults: excellent. Likewise, little benefit is to be expected from ECT in patients, regardless of age, whose chronic nonaffective psychoses are characterized by treatment resistance, emotional blunting, social isolation, and the stigmata of coarse brain disease.

Nonpsychiatric Indications for
Electroconvulsive Therapy

Parkinson's Disease

Parkinson's disease is a neurodegenerative disorder that affects 1% of the population over age 50—approximately half a million Americans. Pharmacologic treatments include dopaminergic agents such as levodopa (usually combined with the peripheral decarboxylase inhibitor carbidopa), amantadine, bromocriptine, pergolide, and selegiline, as well as anticholinergic agents such as benztropine and trihexyphenidyl. When they are first administered, these agents all tend to be effective. However, they are associated with numerous side effects (including psychosis and mood disorders) and typically lose efficacy as the disease progresses. With levodopa—the standard pharmacologic therapy for Parkinson's disease—severe, abrupt, and often incapacitating fluctuations in extrapyramidal symptoms (the ''on-off'' syndrome) ultimately develop in virtually all patients taking the medication who survive long enough.

In addition to these pharmacologic agents, autologous adrenal medullary and fetal brain tissues have been transplanted into the caudate nucleus at considerable risk and expense, but with limited success (Abrams, 1989b; Goetz et al., 1989; Ahlskog et al., 1990).

For over 30 years, ECT has been reported to be helpful in many dozens of patients with Parkinson's disease who received this therapy for a variety of psychiatric indications, including depression, mania, and drug-induced psychosis (Rasmussen and Abrams, 1991, 1992). There is also substantial evidence for the antiparkinsonian effect of ECT in nonpsychiatric patients, leading recent editorials to recommend the use of ECT in selected Parkinson's disease patients (Fink, 1988; Abrams, 1989b).

The first clinical report was from Fromm (1959), who treated 8 patients with Parkinson's disease and unspecified psychopathologic symptoms, who had received various antiparkinsonian medications and showed no sustained improvement. His patients, who ranged in age from 40 to 69 years with a duration of symptoms of 5 to 20 years, all exhibited prominent rigidity, bradykinesia, and bradyphrenia. After 5 to 6 ECT treatments, 5 patients improved markedly, and some previously bedridden patients were able to walk. Improvement generally began after the first treatment, was maximally observed after the second or third, and was sustained for 2 to 3 months before relapse. Prominent tremor was a poor prognostic sign in this sample.

Virtually all subsequent reports have been equally sanguine and have been reviewed in detail elsewhere (Rasmussen and Abrams, 1991, 1992).

In the most systematic clinical presentation to date, Douyon et al. (1989) provided extensive quantitative data for 7 patients treated for depression with ECT. All had received levodopa/carbidopa before ECT and were continued on this regimen during the course of treatment. Ages ranged from 61 to 73 years, with an average duration of Parkinson's disease of about 9 years. Bilateral ECT given at just above seizure threshold yielded substantial improvements in all of five subscales of an extrapyramidal symptoms rating scale that included postural stability, gait, tremor, bradykinesia, and rigidity. These effects appeared after only two treatments and generally continued for up to five more treatments, although one patient had only minimal improvement. Depressed mood improved in all. Two patients developed treatment-emergent dyskinesias that resolved when their levodopa doses were halved. While patients were on maintenance levodopa/carbidopa, relapses occurred at 4 weeks in 1 patient, 6 weeks in another, and not at all in 4 patients during a 6-month follow-up. Interestingly, there was a high positive association ($r = 0.917$) between the age of the patient and the scored degree of ECT-induced improvement.

In addition to the numerous case reports and small series, a group of Swedish investigators has used ECT as the primary treatment for Parkinson's disease without concomitant psychopathologic symptoms. Balldin et al. (1980b, 1981) used bilateral ECT to treat 9 such patients, age 52 to 70 years, with a duration of Parkinson's disease of 6 to 20 years. All patients had been on levodopa and had developed the on-off syndrome. The investigators quantified the percent of "on" and "off" time before and after the courses of ECT. After five to six treatments, a marked reduction in "off" time was observed for 4 to 41 weeks in 5 patients; 4 patients experienced little if any benefit. As in the report by Douyon et al. (1989), there was a high positive correlation between age and degree of improvement. Duration and amount of levodopa treatment also correlated substantially with ECT response.

In the methodologically most compelling study to date, also from the Swedish group (Andersen et al., 1987), 11 nondepressed, nondemented Parkinson's disease patients were randomly assigned to receive either genuine or sham ECT, the latter consisting of anesthesia induction without subsequent electrical stimulation. Patient ages ranged from 54 to 81 years, with a 6- to 32-year history of Parkinson's disease. All patients had been on levodopa and had developed the on-off phenomenon. Patients treated with genuine ECT enjoyed a greater reduction in "off" time than those receiving sham ECT. Most patients were treated with bilateral ECT; of the two who received unilateral ECT, only one experienced substantial reduction in "off" time. For the 9 patients who experienced a marked reduction in extrapyramidal symptoms with genuine ECT, improvement lasted from 2 to 6 weeks.

Thus, numerous case reports of psychiatric patients with Parkinson's disease demonstrate a substantial and occasionally long-lived antiparkinsonian effect of ECT. Additionally, three prospective trials of ECT—one of them placebo-controlled—have confirmed this effect in nondepressed, nondemented Parkinson's disease patients. Although systematic clinical data have not been extensively collected, it appears that advanced age and severe disability (bedridden, on-off syndrome) may actually be favorable prognostic features for a response to ECT. Although treatment-emergent dyskinesias may occur during ECT in patients receiving concomitant levodopa therapy, they respond to levodopa dosage reduction (prophylactic halving of levodopa dosage before starting ECT may prevent this troubling side effect).

Improvement in Parkinson's disease symptoms is reported with both bilateral and unilateral ECT and tends to occur after the first few treatments (Douyon et al., 1989). Few investigators have recorded the stimulus parameters used. Roth et al. (1988) achieved success with right unilateral placement and stimuli that were 150% above threshold, and Douyon et al. (1989) used just-above-threshold bilateral ECT. Although there are virtually no data concerning optimal seizure length in the treatment of Parkinson's disease, it is notable that one of the patients of Douyon et al. (1989) improved substantially after two seizures of less than 15 seconds each.

Although sustained improvement in extrapyramidal symptoms has been described after ECT (Birkett, 1988), patients generally enjoy only a few days' to several months' remission, even with maintenance antiparkinsonian medication (Balldin, 1981; Andersen et al., 1987). The only published allusion to maintenance ECT is from Holcomb et al. (1983), who briefly described a several-month extended antiparkinsonian benefit of monthly ECT treatments.

PRACTICAL CONSIDERATIONS

The primary indication for ECT in Parkinson's disease is demonstrated refractoriness to antiparkinsonian medications or intolerance to their side effects. Thus, patients with severe disability (e.g., bedridden, on-off status) will be the usual candidates for this form of therapy. Patients should be thoroughly informed of the tentative nature of the use of ECT for their condition—the possibilities of limited benefit and rapid relapse—and explicit, written consent should be obtained in each instance. Levodopa doses should be reduced by half to prevent emergent dyskinesias, and adjunctive agents (e.g., anticholinergics, amantidine) should be discontinued before starting ECT.

As is done in the treatment of patients with associated dementia, brief-pulse right unilateral ECT should be used intially, because it has been reported effective in Parkinson's disease and is generally free from significant cognitive side effects. If the patient does not respond to the first three treatments, he should be switched to bilateral electrode placement. An electrical dosage markedly above the threshold should be given (e.g., 75% of the device's maximum charge); seizure length, as in ECT used for psychiatric disorders, should be at least 30 seconds of EEG activity.

Optimal antiparkinsonian medication should be re-instituted as soon as ECT is terminated. This includes return of the levodopa dosages to previous levels (assuming no intolerable adverse effects) and re-starting any previously helpful adjunctive agents. Serious consideration should be given to initiating maintenance ECT at regular intervals to prevent or delay return of extrapyramidal symptoms. This will require a trial-and-error approach of progressively increasing the inter-treatment interval from, say, once a week initially, to the longest interval that will effectively sustain improvement (e.g., monthly).

Neuroleptic-induced parkinsonism also responds to ECT (Shapiro and Goldberg, 1953; Ananth et al., 1979; Gangadhar et al., 1983; Goswami et al., 1989; Chacko and Root, 1983), even in patients who remain on neuroleptic drugs.

Neuroleptic Malignant Syndrome/Lethal Catatonia

The neuroleptic malignant syndrome, a potentially fatal disorder, is characterized by the development of fever, rigidity, dysautonomia, stupor, and elevated creatine phosphokinase levels in a patient receiving neuroleptic drugs. The rationale for treating neuroleptic malignant syndrome with ECT is obscure, but may derive from its resemblance to "febrile" or "lethal" catatonia (a.k.a. pernicious catatonia, delirium acutum, Bell's mania, manic-depressive exhaustion syndrome), a rare and reportedly highly ECT-responsive syndrome (Lotstra et al., 1983). Indeed, Mann et al. (1990) conceive neuroleptic malignant syndrome to be a neuroleptic-induced, iatrogenic form of lethal catatonia.

Several reviews during the past decade have amply demonstrated the often striking efficacy of ECT in alleviating neuroleptic malignant syndrome (Greenberg and Gujavarty, 1985; Casey, 1987; Mann et al., 1990; Pearlman, 1990; Davis et al., 1991): About 80% of cases respond significantly, reducing the untreated mortality rate for this syndrome by about half, a result similar to that obtained with dantrolene, bromocriptine, levodopa, or amantidine (Davis et al., 1991). Several authors report, however, that the procedure is not without risk. Regestein et al. (1971) report a 22-year-old man diagnosed as having catatonic stupor—but who clearly met criteria for neuroleptic malignant syndrome—complicated by thrombophlebitis, atrial tachycardia, pneumonitis, and massive pulmonary embolism that required inferior vena cava clipping. Immediately after his sixth ECT he developed ventricular fibrillation and lapsed into a coma with decerebrate posturing in which he remained at the time the report was written 7 months later. This disastrous outcome was doubtless aggravated (if not caused) by 5 days of parenteral administration of chlorpromazine just prior to the course of ECT in an unsuccessful attempt to treat the "catatonia." Hughes (1986) reported a 33-year-old woman with neuroleptic malignant syndrome who developed cardiac arrest during a session of multiple bilateral ECT, from which she was successfully resuscitated, and Grigg (1988) described a patient who received ECT 2 days after an episode of neuroleptic malignant syndrome with coma and who developed fever, tachycardia, and marked elevation in serum creatine phosphokinase several hours later. Interestingly, none of these three patients experienced significant relief of their neuroleptic malignant syndrome with ECT. Three deaths occurred despite intervention with ECT—two of them in patients who continued to receive high-potency neuroleptic drugs—whereas ECT benefited the syndrome in all cases where concomitant neuroleptics were not used (Davis et al., 1991). Incredibly, a major review article on the pathogenesis and treatment of neuroleptic malignant syndrome (Ebadi et al., 1990) contains but a single reference on the use of ECT for this disorder.

The frequently dramatic efficacy of ECT in patients diagnosed as having lethal catatonia (differing from neuroleptic malignant syndrome only in its temporal proximity to neuroleptic drug administration) has also been thoroughly documented by Mann et al. (1990), although the case they report—as well as the one described by Nolen and Zwaan (1990)—is unconvincing because the patient had developed the initial syndrome after receiving haloperidol. The fact that each patient then enjoyed a prolonged period of improvement—without further administration of neuroleptics—before again developing the syndrome hardly seems an adequate basis for claiming the existence of two separate disorders. More convincing is the recent report of Rummans and Bassingthwaigte (1991), in which 8 bilateral ECTs rapidly reversed a syndrome of severe hyperthermia, bilateral extensor toe reflexes, and decerebrate posturing in a 49-year-old catatonic woman who had not received neuroleptic drugs for over a year.

Lethal catatonia and its equivalents were described and reported to be responsive to ECT long before the introduction of neuroleptic drug therapy. Because its characteristic symptoms—with or without a recent history of neuroleptic therapy—are so often resistant to or aggravated by neuroleptic therapy and are rapidly sensitive to the effects of a few induced seizures, ECT is doubtless the conservative treatment of choice for this syndrome as well as its neuroleptic-induced twin.

Pain Syndromes

The only prospective trial of ECT for pain in nonpsychiatric patients is that of Salmon et al. (1988), who gave 6 right unilateral ECTs to 4 dextral patients with intractable thalamic pain secondary to right hemisphere strokes, none of whom experienced any relief.

3

Prediction of Response to Electroconvulsive Therapy

Prediction in medicine is more aptly termed prognostication and usually constitutes an assessment of variables that determine the likelihood of developing a given illness (e.g., myocardial infarction risk factors), surviving one (e.g., the staging of cancers), or enjoying a favorable outcome following an intervention.

Earlier prognostic methods are now mainly of historical interest. These include physiologic measures, such as the methacholine and sedation threshold tests (Funkenstein et al., 1952; Shagass and Jones, 1958), and personality variables as assessed by the Minnesota Multiphasic Personality Inventory (Feldman, 1951), Rorschach test (Kahn and Fink, 1960), and California F scale (Kahn et al., 1959). These have been reviewed in detail elsewhere (Fink, 1979; Hamilton, 1982) and are not included here because they provide no practical guide to the present-day administration of ECT. Somewhat more relevant to modern practice are the prognostic scales derived from the clinical and psychopathologic features of the depressed state, although, as we shall see, they are also of limited utility.

Hobson (1953) was the first to construct such a predictive index, recording the presence or absence of 121 clinical and historical features in a sample of 127 patients (''almost all'' of them depressed) before they received ECT. Two weeks after the treatment course, patients were classified as having had a ''good'' or ''poor'' response, and each of the 121 features was examined for its correlation with this measure. Thirteen features correlated significantly with the outcome. Five were favorable (sudden onset, good insight, obsessional personality, self-reproach, duration of illness less than 1 year) and 8 were unfavorable (mild-to-moderate hypochondriasis, depersonalization, emotional lability, adult neurotic traits, hysterical attitude, above average intelligence, childhood neurotic traits). By adding three "very suggestive" features (a favorable one of pronounced retardation and two unfavorable ones of ill-adjusted or hysterical personality) to this list, a checklist of 16 features was provided and scored by assigning one point for the absence of a favorable feature or the presence of an unfavorable one. Scores ranged from 1 to 14, the lower the better. A mean score of 7.5 was found to provide the fewest misclassifications into the good and poor outcome groupings, yielding a "hit rate" of 79.7%

Roberts (1959a) found that the Hobson index successfully predicted the outcome in 80% of depressives, and Mendels (1965a) in 78%, whereas Hamilton and White (1960) and Abrams et al. (1973) found it to be of no value. Mendels (1965b) also employed an item analysis (similar to Hobson's method) to construct his own index of all variables associated with a 50% or greater reduction in depression scale score 1 month after ECT. Four favorable items (family history of depression, early waking, delusions, retardation) and four unfavorable ones (neurotic traits, inadequate personality, precipitating event, emotional lability) correctly predicted the outcome in 90% of the cases; a subsequent study with an enlarged sample and slightly different index (Mendels, 1967) yielded a predictive accuracy of 86%. In this study, personality traits (e.g., histrionic) that were associated with reactive or neurotic depression were better predictors of outcome than were the clinical variables (e.g., early waking) that were classically associated with a diagnosis of endogenous depression. Abrams et al. (1973) were unable to confirm the predictive value of Mendels' (1965b) index in a sample of 76 primary depressives studied before and after a course of 4 bilateral or right unilateral ECTs.

Multiple regression analysis is a more sophisticated procedure for weighting the prognostic value of variables. It was first used for this purpose by Hamilton and White (1960). These authors included five pretreatment variables in their regression analysis that were selected for their significant correlation with the Hamilton (1960) depression scale score after ECT: duration of illness, body index, postmethacholine fall of systolic blood pressure, and pretreatment Hamilton depression scale score. The multiple correlation achieved was a modest +0.62, somewhat lower, but in the same general range, as that reported by subsequent investigators using similar techniques. Nyström (1964) selected 24 variables that were correlated with outcome and calculated individual prognostic values for each patient based on the partial regression coefficients of the items. Favorable features included early waking, retardation, and a profoundly depressed mood; unfavorable ones included seclusiveness, ideas of reference, depersonalization, obsessionality, and histrionic behavior. Outcome was correctly predicted in 76% of the cases. Carney, Roth, and Garside (1965) constructed their Newcastle Scale predictive index by applying multiple regression analysis to determine the weights for each of 35 clinical variables that best predicted the outcome 3 months after ECT. Five favorable features (weight loss, pyknic physique, early waking, somatic delusions, paranoid delusions) and five unfavorable ones (anxiety, worsening of mood in evening, self-pity, hypochondriasis, hysterical traits) were selected and yielded a score that had a multiple correlation with outcome of +0.67. Each item that correlated significantly with outcome also did so with a diagnosis of endogenous depression. The Newcastle scale was subsequently tested on a new sample of depressives by Carney and Sheffield (1972) and found to have a predictive accuracy of 76%; Katona et al. (1987) used the scale to predict both immediate and 6-month outcome in response to ECT.

It is also instructive to compare the accuracy of the predictive indices with the results that would have been achieved by simply giving ECT to every depressive referred for treatment (i.e., predicting a favorable outcome in every patient). Such a procedure would have yielded a 62% predictive accuracy in the sample of Hobson (1953), and 60% in the sample of Mendels (1967). Giving ECT to every patient with prominent melancholic symptoms would have increased the predictive yield to 72% (Mendels, 1965b).

Inflation of the prognostic accuracy reported for these various indices is inherent in the statistical procedures used to derive them (Abrams et al., 1973; Hamilton, 1982; Abrams, 1982a): Selecting those items significantly correlated with outcome and combining them in a coefficient of multiple correlation that "predicts" outcome in the sample from which they were derived. Because the item set was derived from the particular sample studied, the same variables and weights are never as effective at predicting outcome in other samples.

Moreover, workers from the University of Iowa have recently had less success in confirming the prognostic value of melancholic/endogenous features. Coryell and Zimmerman (1984) tested the predictive value of a DSM-III diagnosis of melancholia, along with a variety of other response predictors, in a sample of primary unipolar depressives receiving ECT. The presence or absence of melancholia was the only variable of seven tested that bore an inverse relation to any of the three outcome measures employed (Hamilton scale score at discharge, global rating at discharge, and mean weekly follow-up symptom score): Melancholics had insignificantly higher follow-up symptom scores and poorer global ratings at discharge. The presence of delusions was the most favorable predictor variable, followed by increasing age and female sex. The familial subtype of depressive spectrum disease was unfavorable, as was a longer duration of illness prior to admission. In a subsequent analysis of the same data set, Coryell, Pfohl, and Zimmerman (1985) also found secondary depressives to have a worse outcome than primary depressives. Depressed patients with a diagnosable personality disorder, however, do not fare any worse with ECT (Zimmerman et al., 1986). Another study from the same group failed to find any predictive value of a Newcastle scale diagnosis of endogenous compared with reactive depression in predicting ECT respone (Zimmerman et al., 1986).

Although Rich et al. (1984) also failed to find any predictive value of RDC and DSM-III subtypes of major depression—reactive, secondary, nonpsychotic—in 48 depressives receiving bilateral ECT, their sample consisted mostly of patients with endogenous or melancholic depressives, leaving little variance for their predictors to explain.

Abrams (1982a) analyzed retrospectively the data from 97 endogenous depressives who had participated in a series of studies of unilateral and bilateral ECT conducted over a 10-year period (Abrams and Taylor, 1973, 1974, 1976b; Abrams et al., 1983) in which Hamilton depression scale scores were obtained blindly before and after a course of ECT. Hierarchical multiple regression analysis was used to examine the relation between each of the depression scale items at baseline and the post-ECT depression score, which was adjusted to account for the variances of the pretreatment depression score, treatment electrode placement, sex, and the total number of ECTs received. After applying Bonferroni's correction for multiple statistical tests, no significant correlations were obtained.

Similar results were obtained in subsequent prospective studies attempting to predict ECT response in endogenous depression/melancholia. Andrade and associates (1988b) used four different indices (Hobson Index, Mendels Index, Newcastle Prognostic Index, and Newcastle Diagnostic Index) to predict ECT response in 29 endogenously depressed patients and found that, although the Newcastle Prognostic Index identified with high specificity (86.7%) ECT responders among endogenous depressives, it inaccurately classified too many patients as nonresponders, thus gaining specificity at the expense of sensitivity. The response rates of the other indices ranged from 75% to 76.9%, and their predictive accuracies were likewise unimpressive. Similarly, if one applies Bonferroni's correction to the data of Pande et al. (1988), no significant predictors of ECT response emerge from among 17 Hamilton depression scale items in a sample of Research Diagnostic Criteria major depressives. Prudic et al. (1989) also found that, among a group of patients who met research criteria for endogenous depression, endogenous and nonendogenous symptom clusters derived from the Hamilton depression scale were equally responsive to low-dose ECT.

Most recently, we attempted to predict the response of 47 melancholic male patients to 6 unilateral or bilateral ECTs by using individual rating items from the Hamilton depression scale obtained at baseline, as well as 5 depression factors derived therefrom (Abrams and Vedak, 1991). After applying Bonferroni's correction for multiple independent statistical tests, none of the 15 individual Hamilton depression scale items or depression factors significantly predicted the adjusted post-treatment Hamilton depression score, confirming that excluding patients with nonmelancholic syndromes from ECT samples attenuates the predictive value of individual or grouped clinical psychopathologic features of depression, presumably by truncating the variance to be explained (Abrams, 1982a).

Diverse individual clinical and demographic items have been reported to exhibit an association with ECT reponse. A favorable effect of increasing age on outcome with ECT was found by several earlier investigators (Roberts, 1959b; Mendels, 1965a; Carney et al., 1965), as was a shorter duration of illness (Hamilton and White, 1960; Hobson, 1953; Carney et al., 1965; Herrington et al., 1974). Although there are disparate results (Hamilton, 1982), two studies in addition to that of Coryell and Zimmerman (1984) also report better results in women than in men (Herrington et al., 1974; Medical Research Council, 1965). Other variables predicting a favorable response to ECT include cyclothymic personality (Ottosson, 1962a; Abrams and Taylor, 1974), pyknic physique (Abrams and Taylor 1974), diminished salivary flow (Weckowicz et al., 1971), and psychomotor retardation (Hickie et al., 1990). The report of a better ECT reponse in bipolar than in unipolar depressives (Perris and d'Elia, 1966) was not confirmed by Abrams and Taylor (1974) or by Heshe et al. (1978). Although there are contradictory data, the presence of precipitating social stressors does not appear to predict the response of depressed patients to ECT (Zimmerman et al., 1987).

The presence of delusional or psychotic depression has long been considered a useful clinical predictor of a favorable response to ECT; indeed, the largest between-group differences in the controlled, random-assignment prospective studies of genuine compared with sham ECT have occurred in the subgroup of patients with delusional depression (Clinical Research Centre, 1984; Brandon et al., 1984). The remaining literature is divided on this point, however, with several studies reporting a more favorable response in psychotic than non-psychotic depressives (Kantor and Glassman, 1977; Dunn and Quinlan, 1978; Charney and Nelson, 1981; Coryell and Zimmerman, 1984; Lykouras et al., 1986) and others failing to find such a difference (Abrams et al., 1973; Avery and Winokur, 1977; Avery and Lubrano, 1979; Rich et al., 1984, 1986; Solan et al., 1988; Hickie et al., 1990; Sobin et al., 1997). Clinically speaking, however, one retains the firm impression—shared by many other clinical investigators—of a particularly favorable response to ECT in patients with delusional/psychotic depression.

Schizophrenia

To my knowledge, Dodwell and Goldberg (1989) have reported the only prospective study of clinical factors associated with the response of schizophrenic patients to ECT. In 17 patients who satisfied Research Diagnostic Criteria for schizophrenia or schizoaffective disorder, short total and present illness durations, a paucity of premorbid schizoid or paranoid personality traits, and the presence of perplexity, were all associated with a favorable treatment response—a finding entirely in keeping with the known prognostically favorable features in untreated schizophrenia.

Dexamethasone Suppression Test

The dexamethasone suppression test has received special interest as a possible predictor of treatment response in depressed patients receiving biological treatments (Fink, 1986a). In an analysis of pooled data from studies that assessed the value of this test in predicting treatment response of major depressives to adequate doses of an antidepressant or to ECT, Arana et al. (1985) found that more than 70% of responders had a positive (nonsuppression) response compared with fewer than

50% of nonresponders, a modest but highly significant difference. ECT response was not examined separately in this analysis, and several investigators have now conducted prospective studies specifically relating suppressor status to ECT response. Coryell (1982) obtained dexamethasone suppression tests within one week of admission in 42 DSM-III major depressives who subsequently received ECT for clinical reasons. Blindly assigned global ratings of improvement based on a review of nursing and progress notes for the final 3 days of hospitalization were greater for nonsuppressors than for suppressors, a difference not found for Hamilton Depression Scale scores. At follow-up 6 months later (Coryell and Zimmerman, 1983), no between-group differences were found on any measures. In a subsequent and different sample of unipolar depressives receiving ECT, these authors (Coryell and Zimmerman, 1984) again found a significant correlation in the predicted direction between the suppressor status and the globally rated outcome, but not in the outcome as determined by Hamilton Scale scores.

Subsequent studies have, however, generally failed to confirm these initial sanguine results (Ames et al., 1984; Katona and Aldridge, 1984; Coppen et al., 1985; Lipman et al., 1986a, 1986b; Devanand et al., 1987; Katonah et al., 1987; Fink et al., 1987), and one can only agree with Scott (1989) that "there are no physiological measures or tests which are superior to clinical criteria in the selection of depressed patients for whom ECT would be an effective treatment."

Individual clinical features may, however, lack utility (Sobin et al., 1997). The observation that a given depressed patient is female, or older, or has a stocky build, or is agitated, is unlikely to influence the decision to give ECT. The fact is that favorable and unfavorable features do not exist independently of ill patients but tend to group together naturally into depressive syndromes, unfortunately often with substantial overlap. Favorable features generally characterize patients with endogenous or melancholic syndromes, and these are the patients who recover rapidly with ECT. The unfavorable features characterize patients with long-standing anxiety, hypochondriacal, and somatization symptoms—often dating from childhood—and personality traits of hysteroid dysphoria, dependency, and inadequacy. Such patients typically respond briefly or not at all to ECT and may even be made worse by the treatment. In practice, it is not so difficult to identify patients who are likely to benefit from ECT. For example, it is rare for a retarded patient with guilty delusions and suicidal intent not to respond favorably to ECT. The difficulty usually arises in patients who would not generally be considered prime candidates for ECT but whose atypical depressive features resist adequate treatment with antidepressant drugs. In such instances there is little help to be derived from the predictors, and the administration of a trial course of ECT results in improvement with a frequency that is sufficient to maintain the strategy in clinical practice.

4

The Medical Physiology of Electroconvulsive Therapy

Cardiovascular Physiology and Metabolism

Heart Rate

Anesthesia induction by itself increases baseline heart rate by about 25% (Usubiaga et al., 1967; Rollason et al., 1971; Kitamura and Page, 1984; Wells and Davies, 1987). During and immediately after administration of the electrical stimulus there is a sharp vagal parasympathetic outflow that is both neurally mediated and consequent to a Valsalva effect induced by forced expiration against a closed glottis. Without anticholinergic premedication (e.g., atropinization), an intense but transient sinus bradycardia occurs (Bellett et al., 1941; Perrin, 1961; Clement, 1962), with periods of sinus arrest (cardiac asystole) averaging about 2 seconds but occasionally recorded in excess of 7 seconds (Clement, 1962; Gravenstein et al., 1965; Welch and Drop, 1989). The fact that even longer periods of bradycardia/asystole can occur in association with subconvulsive stimuli (Decina et al., 1984; Wells et al., 1988) demonstrates that the electrical stimulus— rather than the induced seizure—is responsible for this vagal effect. Wyant and MacDonald (1980), who were unable to demonstrate significant bradycardia during ECT, reported the phenomenon in only 1 of 39 patients observed during 297 seizures; however, they did not specifically focus on heart rate during or immediately after stimulus administration—which is the point of maximum bradycardia—but inexplicably took mean highest heart rate during the induced seizure as their primary measure of interest.

49

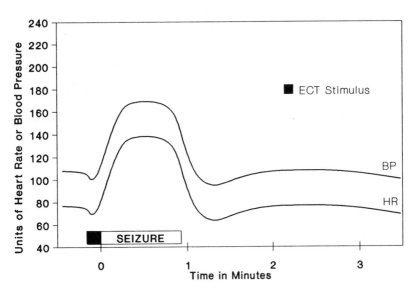

Figure 4-1   Heart rate and blood pressure changes with ECT.

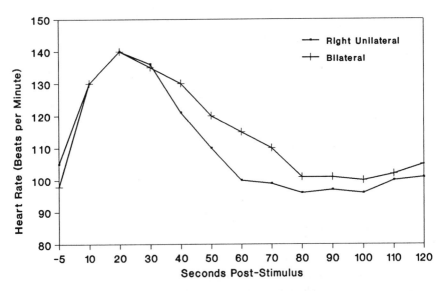

Figure 4-2   Effects of bilateral compared with right unilateral
ECT on heart rate. (Adapted from Lane et al., 1989.)

A sympathoadrenal tachycardia then supervenes (Figure 4-1), which is initially driven predominantly by direct sympathetic neural outflow of discharging cardioaccelerator areas in the hypothalamus, descending ipsilaterally by way of the medulla, upper thoracic cord, paravertebral stellate ganglia, and postganglionic cardiac nerves to the heart (Berne and Levy, 1981; Welch and Drop, 1989). Adrenal medullary catecholamine release later in the seizure may contribute to maintaining heart rate above baseline during the late ictal and postictal phases, although the mean duration of the maximal phase of the ECT-induced tachycardia is significantly shorter than that of total paroxysmal EEG seizure activity (Larson et al., 1984). Most authors (Gravenstein et al., 1965; Jones and Knight, 1981; Mulgaokar et al., 1985; Griffiths et al., 1989; Cuche et al., 1990) find plasma catecholamine levels in patients receiving ECT to be higher during the first poststimulus minute (presumably during the seizure) than at baseline or 5 to 10 minutes later. Contrary data are provided by Khan et al., (1985), who found that plasma catecholamine levels measured during two seizures in their patient reached a peak 9 minutes poststimulus during one seizure and were still rising after the patient had fully awakened from the other; the increases observed during the first poststimulus minute were only a tiny fraction of those recorded afterwards.

The relevance of plasma catecholamine levels to the ECT-induced tachycardia, however, is nullified by the report of Liston and Salk (1990) of a 73-year-old woman with bilateral adrenalectomy who nonetheless exhibited a classic hemodynamic response to ECT despite concurrent nifedipine administration: The mean rate-pressure product increased by more than 50%, from a baseline value of 13 897 to a postseizure peak of 21 069, and returned to baseline over several minutes postseizure. The authors concluded that ''a functionally intact adrenal medulla is not necessary for the pressor response to ECT.''

A neural-neurohumoral model of the effects of ECT on heart rate is consistent with the results of three separate studies from our group. In the first, Larson, Swartz and Abrams (1984) found a close correspondence between the durations of the ECT-induced tachycardia and the concurrent paroxysmal EEG activity; the correlation between the point of maximal heart rate deceleration and cessation of paroxysmal EEG activity was 0.75 ($p < 0.001$), a result consistent with primarily neural chronotropic effects during the ictal phase of ECT. In a second study (Figure 4-2), Lane et al. (1989) found greater postictal heart rates with bilateral compared with right unilateral ECT and attributed this

result to greater brain-stem stimulation—and resultant greater induced
adrenal catecholamine release—with the former method.

In the most recent of the three studies (Swartz et al., 1994b), ECT-
induced heart rate elevations after occurrence of the peak heart rate
were greater following right compared with left unilateral ECT (Figure
4-3), a result consistent with reports of asymmetric autonomic inner-
vation of the human heart, with lateralization of sympathetic control
of heart rate—specifically, cardioacceleration—to the right cerebral
cortex, diencephalon, medulla, spinal cord, and stellate ganlgion (Rogers et al., 1978; Berne and Levy, 1981; Rosen et al., 1982; Cinca
et al., 1985; Lane et al., 1988; Zamrini et al., 1990). This is the first
study in neurologically intact humans to demonstrate right-hemisphere
superiority in the control of heart rate within a paradigm of neuronal
activation, and it demonstrates that lateralization of electrode placement during ECT is reflected in lateralization of brain-stem as well as
cortical stimulation.

Heart rate drops rapidly at the termination of the seizure (Larson,
Swartz and Abrams, 1984)—falling to 50% of the ictal rate within 5
seconds (Welch and Drop, 1989)—and generally returns to baseline

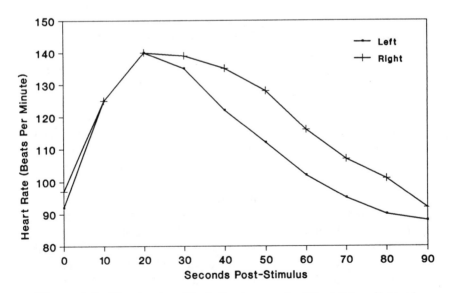

Figure 4-3   Heart rate after left compared with right unilateral
ECT.

or below it within minutes after the seizure ends (Tewfik and Wells, 1957; Perrin, 1961; Deliyiannis et al., 1962; Kitamura and Page, 1984; Wells and Davies, 1987; Huang et al., 1989), concomitant with declining plasma catecholamine levels (Gravenstein et al., 1965; Jones and Knight, 1981; Mulgaokar et al., 1985; Griffiths et al., 1989).

Blood Pressure

Blood pressure generally parallels heart rate throughout the treatment (Figure 4-1), dropping sharply during the initial vagal hypertonic phase and then rapidly increasing 30% to 40% over baseline to reach peak systolic values that often exceed 200 mm Hg in the presence of atropine premedication (Perrin, 1961; Bodley and Fenwick, 1966; Rollason, Sutherland, and Hall, 1971; Mulgaokar et al., 1985; Prudic et al., 1987; Wells, Davies, and Rosewarne, 1989). The fact that intra-arterial systolic pressures peak within 7 seconds of the first poststimulus heartbeat (Welch and Drop, 1989) suggests that—as for heart rate—the first phase of the ECT-induced hypertensive response is neuronally mediated. The initial rise in systolic pressure is proportionately greater than the initial rise in diastolic pressure, is more pronounced in hypertensive than normotensive patients, and in males than females (Prudic et al., 1987). Although much more epinephrine than norepinephrine is released during ECT (Jones and Knight, 1981), the norepinephrine levels correlate best with the hypertensive response (Gravenstein et al., 1965).

Early reports that the hypertensive response to ECT was related to its cognitive side effects (Hamilton et al., 1979; Stoker et al., 1981) were not confirmed in subsequent studies of the hemodynamic response to ECT (Taylor et al., 1985; O'Donnell and Webb, 1986; Webb et al., 1990).

Rate Pressure Product

The rate pressure product (RPP), systolic arterial pressure $\times$ heart rate, is a rough indicator of myocardial oxygen consumption. It increases 30% to 140% during the seizure (Jones and Knight, 1981; Mulgaokar et al., 1985; Huang et al., 1989; Webb et al., 1990), reaching its maximum about 30 seconds after the ECT stimulus; this response is substantially attenuated by beta adrenergic receptor blockade (Jones and Knight, 1981). The RPP and, of course, heart rate and blood pressure, varies inversely with age and baseline RPP (Huang et al., 1989; Webb et al., 1990).

Cardiac Output

Wells and Davies (1987) used noninvasive electrical bioimpedance monitoring in 10 patients to determine that cardiac output (ventricular stroke volume × heart rate) immediately following the ECT-induced seizure increased over preanesthesia baseline by an average of 81% and returned to baseline within 2 minutes. Using the same make and model of equipment, however, Huang et al. (1989) found that cardiac output divided by body surface area (the Cardiac Index) remained unchanged throughout the ictal and postictal period in 13 patients receiving ECT. These authors postulated an increase in peripheral vascular resistance as an explanation for their findings.

Electrocardiographic Effects

Abnormalities of cardiac rhythm and conduction are recorded much more frequently just after the induced seizure than during it, and are classified as either vagal or sympathetic. The vagal arrhythmias are of atrial, junctional, or nodal origin and include sinus bradycardia, sinus arrest, atrial premature contractions, paroxysmal atrial tachycardia (atrioventricular junctional tachycardia), atrial flutter, atrial fibrillation, atrioventricular block (first-, second-, and third-degree), and premature ventricular contractions during periods of sinus bradycardia. The sympathetic arrhythmias originate in the ventricles as premature contractions occurring during sinus tachycardia, bigeminy, trigeminy, ventricular tachycardia, and ventricular fibrillation (Perrin, 1961; Elliot et al., 1982; Pitts, 1982; Dennison and French, 1989).

Electrocardiographic (ECG) repolarization abnormalities reported during and immediately after ECT include increased T-wave amplitude, T-wave inversion, and ST-segment depression of nonischemic and ischemic types (Lewis et al., 1955; Green and Woods, 1955; Deliyiannis et al., 1962; Graybar et al., 1983; Dec et al., 1985; Khoury and Benedetti, 1989), all of which are reported to be entirely benign. The prevalence of ECT-induced ECG abnormalities is increased in patients with preexisting cardiac pathology and was reported by Pitts et al. (1965) to be significantly greater after thiopental than after methohexital barbiturate narcosis. Although this latter point has been repeatedly stressed in the ECT literature (Fink, 1979; Abrams, 1988;

APA, 1990), it is far from universally accepted (Selvin, 1987), and was not confirmed in the recent study of Pearlman and Richmond (1990). The occurrence of ECG abnormalities is essentially limited to the ictal and immediate postictal periods. Extensive examinations—including Holter monitoring—conducted up to 24 hours post-ECT do not reveal persistent ECG changes, even in patients with preexisting cardiovascular disease (Troup et al., 1978; Kitamura and Page, 1984; Dec et al., 1985). These latter authors have also stressed the neural origin of these phenomena, attributing them to direct electrical stimulation of brain-stem subcortical structures and thalamic and hypothalamic nuclei. Many of these phenomena (e.g., ectopy, repolarization abnormalities) are so regularly observed in young patients with no history or symptoms of cardiovascular disease that they must be considered normal physiologic concomitants of ECT and not in any way contraindications to continuing it (Deliyiannis et al., 1962).

Cardiac Enzymes

During the hours after ECT, significant elevations occur in serum levels of creatine phosphokinase and lactate dehydrogenase, but not in glutamic oxalaminase transaminase (Rich et al., 1975a,b; Braasch and Demaso, 1980; Dec et al., 1985). Creatine phosphokinase is found in the skeletal muscle, myocardium, brain, and gastrointestinal tract; only the creatine phosphokinase–muscle-brain isoenzyme is specifically elevated after myocardial damage (and the brain creatine phosphokinase isoenzyme does not cross the blood-brain barrier in the absence of brain damage). Lactate dehydrogenase is found in most human tissues, including skeletal muscle and myocardium; its lactate dehydrogenase-1 and lactate dehydrogenase-2 isoenzymes are considered fairly specific for myocardial damage. None of the myocardiospecific isoenzymes are significantly elevated when tested at multiple intervals up to 96 hours after ECT (Braasch and Demaso, 1980; Taylor et al., 1981; Dec et al., 1985).

Cerebral Physiology and Metabolism

The combined physiological effects of the electrical stimulus for ECT and the resultant generalized seizure discharge are immediate and powerful and may be detectable days or weeks after the treatment course terminates.

Cerebral Electrographic Events

If an electrical stimulus depolarizes a sufficient number of neurons, a generalized, paroxysmal, cerebral seizure ensues (Figure 4-4), the threshold for which is defined as the electrical dose (in millicoulombs, mC) that produced it. Subconvulsive stimuli elicit only an electroencephalographic (EEG) "arousal" response of low-voltage fast activity that is indistinguishable in appearance from that seen in the earliest phases of ECT-induced seizures (Penfield and Jasper, 1954; Chatrian and Petersen, 1960; Staton et al., 1981) and that Weiner (1982) has dubbed the "epileptic recruiting" stage. With substantially suprathreshold stimuli, this initial low-voltage, 18- to 22-Hz activity is rapidly replaced by a crescendo of high-voltage 10- to 20-Hz hypersynchronous polyspikes occurring simultaneously throughout the brain and corresponding to the tonic phase of the motor seizure. This discharge gradually decreases in frequency as the seizure progresses, evolving into the characteristic polyspike and slow-wave complexes of the clonic motor phase, which slow to 1 to 3 Hz just before seizure termination, and are often abruptly replaced by EEG flattening ("postictal suppression").

The degree of postictal suppression immediately following termination of the clonic phase of the seizure varies. Although it occurs abruptly in about one third of the cases and more often after bilateral than after unilateral ECT (Abrams et al., 1973; Daniel et al., 1985), many records show a less precise end point, with polyspike and slow-wave activity apparently stopping for a second or two and then resuming (Daniel et al., 1985; Swartz and Abrams, 1986) or gradually and imperceptibly blending into a mixture of alpha and beta activity (Small et al., 1970; Abrams et al., 1973). In about 10% of instances, however, the seizure end point is indeterminate (Larson et al., 1984). When it is clearly observed, the phase of postictal suppression lasts up to about 90 seconds, when high-voltage, irregular delta waves of 1 to 3 Hz gradually appear, followed by increasingly rhythmic theta waves that progressively merge into the preseizure rhythms by about 20 to 30 minutes after seizure termination. As discussed elsewhere in this volume (p. 132), the degree of EEG postictal suppression may reflect the extent of intracerebral generalization—and the therapeutic quality or impact—of the ECT-induced seizure.

The abruptness with which a seizure ended was attributed by Blachly and Gowing (1966) to a hypothetical "fit switch" that they believed became less precise with increasing numbers of treatments. They reported this phenomenon in patients receiving multiple electrically induced seizures in a single treatment session (this volume, p. 187) with concomitant EEG and ECG monitoring. They also claimed that successive seizures induced during a single treatment session tended to increase in duration, in contrast to the reverse trend observed for seizures administered at the usual rate (Holmberg, 1955; Sackeim et al., 1986b).

Our own data (Abrams et al., 1973) are at variance with theirs. We recorded the EEG during 45 sessions of multiple unilateral or bilateral ECT in 18 depressed patients. Most of the 160 seizures that we blindly rated terminated precisely and abruptly on both sides of the head, regardless of treatment electrode placement, a finding consistent with that of Bridenbaugh et al. (1972) and Kurland et al. (1976). When we considered the ordinal position of seizures in a treatment session relative to the clarity of their end points, we found that the final seizure tended to terminate more precisely than the first. In fact, in only 19% of the sessions did the final seizure terminate less abruptly than the first. We also examined the characteristics of the postseizure EEG by dividing the records into those that were flat and those that exhibited mixed rhythms in the alpha/beta range; virtually all of the latter records occurred after unilateral ECT. When postictal flattening occurred after unilateral ECT, it was always over the treated hemisphere. We did confirm an increasing duration of seizures within a single session, a phenomenon also reported by Bidder and Strain (1970).

The tendency for unilaterally induced seizures to terminate in mixed alpha/beta activity was also observed by Small et al. (1970), and may reflect a seizure for unilateral ECT that is incompletely generalized. A similar pattern of the immediate postictal activity was also observed by Kirstein and Ottosson (1960) for lidocaine-modified seizures, which were shorter in duration and less therapeutically active than those produced by conventional ECT.

At the level of the scalp-recorded EEG, the seizure appears to be an all-or-none phenomenon. The titration procedures developed by Sackeim et al. (1987a) show that it only takes a small increment in electrical dosage to convert an entirely subconvulsive stimulus into one that yields a generalized seizure of adequate duration; moreover, substantial increases in stimulus intensity above threshold do not further lengthen the seizure (Ottosson 1960). In the brain, however, seizure

EEG Seizure Phase 1
Buildup (Recruitment)

EEG Seizure Phase 2
Hypersynchronous Polyspikes (Tonus)

EEG Seizure Phase 3
Polyspike-and-Slow Wave (Clonus)

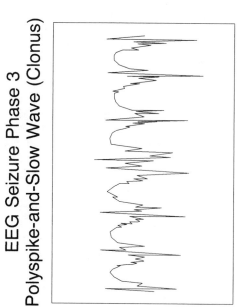

EEG Seizure Phase 4
Suppression (Electrical Silence)

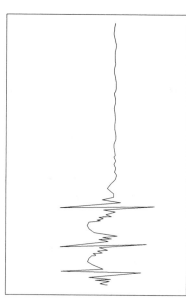

Figure 4-4   The 4 EEG seizure phases (diagrammatic representation).

threshold, frequency, amplitude, and duration may vary according to the structures involved. Chatrian and Petersen's (1960) depth electrode recordings in patients receiving inhalant- or chemically induced seizures also clearly demonstrate the polyspike phase starting at variable postinduction intervals:

> A high-voltage, rhythmic discharge already may be well developed in one area of the brain, while in other areas a similar discharge is only at the outset or the recording is still apparently flat.

The induced seizure activity described often terminated separately in different parts of the brain.

Seizure duration is variable in relation to stimulus wave-form and treatment electrode placement. Using a sine-wave stimulus, Abrams et al. (1973) found significantly shorter seizures with unilateral than with bilateral ECT, but the same method in a younger population (Abrams et al., 1983) revealed slightly longer seizures with unilateral ECT. Moreover, when brief-pulse ECT was studied in a smaller sample at the same center, seizure length was equal for both methods (Swartz and Abrams, 1984). In a four-cell comparison of unilateral, bilateral, sine-wave, and brief-pulse techniques, Weiner (1980) reported significantly longer seizures with bilateral than with unilateral ECT overall, a difference much more clearly seen with sine-wave stimuli. Although Horne et al. (1985) reported no statistically significant difference in seizure duration between unilateral and bilateral brief-pulse ECT, their raw data reflect about 30% more total seizure activity with bilateral than with unilateral placement. The most recent brief-pulse ECT studies (Weiner et al., 1986a; Sackeim et al., 1987a) find no differences in seizure length for the two methods when they are administered with just- or moderately-above-threshold stimulation. To summarize these disparate results: It seems that a tendency for seizures to last longer with bilateral than unilateral ECT is augmented by sine-wave stimulation administered at substantially suprathreshold levels.

Seizure monitoring during ECT has also provided the interesting observation that paroxysmal EEG seizure activity variably continues for about 10 to 15 seconds after all visible motor activity ends (this volume, p. 172), a discrepancy that may reflect incomplete intracerebral seizure generalization.

Intraseizure EEG patterns are usually symmetric in both hemispheres with conventional bilateral ECT but not with unilateral ECT. Small et al. (1970) reported asymmetric paroxysmal EEG activity during the late clonic phase, with greater amplitude and persistence in the nonstimulated hemisphere. D'Elia and Perris (1970) also observed a variable amplitude of EEG seizure activity with unilateral ECT: Their findings toward the end of the seizure were similar to those of Small et al. (1970), but were reversed at the beginning of the seizure. Kriss et al. (1978) continuously recorded the EEG for 30 minutes during left- or right-sided unilateral ECT and subjected the data to frequency analysis. During the seizure, paroxysmal slow-wave activity had significantly greater power over the stimulated hemisphere, contradictory to the findings by Small et al. (1970). This asymmetry extended to the immediate postictal period, with the treated side producing significantly more delta and less alpha and beta activity than the contralateral side. Confirmation of this finding comes from an EEG study of unilateral ECT (Gerst et al., 1982) that found that polyspike activity on visual analysis was more prominent and of higher voltage over the stimulated hemisphere, where digitally analyzed seizure activity also showed the greatest energy content.

In a series of studies utilizing computer algorithms to analyze patterns of EEG activity during ECT, Krystal et al. (1992, 1995, 1996) have focused on the variables of EEG spectral amplitude (power) and coherence (interhemispheric cross-correlations) in their search for measures of intracerebral seizure generalization and correlates of clinical improvement.

In the first study, involving 9 patients (Krystal et al., 1992), brief-pulse right unilateral and bilateral ECT were compared for the variables of EEG amplitude, symmetry, regularity, coherence, and envelope form. Although seizure duration was the same for both treatment groups, bilaterally induced seizures were associated with greater ictal amplitude (most pronounced in the 2- to 5-Hz bandwidth during mid-seizure), greater postictal amplitude suppression, and greater coherence during the ictal period. In contrast, unilateral ECT showed greater coherence in the immediate postictal period. Based on these data, the authors concluded that bilaterally induced seizures were more intense and better-generalized in both hemispheres than seizures induced with unilateral placement.

The finding of greater ictal coherence for bilateral ECT, yet greater postictal coherence for unilateral ECT, is consistent with the view that interhemispheric coherence should be maximized during well-generalized seizures, when all areas of the brain are discharging synchronously in response to the intense excitatory driving by a central pacemaker, and minimized immediately postictally, when driving has terminated. Postictal coherence should be lower after well-generalized than after less well generalized seizures (i.e., with unilateral ECT) because inhibitory processes are greater in the former.

In the second study, 25 patients were randomly assigned to just-above-threshold or 2.5-times-threshold right unilateral ECT, employing similar computer algorithms for the EEG analyses as in the 1992 study. The high-dose condition was associated with significantly greater spectral amplitude, coherence, and postictal suppression than the low-dose condition, and a shorter latency to slow-wave onset. The relation of these EEG variables to clinical response (and the implications thereof) are described on p. 131 of this book; suffice it to say here that the authors concluded that high-dose stimuli were characterized by greater ictal EEG evidence for more intense, rapidly- and well-generalized seizure activity, confirming and extending their earlier study.

The third study (Krystal et al., 1996) re-analyzed the data from the two earlier studies in terms of the relation of EEG variables to treatment response, and is discussed in more detail on p. 133 of this volume.

These considerations led Weiner and Krystal (1993) to call for the development of effective computer-automated physiologic assays of seizure adequacy that could be used on-line to provide real-time feedback on the quality of the induced seizure. Such assays for EEG delta power and coherence have now been developed for incorporation into an ECT device (Abrams and Swartz, 1989, 1997; Swartz and Abrams, 1993) and are awaiting independent experimental validation.

Because seizures induce physiologic effects related to the activation of different regions of the brain, the duration of these effects should correlate highly for well-generalized seizures. Swartz and Larson (1986) calculated the correlation coefficients between pairs of four different measures of seizure duration (motor activity, EEG spike activity, total paroxysmal EEG activity, and tachycardia duration) and found them to be significantly higher with bilateral compared with unilateral ECT, suggesting greater generalization throughout the brain with the former technique. Using the same method, Larson and Swartz (1986) also demonstrated greater intracerebral generalization with the first than with the second of two seizures given consecutively in a single treatment session. Because less well generalized seizures may be expected to spread more slowly and therefore last longer (indeed, the duration of total paroxysmal EEG activity was significantly longer for the second ECT), the authors' finding may help explain the increased occurrence of prolonged seizures with multiple-monitored ECT.

Following a single ECT, very little EEG change persists after the seizure patterns have terminated and been gradually replaced by the pretreatment rhythms. As the numbers of treatments increase, however, the EEG slowing persists into the postconvulsive period, accumulating as a function of the total number of ECTs and their rate of administration (Fink, 1979; Sackeim et al., 1996). This EEG activity increases in amplitude and duration and decreases in frequency with each additional treatment as long as the rate of administration remains above one per week. These changes are accompanied by a decreased mean frequency and total beta activity and an increased mean EEG amplitude, total power, and total paroxysmal activity (Fink, 1979; Kolbeinson and Petursson, 1988). Total EEG power reaches its peak 1 week following a course of ECT and then diminishes rapidly over the following weeks (Kolbeinsson and Petursson, 1988).

With the usual three treatments per week, the EEG obtained 24 to 48 hours after six to eight seizures given with sine-wave bilateral ECT is often dominated by theta/delta activity (Figure 4-5) with a marked reduction in the abundance of normal alpha/beta rhythms. This

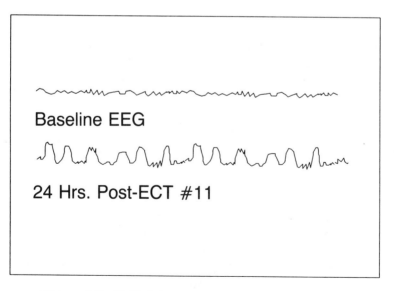

Baseline EEG

24 Hrs. Post-ECT #11

Figure 4-5   EEG delta activity 24 hours after ECT.

postconvulsive (interictal) EEG slowing is also related to the pretreatment EEG, age, and method of seizure induction (Volavka et al., 1972). Following the final treatment of a series of ECT, the cumulative EEG slowing typically diminishes gradually over time and eventually disappears (Weiner, 1980). The time required for this to occur varies directly with the total number of treatments received (Pacella et al., 1942; Mosovich and Katzenelbogen, 1948; Roth, 1951). Most studies show a return to baseline by 30 days post-ECT (Moriarity and Siemens, 1947; Roth, 1951; Bergman et al., 1952; Kolbeinsson and Petursson, 1988), although a few patients are described with persistent slowing up to 1 year later (Proctor and Goodwin, 1943; Taylor and Pacella, 1948; Klotz, 1955; Small, 1974). The most recent study (Sackeim et al., 1996) found no evidence of EEG slowing 8 weeks after ECT. Similar findings have been reported with chemically induced seizures (Weiner, 1980). In a study of patients who had received ECT 6 to 94 months earlier (mean, 26 months), Kolbeinsson and Petursson (1988) found combined theta/delta activity to account for 39.5% of total EEG power, compared with values of 37.6% in healthy volunteers, 33.1% in comparable patients without a history of ECT, and 34.7% in patients receiving 150 mg/day amitriptyline.

The pretreatment EEG is a significant predictor of postconvulsive patterns. In our own work (Volavka et al., 1972), we subjected the pre- and post-ECT EEGs to computer analysis and found that the pretreatment EEG accounted for 14% of the variance of the total post-ECT slowing and for 41% of the variance of the pooled average frequency. ECT-induced EEG slowing was directly proportional to the number of treatments given and consisted mainly of an increase in delta activity. We also reported a significant correlation between increasing age and decreasing average frequency. The failure of Strömgren and Juul-Jensen (1975) and Weiner (1983a) to find a significant correlation between the number of ECTs administered and the degree of EEG slowing may be a statistical artifact caused by the small range of treatments given (Weiner, 1983a).

With sine-wave bilateral ECT, the induced EEG slowing is either symmetric or accentuated over the left hemisphere (Green, 1957; Abrams et al., 1970; Volavka et al., 1972; Marjerrisson et al., 1975; Strömgren and Juul-Jensen, 1975; Weiner et al., 1986a; Abrams et al., 1987; Sackeim et al., 1996). Schultz et al. (1968) found a similar asymmetry in patients receiving pentylenetetrazol convulsive therapy. Sine-wave unilateral ECT also frequently induces asymmetric postconvulsive EEG slowing (Martin et al., 1965; Zamora and Kaelbling,

1965; Sutherland et al., 1969; Abrams et al., 1970; Volavka et al., 1972; Abrams et al., 1987; Sackeim et al., 1996) that is accentuated over the stimulated (usually, right) hemisphere. Using brief-pulse ECT, however (Abrams, Volavka, and Schrift, 1992), we found no tendency for any treatment electrode placement—bilateral or left or right unilateral—to induce lateralized interictal EEG patterns (see below). The differential lateralization of EEG slowing with sine-wave right unilateral and bilateral ECT is age-related, with increasing age associated with a relative reduction of left versus right hemisphere frequencies (Volavka et al., 1972). The visual evoked potential is also asymmetric after unilateral ECT (Kriss et al., 1980), with the major positive component being significantly smaller and later on the treated side.

Electroencephalographic Change and Treatment Response

Some early studies reported a direct relation of ECT-induced EEG slowing to the therapeutic response in depressed patients. Roth (1951) used quantitative measures to assess the EEG delta activity elicited by intravenous thiopental in endogenous depressives after a course of ECT. He found that the greater the amount of delta activity elicited, the less was the likelihood of a relapse 3 and 6 months later, but he detected no relation between therapeutic outcome and thiopental-elicited delta activity 3 days after ECT. Fink and Kahn (1957) also used objective methods to measure the ECT-induced delta activity in a large sample of patients and related this activity to clinical response as evaluated during at least 8 weeks of follow-up. They found the greatest clinical improvement in patients with the most EEG slowing and also reported that the early appearance of such slowing was related to assessments of global improvement. Other early workers reported either no relation between EEG slowing and improvement (Hughes et al., 1941; Taylor and Pacella, 1948; Bergman et al., 1952; Johnson et al., 1960; Ulett, 1962) or an inverse one (Honcke and Zahle, 1946; Mosovich and Katzenelbogen, 1948).

In a subsequent study from Fink's laboratory (Volavka et al., 1972) computer-derived frequency and power spectral analyses were used to measure EEG delta activity after ECT. No relation was found between these measures and clinical improvement in depression as assessed by reduction in Hamilton Depression Scale scores. This study differed from the earlier ones both in its use of computer EEG analysis and a multiple regression data-analytic procedure that covaried the total number of treatments given out of the equation before calculating the correlation between EEG slowing and therapeutic response. This finding suggested that global EEG slowing and therapeutic response were both a function of the number of ECTs given, but were not themselves causally related. Indeed, recent EEG data from patients receiving brief-pulse unilateral ECT indicated that full recovery was possible in the absence of demonstrable slowing (Weiner et al., 1986a; Abrams Volavka, and Schrift, 1992).

The previous studies, however, were concerned primarily with measuring global EEG slowing, whereas our own data (Abrams et al., 1987) initially suggested that an existing relation between lateralized EEG slowing and improvement might have been obscured in global analyses because it was opposite in direction for each hemisphere. In that study, we obtained Hamilton Rating Scales for depression and research EEGs for visual and computer analysis in a sample of 34 melancholics before and after 6 right unilateral or bilateral ECTs. Depression scale ratings and EEG analyses were done blindly and independently. The two ECT methods were equally effective in patients who did not develop asymmetrical EEG slowing after ECT; however, a substantial therapeutic advantage was observed for bilateral ECT in patients who developed asymmetrical EEG slowing: a right-sided asymmetry was associated with unilateral ECT and a lesser treatment response, and a left-sided asymmetry, with bilateral ECT and a greater treatment response. Computer EEG analysis using a right-to-left ratio of the EEG slowing supported this relationship, which was not a function of age, handedness, pre-ECT EEG asymmetry, or drug administration.

In a later attempt to confirm this study, we used a brief-pulse stimulus and the wide temporoparietal d'Elia unilateral placement instead of the sine-wave stimulus and the narrow Lancaster placement originally used. This time, however, a visual analysis of EEGs obtained in 33 melancholic men before and after 6 ECTs failed to reveal the previously detected relation between therapeutic outcome and differential hemispheric lateralization of ECT-induced EEG slowing (Abrams, Volavka and Schrift, 1992). These results are likely related to differences in stimulus site or waveform—consistent with reduced neurotoxicity of the brief-pulse compared with the sine-wave stimulus—and do not support the hypothesis that lateralization of ECT-induced EEG slowing is central to the antidepressant effects of ECT. Thus, a simple therapeutic advantage for bilateral over right-unilateral ECT—rather than a specific relation between induced EEG asymmetry and treatment response—is the most parsimonious explanation for our earlier results.

Considering the foregoing, it is striking that the methodologically sophisticated and meticulous study of Sackeim et al. (1996) has nevertheless finally confirmed the original suggestion of Fink and Kahn (1957) that increased frontal delta activity is related to improvement with ECT. In a sample of 62 inpatients with major depressive disorder who were randomized to receive right unilateral or bilateral ECT given at high or low dosages, effective forms of ECT (i.e., both forms of bilateral ECT, plus high-dose unilateral ECT) increased interictal delta power in prefrontal brain regions, an increase that correlated significantly with the degree of clinical improvement. Confirming earlier studies (Abrams et al., 1970; Volavka et al., 1972; Abrams, Taylor, and Volavka, 1987) Sackeim et al. (1996) found differential lateralization of ECT-induced delta power for bilateral and right unilateral ECT, with an accentuation over the right hemisphere with right unilateral ECT, and the left hemisphere with bilateral ECT. As in the study of Abrams, Volavka, and Schrift (1992), no relation was found between lateralized delta power increases and treatment response.

The results of Sackeim et al. (1996) are especially interesting in view of that group's corollary finding (this volume, p. 70) that reduced prefrontal cerebral blood flow immediately following ECT was strongly related to clinical response (Nobler et al., 1994). Because both increased delta power and reduced cerebral blood flow reflect increased cortical inhibition, the two studies taken together provide substantial support for the theory that inhibitory processes are central to the mechanism of action of ECT in major depression (Sackeim, 1994a,b).

The Sleep Electroencephalogram

Abnormalities in the all-night sleep EEG have been described in depressed patients, the most consistently reported of which is a reduction in the speed of onset (latency) of rapid-eye-movement (REM) sleep, which also correlates with the severity of the depression (Kupfer, 1986). Although ECT is generally reported to increase mean REM latency in samples of drug-free depressives (Hoffman et al., 1985; Linkowski et al., 1987; Coffey et al., 1988b), the data have been characterized by marked individual variability, perhaps as a result of the small samples studied and their diagnostic heterogeneity (Coffey et al., 1988a). Even more problematic is the relation between ECT-induced

REM latency increase and relief from depression, because several instances of full recovery without restoration of REM latency to the
normal range, and vice versa, have been reported. Characterization of
the specific effects of ECT on EEG sleep stages and the resultant
effects, if any, on clinical symptoms, awaits the study of larger samples
of drug-free melancholic patients.

Cerebral Metabolism, Oxygenation, and Blood Flow

The induced cerebral electrical discharges during ECT and the subsequent changes in electrical rhythms are accompanied by changes in
cerebral blood flow, oxygenation, and glucose utilization. Penfield et
al. (1939) studied cerebral blood flow during induced seizures in animals and humans and reported that vasospasm played no role during
a seizure and that blood flow increased. They did not study oxygenation, however, and noted that it would have been possible for oxygen
consumption to outstrip supply during a seizure, despite increased
blood flow. Posner et al. (1969) studied patients undergoing ECT with
general anesthesia, oxygenation, and muscle relaxation, and measured
oxygen, carbon dioxide, and lactate concentrations in blood samples
drawn throughout the procedure simultaneously from the femoral artery and the jugular vein. Probably because all patients were ventilated
with oxygen, the pO_2 always remained above 100 mm Hg. The most
striking finding was the consistency of the cerebral venous oxygen
tension, which remained steady at approximately 63 mm Hg throughout the seizure. At no time in any patient did pO_2 fall near the 20 mm
Hg level, which is usually taken to indicate cerebral hypoxia. Arterial
pCO_2 did not change during the seizure, but cerebral venous pCO_2
increased significantly and returned to baseline during the postictal
period. There were no significant changes in lactic or pyruvic acid
during the procedure.

Intracerebral cannulation studies in dogs and monkeys have confirmed the substantial increases—averaging 74% in monkeys—in
brain pO_2 for at least 40 minutes after induced seizures (Reed et al.,
1971; Roberts et al., 1972)

Brodersen et al. (1973) studied cerebral blood flow and metabolism in patients undergoing ECT with anesthesia, muscle relaxation,
and oxygenation. They found that blood flow, oxygen consumption,
and glucose uptake doubled during seizures, with modest increases in
both cerebral venous pO_2 and pCO_2. In contrast to the findings of

Posner et al. (1969) these authors found a very slight but significant arteriovenous lactate difference during the seizure, amounting to 0.08 mMol/L 1 minute after ECT. Bolwig et al. (1977) used a xenon 133 (^{133}Xe) inhalation technique to demonstrate increased cerebral blood flow during ECT and postulated that a simultaneously observed increased permeability of the blood-brain barrier was secondary to capillary hyperperfusion consequent to the increased flow. Bajc et al. (1989) used single-photon emission computerized tomography (SPECT) with Tc99m-hexamethylpropyleneamineoxime to study 11 patients before and during bilateral ECT, starting with stimulus administration. Relative isotope uptake—and therefore brain perfusion —increased significantly during the seizure over the right, but not over the left, frontal and frontotemporal areas, increases that were much smaller in magnitude (e.g., only about 10%) than those reported by Broderson et al. (1973). The close coupling of regional blood flow and oxygen utilization in the brain (Raichle et al., 1976; Lebrun-Grandie et al., 1983) permits the interpretation of cerebral blood flow changes in terms of regional metabolic activity.

Using impedance plethysmography in patients receiving ECT under oxygenation, anesthesia, and muscle relaxation, Lovett-Doust and Raschka (1975) confirmed the marked increase in cerebral blood flow during ECT. Changes in blood gases during ECT are also associated with changes in brain electrical activity. Szirmai et al. (1975) measured femoral arterial and cerebral venous oxygen saturation, pO_2 and pCO_2 in patients receiving modified ECT and correlated changes in these gases with changes in the EEG, recorded simultaneously and divided into six phases: pretreatment, seizure, electrical silence, delta, theta/alpha, and alpha. Cerebral venous oxygen saturation did not change significantly during any of the EEG phases and remained more than 90% at all times. The venous pO_2 did fall significantly during the seizure, but rose above pre-ECT levels during the period of electrical silence, returning to baseline thereafter. The venous pCO_2 increased significantly during the seizure, remained elevated during the postictal slowing, and returned to baseline with the return of normal rhythms. These authors concluded, as did the others quoted previously, that there was no evidence of cerebral anoxia during modified ECT in humans. This conclusion was attributed in part to the small amount of oxygen used by the paralyzed muscles.

The increased cerebral blood flow reported during the induced seizure contrasts with consistent reports of its postictal suppression. Early studies using the nitrous oxide technique (Kety et al., 1948;

Wilson et al., 1952) reported modest reductions in flow during the postictal phase. Silfverskiöld et al. (1986) used the ^{133}Xe technique to study depressed patients before and after unilateral or bilateral ECT. They found cerebral blood flow significantly reduced for 1 to 2 hours after ECT with both treatment methods, more with bilateral than with unilateral ECT. Moreover, there was a significant accentuation of suppression of flow in the stimulated (right) hemisphere with unilateral ECT. All differences were more pronounced earlier than later in the treatment course.

Similar findings were reported by Prohovnik et al. (1986), who examined depressed patients 25 minutes before and 50 minutes after inductions with low-dose unilateral or bilateral ECT. Bilateral ECT resulted in symmetric frontal flow reductions of about 15%, and right unilateral ECT resulted in similar reductions over the stimulated hemisphere but only about 5% reductions over the nonstimulated hemisphere. These reductions in blood flow were greatly attenuated after the first ECT in a series, analagous to the attenuation over time of the increased flows observed during the seizure itself (Brodersen et al., 1973). Rosenberg et al. (1988) obtained similar results using SPECT with ^{133}Xe inhalation, reporting that cerebral blood flow dropped 8% after the third ECT and a further 13% after the last treatment.

In an extension and amplification of the earlier study of Prohovnik et al. (1986), Nobler et al. (1994) examined the effects of ECT on rCBF in both depressed (N = 54) and manic (N = 10) patients, using the ^{133}Xe technique, and specifically relating the blood flow changes to clinical improvement. Cortical blood flow was assessed 30 minutes before and 50 minutes after a single ECT for both depressed and manic patients, and again during the week following ECT for depressed patients. At baseline, both patient groups exhibited deficits in global and topographic blood flow (e.g., hypofrontality); nevertheless, ECT unexpectedly induced even further global and regional blood flow reductions, which in turn were associated with greater clinical improvement following the course of ECT. In particular, anterior cortical (prefrontal) blood flow reductions were strongly associated with a positive outcome.

Together with the EEG findings described earlier (p. 67) of a positive relation between ECT-induced EEG delta power and a favorable treatment response in depression, these findings support the view that enhanced cortical (and specifically, prefrontal) inhibition is associated with the clinical efficacy of ECT. Of several hypotheses offered by the authors to account for the fact that ECT augmented, rather than reduced, the preexisting baseline abnormalities in cortical blood flow, I prefer the one that views those baseline abnormalities as inadequate endogenous cerebral efforts to counteract the physiology of major depression; when this effect is sufficiently amplified by ECT, it achieves the result obtained.

Positron emission tomography (PET) employing various forms of labeled deoxyglucose provides a measure of local glucose metabolism during seizures (Engle, 1984). Unfortunately, the present level of technology of this procedure, which only measures utilization over relatively prolonged periods of time (e.g., 20 to 30 minutes), does not allow discrimination of ictal from postictal phases. Within this constraint, however, Engle et al. (1982) were initially able to demonstrate increased 2-deoxyglucose utilization over baseline during ECT-induced seizures and a sharp drop in utilization below baseline during postictal suppression. They were, however, unable to confirm such a relation in the next series of patients they studied (Ackermann et al., 1986), perhaps because of technical and methodologic difficulties. Volkow et al. (1988) found statistically nonsignificant reductions in bifrontal cortical uptake of fluorodeoxyglucose on PET scans obtained in four depressed patients before and 24 hours after 6 to 11 bilateral ECTs, but Guze et al. (1991) were unable to confirm such a reduction in 3 patients studied 24 hours after courses of 6 to 11 right unilateral ECTs. Although the sample sizes and effects observed were small, it is notable that greater reductions in glucose uptake after bilateral compared with unilateral ECT are consistent with similar observations described previously for cerebral blood flow.

Cerebral permeability (the blood-brain barrier) is also affected by ECT. Bolwig and his associates (Bolwig, 1984, 1988), used a double-isotope technique to study both transcapillary escape and the capacity for capillary diffusion of small tracers (e.g., urea) into the brain during ECT. No increase in transcapillary escape occurred (e.g., as might be expected in a ''breakdown'' of the blood-brain barrier), but a net increase in passive diffusion of these small molecules across capillary endothelial cells was observed during a seizure, perhaps as a result of increased available capillary area caused by stretching (hyperperfusion) or by recruitment of underperfused capillaries. The fact that the same results were obtained during a period of increased cerebral blood flow that was deliberately induced by hypercapnia 15 minutes postictally suggests that hyperperfusion is the mechanism through which seizures increase cerebral permeability.

Mander et al. (1987) used MRI to study cerebral and brain-stem changes after bilateral or unilateral ECT in 14 patients. Scans were obtained before and after the first and a later treatment in the course in 11 patients and before and after the last treatment—followed by 6 additional scans at hourly intervals—in 3 patients. Immediate posttreatment scans were obtained as soon as possible after the patient emerged from anesthesia. T1 (spin lattice relaxation) times—reflecting tissue water content—rose immediately after the seizure, peaked at 4 to 6 hours, then returned to baseline; no long-term increases occurred across the treatment course. The rise in T1 time was 83% greater after bilateral compared with unilateral ECT, but not significantly so. These authors interpreted their data to support the hypothesis of Bolwig and associates (Bolwig, 1984,1988) that ECT induces a temporary, functional breakdown of the blood-brain barrier through increased cerebrovascular permeability.

Scott et al. (1990) generally confirmed these MRI findings in 20 unipolar depressives studied immediately before and 25 minutes after right unilateral ECT, with follow-up scans obtained 24 hours later in 13 subjects. The maximal increase in T1 relaxation times occurred between 25 minutes and 2 hours post-ECT; the largest fall was observed from 2 to 6 hours post-ECT; and all values returned to baseline by 24 hours post-ECT.

Seizure Threshold

Electrically induced seizures themselves exert a major effect on seizure threshold and duration. Early clinical observations of a progressive rise in seizure threshold across a course of treatments (Kalinowsky and Kennedy, 1943; Finner, 1954; Holmberg, 1954a; Brockman et al., 1956; Green, 1960) have been amply confirmed by the study of Sackeim et al. (1987b). These authors used a titration procedure of graduated electrical dosages to determine the seizure threshold at the beginning and end of a course of brief-pulse ECT; they observed a progressive increase in seizure threshold averaging 65% over the treatment course, an effect that was significantly more pronounced with bilateral compared with unilateral electrode placement. A progressive reduction in seizure duration from treatment to treatment was also found, likewise confirming earlier clinical observations (Holmberg, 1954a; Small et al., 1981). These anticonvulsant effects of ECT have also been used clinically in the treatment of epileptic patients (Caplan 1946; Kalinowsky, 1947; Sackeim et al., 1983).

Although it has been suggested that ECT may itself kindle (create by repeated low-dose intracerebral electrical stimulation) epileptic foci (Pinel and Van Oot, 1975, 1977), several studies show that electroconvulsive shock (ECS) exerts a pronounced anticonvulsant effect on amygdala-kindled seizures in animals. Babington and Wedeking (1975) showed that one electrically induced seizure administered from 15 minutes to 2 hours before an amygdala-kindled seizure markedly reduced its duration, an effect confirmed by Handforth (1982), who found that the anticonvulsant effects of multiple ECS lasted 1 to 2 days. Post et al. (1984) found no effect on amygdala-kindled seizures 6 days after a single ECS, but demonstrated a marked protective effect lasting up to 5 days after a 7-day course of once-daily ECSs. Moreover, these authors found that when ECSs were administered before stimulation given to induce kindling, this phenomenon was completely prevented.

Although no prospective studies have been done to determine whether ECT induces kindling in humans, a survey of 1000 patients who had received ECT in the past failed to reveal any clinical or EEG evidence of ECT-induced epileptogenic activity (Small et al., 1981). This is scarcely surprising, because direct intracerebral stimulation— a prerequisite for inducing kindling—does not occur during ECT.

Do Persistent Brain Changes Occur?

In view of the large and diverse effects of ECT on cerebral physiology and metabolism described previously, is there convincing evidence that ECT is capable of permanently damaging the brain? Although there are no data suggesting the possibility of such an occurrence, it remains a question of concern among many patients who receive ECT (see Chapter 11) as well as among two outspoken medical opponents of this form of therapy (Friedberg, 1977; Breggin, 1979). For obvious reasons, the question must be considered in light of the present-day practice of ECT, using barbiturate anesthesia, muscle relaxation, and oxygenation, sharply truncating the available body of data that addresses the topic, much of it obtained before modern treatment techniques became standard. Might ECT given in the era before these advances were introduced have caused brain damage in certain patients under certain circumstances? Conceivably, because patients often became cyanotic during treatment, generally received substantially longer courses of treatment than are administered today, and may possibly—although rarely—have developed tardive seizures long after the treatment course was terminated (Fink, 1979). Even in the absence of oxygenation and muscular relaxation, however, studies of electrically induced seizures in animals demonstrate that cerebral lesions do not occur unless seizures are prolonged for many multiples of the duration of those encountered during the administration of ECT (Weiner, 1981).

ECT could only cause brain damage through the electrical stimulation or the induced seizure. Because an electrical stimulus can only damage brain tissue by burning, the calculations of Swartz (1989a), which show that even under a worst-case scenario, the maximum output of modern brief-pulse ECT devices is incapable of elevating brain tissue temperature by even one tenth of a degree centigrade, effectively eliminate the possibility of stimulus-induced damage.

In reviewing his own and other studies of the neuropathologic consequences of induced seizures (primarily in baboons), Meldrum (1986) pointed out that selective brain damage involving neuronal loss and gliosis in the hippocampus (the brain region most susceptible to anoxia) requires sustained generalized seizures lasting more than 90 minutes, or more than 26 recurrent seizures in an 8-hour interval, or continuous limbic seizures lasting longer than 3 to 5 hours. These figures are for unmodified seizures; when curarization and oxygenation are employed during the procedure, continuous seizures for 3 to 7 hours are required to produce permanent damage. Although he raises the possibility that a prolonged period of limbic status epilepticus might conceivably be triggered in a susceptible patient, Meldrum also acknowledges that the potent anticonvulsant effects of ECT render such an occurrence extremely unlikely.

O'Connell et al. (1988) used mercaptopropionic acid to produce status epilepticus in paralyzed, ventilated rats under EEG monitoring and found that, compared with controls, lesions in the substantia nigra occurred after as little as 10 minutes of continuous seizure activity. Although this paper is the first to demonstrate neuronal damage in animals subjected to continuous seizures of less than 30 to 60 minutes' duration, its use of a neurotoxic chemical to induce seizures makes its relevance to ECT questionable.

Virtually all of the animal studies literature reviewed by Weiner (1984) had to be rejected because of the excessive electrical doses used, the fact that the seizures studied were unmodified by muscle-paralysis and oxygenation, the lack of unshocked control animals for comparison, and—most importantly—the inappropriate tissue fixation methods used. Two methodological features particularly characterize the animal studies of the 1940s that purported to find that electrically induced seizures could cause neuropathologic changes (Alpers and Hughes, 1942; Heilbrunn and Weil, 1942; Neuberger et al., 1942; Lidbeck, 1944; Winkelmann and Moore, 1944; Ferraro et al., 1946): All used the technique of immersion fixation in formalin to preserve the brains for study, and none used unshocked control animals.

Because postmortem cellular degeneration begins within 30 minutes after death, studies in which the brain is removed and fixed by immersion in formalin require a control group of untreated animals examined after the same postmortem interval to ensure that any neuronal changes observed in the experimental animals are the result of ECS rather than nonspecific postmortem degeneration. Moreover, crucial data on the lapse of time between death and fixation are lacking in each of the uncontrolled immersion-fixation investigations of ECS-induced neuropathology. The fact is, that in immersion fixation the formalin penetrates the tissues so slowly that autolytic changes take place before the tissue elements are adequately fixed. The definitive method for avoiding this problem is in vivo formalin *perfusion* fixation, a technique that rapidly and simultaneously fixes the entire brain in the living, anesthetized, animal: The formalin is injected arterially, under pressure, in combination with other agents to prevent tissue shrinkage (Windle et al., 1945; Cammermeyer 1972). None of three studies using the in vivo perfusion fixation method found any evidence for ECS-induced brain damage in animals (Fetterman, 1942; Windle et al., 1945; Siekert et al., 1950). It is further noteworthy that the same perfusion fixation technique was sensitive enough to detect the subtle neuronal damage in animals subjected to cerebral concussion (Windle et al., 1944), asphyxiation (Jensen et al., 1948), and inanition (Liu, 1949).

Unshocked animals, prepared and handled identically to experimental animals after the same postmortem interval, provide a critical control for the problems encountered with immersion fixation. Thus, Globus et al. (1942) were able to correctly characterize as ''pseudo-defects'' the minimal changes they found after electrically induced seizures in dogs because such changes were as common in the control as in the experimental animal. Likewise, Dam and Dam (1986) performed a meticulous cell-counting study in a group of rats given 3 electrically induced seizures a day up to 140 seizures and found no difference in hippocampal and Purkinje cell densities compared with unshocked control rats.

Friedberg (1977) and Breggin (1979) have made much of the petechial hemorrhages noted in the brains of animals given ECS in some uncontrolled studies (Alpers and Hughes, 1942; Heilbrunn and Weil, 1942; Neurberger et al., 1942; Lidbeck, 1944). Because these authors found no neuronal changes outside of the immediate petechial areas, which would have indicated electrically- or seizure-induced damage, it is likely that these hemorrhages resulted from craniocerebral trauma caused by the unrestrained muscular movements in the non-paralyzed animals studied (Windle et al., 1945; Siekert et al., 1950). When Siekert et al. (1950), during administration of ECS restrained their monkeys in a special chair in which the monkeys' heads projected through an adjustable aperture, they found no such hemorrhages. Moreover, when studies include unshocked control animals for comparison (e.g., Hartelius, 1952), hemorrhages appear in the control animals as well.

Hartelius (1952) was the sole investigator to use careful methods—albeit immersion fixation—and a control group to report any ECS-induced neuronal changes. He gave cats either 4 ECSs at 2-hour intervals or 11 to 16 ECSs, administered 4 per day for 3 to 4 consecutive days. He found what he characterized as "fairly subtle" neuronal changes in the brains of the shocked cats compared with those of unshocked controls, especially a greater variability in the affinity of cells for the stain and a tendency for the cells to show more darkly stained nuclei. The significance of these changes is unclear, because, as Hartelius was well aware, darkly staining cells are widely considered to be postmortem artifacts (Cammermeyer, 1961, 1972). In fact, Hartelius warns that "the risk of faulty and biased evaluation is still greater in the case of the nerve cell changes in question, since they are less distinct." Dam and Dam (1986) agree, characterizing Hartelius' (1952) findings as slight and mostly reversible.

Autopsy material from patients dying during or just after ECT is rare to begin with, considering the low mortality rates (see Chapter 5), and almost impossible to interpret because of the lack of any information on the structure of these patients' brains before ECT. There is, in addition, a great likelihood of extensive coexisting agonal changes because most ECT deaths are cardiovascular in origin and therefore likely to produce severe anoxic changes.

The recent and widespread availability of brain imaging techniques, however, now makes it possible to study directly the effects of

ECT on ventricular size and cortical structure. Several investigators have attempted to relate lateral ventricular size on CT scans to a history of ECT in different patient samples, a procedure fraught with methodological problems (Schwartz, 1985), especially selection bias. It is difficult to see what useful information might be obtained from demonstrating an association (or lack of one) between lateral ventricular size and a history of ECT in a particular sample of patients, because preexisting cortical atrophy (or the lack of it) may well have influenced the initial decision to administer (or withold) ECT. The problem is even further complicated when the patients studied (often schizophrenic) have also received a variety of other treatments (e.g., neuroleptic drugs) and have a greater-than-normal risk for cerebral atrophy for reasons presumably unrelated to the use of ECT.

Owens et al. (1985) nevertheless found no relation between lateral ventricular size and a history of ECT in their sample of schizophrenic patients, whereas Weinberger et al. (1979) did find such a relation for cortical atrophy. More relevant, because depressives comprised the sample, is the study of Calloway et al. (1981) in 37 elderly patients who had CT scans and were then assessed for a history of ECT. Ventricular measures did not differentiate those who had received ECT ($n = 22$) from those who had not ($n = 15$), but a significant association between frontal atrophy and a history of ECT was demonstrated: It occurred in 68% of those who had ECT compared with 27% who had not. As the authors correctly point out, the possibility that preexisting atrophy produced symptoms that preferentially suggested the use of ECT makes the data difficult to interpret.

Kolbeinsson et al. (1986) retrospectively compared the CT scans of 22 patients with a history of ECT to those of two age- and sex-matched no-ECT control groups: one of comparably ill patients and one of normal, healthy volunteers. Although both patient groups had significantly larger ventricular-to-brain ratios and cortical atrophy scores than did normal controls, they did not differ significantly from each other. In a subsequent computer-analyzed EEG study of patients who had received ECT 6 to 94 months earlier (mean = 26 months), Kolbeinsson and Petursson (1988) found no difference compared with controls for the percent of total EEG power attributed to combined theta/delta activity—which is the typical ECT-induced postictal slowing (this volume, p. 64).

Bergsholm et al. (1989) reported CT scan findings in a nonblind study of 40 patients treated with right unilateral ECT who were initially scanned weeks to years before receiving ECT and again 5 to 10 months after completing their treatment course. The authors do not explain the rationale for their nonsystematic method, which seems best described as inadvertently prospective. With one exception, no CT changes occurred following ECT, despite the fact that 9 of the patients had preexisting definite or possible organic brain disease; several patients had prolonged seizures (up to 6.5 minutes), and 29 received 16 or more ECTs (maximum = 46). A questionable dilatation of the left temporal horn was observed during the 6 months between the first and second CT scan in a 69-year-old hypertensive man who recovered completely after only 3 treatments. The authors felt this was probably unrelated to ECT, because relapses occurring 12 and 18 months later responded completely to ECT and lithium, respectively.

Most important are the several recent prospective brain-imaging studies of patients undergoing ECT. The magnetic resonance imaging (MRI) studies of Mander et al. (1987) and Scott et al. (1990) already cited both showed a return of functional brain changes to baseline by 24 hours post-ECT, providing no support for the existence of long-term or persistent damage. Coffey et al. (1988a) reported their interim results in the first 9 patients to enter a prospective follow-up study of the effects of unilateral or bilateral ECT on brain structure. Blind analysis of brain MRIs obtained at baseline and 2 to 3 days after completing the treatment course revealed no changes in global or cortical atrophy ratings or in ventricle-to-brain ratio, despite the fact that 6 of the 9 patients exhibited abnormal MRIs at baseline, with cortical atrophy or foci of periventricular or deep white matter hyperintensity. Now completed (Coffey et al., 1991), this is the definitive prospective study of the brain anatomic effects of ECT. Blindly analyzed serial MRIs obtained in 35 patients at baseline, 2 to 3 days post-ECT, and 6 months later, revealed no acute or delayed changes in total volumes of the third or lateral ventricles, frontal or temporal lobes, or the amygdala-hippocampal complex. Pairwise global comparisons in 5 subjects revealed an apparent increase in preexisting subcortical white matter hyperintensity, which the authors attributed to progression of ongoing cerebrovascular disease.

Pande et al. (1990) presented preliminary results of a prospective, blind MRI study of seven major depressives who received right unilateral ECT. MRIs obtained within 1 week after the course of ECT revealed no differences from baseline; as in the study by Coffey et al. (1988a), about two thirds of Pande's patients showed multiple areas of signal hyperintensity in the periventricular white matter at baseline, which remained unchanged after ECT.

In a prospective single case study, Scott and Turnbull (1990) followed a 77-year-old hypothyroid woman with MRIs obtained at baseline and seriatim across several courses of ECT. Despite the emergence of significant cognitive impairment following the last course, no evidence for brain damage was detected with MRI. Adding 4 more consecutive prospectively studied cases using quantitative MRI, Scott et al. (1991) found that 2 or 3 courses of ECT showed no consistent effect on brain structure, a result that is quite consistent with the report of Coffey et al. (1991) in patients receiving single courses of ECT. As in the latter study, Scott et al. (1991) recorded the development of a 2-mm subcortical focus of increased signal intensity between the first and second MRI in one patient, an occurrence that is quite frequent in healthy elderly subjects (Scott, 1995).

Although little definitive scientific information can be gleaned from individual cases, it is nevertheless reassuring to note that a 63-year-old woman described by Kendell and Pratt (1983) received 325 ECTs over 4 years without any evidence of brain atrophy on CT scans obtained after a few treatments and at the end of the 4 years. In a similar vein, Menken et al. (1979) reported that a 30-year-old woman who received 10 ECTs in a single 45-minute session showed no brain changes as measured by CT scans obtained before the session and 3 hours afterward. Most striking, however, is the report by Lippmann et al. (1985) of a patient who received 1,250 documented bilateral ECTs over 26 years, with an additional 800 ECTs claimed by her without supporting records. When she came to autopsy after her death at 89 years of age, the results of the neuropathologic examination were normal. Also impressive are the long-term follow-up neuropsychological test data from patients who have received large numbers of ECTs (this volume, p. 245).

Myelin basic protein is an antigen that constitutes 30% of the myelin sheath, and its immunoreactivity in serum and cerebrospinal fluid has been correlated with the degree of central nervous system damage that occurs with stroke and cerebral trauma. Hoyle et al. (1984) found no difference in serially sampled serum myelin basic protein immunoreactivity between a sample of 13 patients undergoing ECT and a sample of 14 normal controls, nor was any pre- to post-ECT increase in mean reactivity observed in the patient sample.

Devanand et al. (1994) reviewed the same material and reached the same conclusion: There is simply no evidence—and virtually no chance—that ECT as presently administered is capable of causing brain damage. Although ''absence of proof does not constitute proof of absence,'' proof of absence is precisely that which science is incapable of providing: No experiment can prove that something does not exist. What remains to be determined, however, is the basis for the reliable observations (Janis 1950a,b; Weiner et al., 1986b) that some patients may have persistent amnesia for selected autobiographical information for months or longer after a course of bilateral ECT. The fact that this amnesia does not occur with right-sided unilateral ECT when administered with the same electrical dosage implies that it has a functional, rather than an anatomical, basis. Studies extending beyond 6 months are now needed to specify the duration of the phenomenon.

Even if they are permanent, however, such memory deficits by no means demonstrate permanent structural changes, at least not as commonly understood (e.g., gross alterations of defined anatomic structures or cell fallout). More likely to occur, if at all, are changes in those microstructures (synaptic vesicles and terminals) that daily wax and wane as new material is learned or forgotten. Interference with protein synthesis can prevent consolidation of newly learned material, and neurotransmitter release at critical phases can enhance or impair memory acquisition and storage. That ECT, with its multiform effects on neurohumors, neuropeptides, and neurohormones, might exert long-term influences on such processes is entirely possible, particularly when it is understood that memory consolidation is an evolving, rather than a discrete, phenomenon (Squire et al., 1975). The question, then, is not to determine whether ECT does or does not cause ''brain damage'' in the sense of gross anatomic pathologic damage—it clearly does not—but to define those short- and long-term (if any) effects that ECT exerts on the acquisition and retention of information, understanding that according to our present view, it is microstructural events that are involved.

5

Electroconvulsive Therapy in the High-Risk Patient

ECT is a low-risk procedure. Its inherent safety, combined with an increasingly precise understanding of its medical physiology and the widespread availability and application of advanced monitoring techniques, now enables its routine and successful application in a group of patients previously believed to be too old or too physically ill to undergo the stress of induced convulsions: the ''high-risk'' patient to whom this chapter is devoted. The most recently published mortality statistics of about two deaths per 100,000 treatments (Kramer, 1985; 1996) places ECT at the low end of the risk range reported for anesthesia induction alone (Fink, 1979)—lower, in fact, than for childbirth—a development that is all the more gratifying in view of the steadily increasing average age of patients for whom ECT is prescribed.

It is instructive to compare these figures with recently published spontaneous death rates in an age range compatible with that of typical ECT samples. In a 10.5-year follow-up of 3,657 community residents aged 65 and older, Glynn et al. (1995) found that 1,709 had died, equivalent to a rate of 4.45% per year, or 1 in 195 over each 6-week interval, a death rate that was linearly related to resting blood pressure. It is thus apparent that, for whatever reason, the death rate reported for patients undergoing ECT is orders of magnitude smaller than the spontaneous death rate of a comparably aged sample. It would be tempting to speculate that the routine medical screening procedures for ECT are effective in eliminating the high-risk patients, were it not for the fact that the high-risk, geriatric cardiac patient is fast becoming the modal candidate for ECT. Far more likely is the possibility that ECT itself actually reduces the age-specific mortality rate in these older patient samples, a hypothesis that is supported by the studies of Avery and Winokur (1976), who found reduced mortality rates in patients treated with ECT compared with those treated with drugs; Philibert et al. (1995), who found that geriatric patients who received ECT were more likely to be alive at follow-up than those who had not received ECT; and Swartz and Inglis (1990), who found that a course of ECT reduced resting blood pressure.

It is further instructive to view the ECT-specific mortality rates cited above in light of the report of a 17-fold overall increase in the risk of fatal myocardial infarction, and a threefold increase in the risk of subarachnoid hemorrhage, in young women (aged 16 to 39 years) currently taking psychotropic drugs, particularly tricyclic antidepressants and benzodiazepines (Thorogood et al., 1992).

As noted in the previous chapter, the brain, heart, and blood vessels bear the brunt of the physiologic impact of ECT, hence it is patients with compromised cerebral and cardiovascular function who constitute the population at greatest risk during the procedure.

Management of Cardiovascular Risks

The gravest potential cardiovascular complications of ECT virtually never occur during the procedure; these include acute myocardial infarction, acute coronary insufficiency, ventricular fibrillation, myocardial rupture, cardiac arrest, cardiovascular collapse, stroke, and ruptured cerebral or aortic aneurysm. They are so rare, in fact, that none were reported in a multihospital study in Denmark of 22,210 consecutive ECT treatments (Heshe and Roeder, 1976).

The detection and management of significant cardiovascular disease before administering ECT is overwhelmingly the most important factor in reducing consequent cardiovascular morbidity and mortality: One need only contemplate the difference in the risk of ECT to a patient in acute congestive heart failure before and after he has been stabilized on digitalis and diuretics. The increasing number of older individuals with significant cardiovascular disease is amply represented among patients referred for ECT, and a great deal of experience has been accumulated in recent years in the pharmacologic management of such "high-risk" patients (Elliot et al., 1982; Weiner, 1983b; Alexopolous et al., 1984a; Dec et al., 1985; Regestein and Reich, 1985; Welch and Drop, 1989). The management of ECT-induced alterations in cardiac rate, rhythm, and blood pressure has received the most attention because these phenomena have multiform potential adverse effects in the presence of preexisting cardiovascular disease.

Vagal Cardiovascular Effects

Although it has been routine practice for many years to attempt to attenuate or abolish the vagal effects of ECT by administering an anticholinergic agent (e.g., atropine) before treatment, some authors have recently suggested that such drugs might best be reserved for patients with hypodynamic cardiac states or a tendency to prolonged asystole during ECT and should be avoided in patients with hyperdynamic states, such as hypertension or tachycardia (Bouckoms et al., 1989; Shettar et al., 1989). Atropine remains the drug of choice, however, for attenuating or blocking the direct vagal effects on the heart during and immediately after the passage of the electrical stimulus and in the immediate postictal period: sinus bradycardia and arrest (and the consequent sharp drop in blood pressure), the atrial and junctional arrhythmias, and ventricular premature contractions during sinus bradycardia.

Glycopyrrolate is an anticholinergic alternative to atropine that does not cross the blood-brain barrier and is therefore potentially less likely to exacerbate post-ECT confusion than atropine, a known deliriant when given at higher doses than generally used during ECT. However, although one prospective comparison of these two agents for ECT premedication (Kramer et al., 1986) found glycopyrrolate to be associated with less post-ECT confusion than atropine, a cognitive advantage of glycopyrrolate was not confirmed by other investigators (Kelway et al., 1986; Sommer et al., 1989; Saheba and Swartz, 1989). Moreover, Calev et al. (1991a), in an open clinical trial, were unable to detect any adverse cognitive effects of atropine, 0.5 mg intravenously, on a comprehensive test battery administered at baseline and sequentially over 110 minutes postictally.

Although Cropper and Hughes (1964) recommend no less than a vagolytic dose of atropine (2.0 mg), a systematic study of the cardiac effects of four dosage levels of atropine (1.0 mg, 1.5 mg, 2.0 mg, and 2.5 mg) for ECT premedication revealed no advantage of exceeding a 1.0 mg dose, administered intramuscularly 45 to 60 minutes before treatment (Rich et al., 1969).

Prolonged Asystole / Cardiac Arrest

The unopposed vagotonicity of subconvulsive stimuli has long been known (Perrin, 1961) and is responsible for the admonition (Wells et al., 1988; Welch and Drop, 1989) that such stimuli may represent a threat to the cardiac patient by inducing a strong parasympathetic stimulus that remains unopposed by a seizure-induced sympathetic response. In the case reported by Wells et al. (1988), a 15-second asystole occurred despite premedication with 0.4 mg atropine intravenously during the first ECT given to a 75-year-old hypertensive man who had sustained an inferior myocardial infarction a year earlier. McCall (1996) described a 55-year-old woman who sustained a 30-second asystole immediately following a subconvulsive stimulus, despite pretreatment with 0.2 mg glycopyrrolate intramuscular 1 hour before ECT.

These instances of prolonged asystole/cardiac arrest following subconvulsive stimulation suggest that the "method of limits" titration procedure for determining the ECT seizure threshold (Sackeim et al., 1987a)—which requires the administration of up to several subconvulsive stimuli in a single treatment session—provides a degree of cardiac risk. As Wells et al. (1988) found during subsequent treatments of their patient, even maximal doses of atropine (e.g., 2.0 mg intravenously) may not prevent the severe bradycardia that can result from subconvulsive stimuli.

Although the chart-review study of Zielinski et al. (1993)—who compared 40 patients with and 40 without cardiac disease who underwent ECT—found no excess in the overall rate of cardiac complications for sessions in which subconvulsive stimuli were used, all 5 episodes of bradycardia occurred in association with subconvulsive stimuli ($p = 0.016$). Two of the episodes required medical intervention, and one (see Decina et al., 1984) resulted in a code 99 being called for cardiac arrest. (It is further notable that an anticholinergic had not been given in 4 of the instances.)

In a prospective study of ECG and cardiovascular effects of subconvulsive stimulation during titrated ECT in 40 patients (22 with a history of active cardiovascular disease), McCall et al. (1994) found that despite intramuscular premedication with low-dose glycopyrrolate 90 minutes prior to ECT, subconvulsive stimuli prolonged the R-R interval and slowed the heart rate compared with baseline, and were associated with occasional junctional block and "brief sinus pauses," otherwise unspecified. (However, convulsive stimuli had an even greater effect on the R-R interval.)

Bradycardia/cardiac arrest can also occur following the administration of beta-adrenergic blocking agents, which prevent the tachycardia response of the induced seizure from reversing the initial vagal bradycardia. The cases reported by Liebowitz and El-Mallakh (1993) and Kaufman (1994), and two of those reported by McCall (1996), clearly illustrate this phenomenon because none was associated with a subconvulsive stimulus.

Liebowitz and El-Mallakh (1993) reported a 15-second asystole (characterized as cardiac arrest) during the fifth ECT of an 80-year-old man with hypertension, coronary artery disease, and an old anterior myocardial infarction, who had received premedication with a 10-mg dose of labetalol intravenously without concomitant anticholinergic premedication. Kaufman's (1994) patient tolerated the first 4 ECTs without difficulty, but then unaccountably received 15 mg of labetalol intravenously just prior to the fifth ECT stimulus (given without anticholinergic premedication), which was immediately followed by a 30-second asystole. McCall (1996) described 2 cases of prolonged asystole occurring in the absence of subconvulsive stimulation. These occurred in association with administration of the beta-blocker esmolol, despite intramuscular premedication with 0.1 mg glycopyrrolate 1 hour before pretreatment in one instance, and atropine, 0.2 mg intravenously, immediately before treatment in the other.

The 15-second asystole reported by Decina et al. (1984), also cited by them as an instance of cardiac arrest, could have resulted from either mechanism, as the patient received both a beta-blocker and a subconvulsive stimulus (again, in the absence of anticholinergic premedication).

The fact that several instances of prolonged asystole occurred despite premedication with 0.2 mg of atropine intravenously, or intramuscular administration of 0.2 mg glycopyrrolate 1 hour before ECT, suggests that these anticholinergic regimens are insufficient for the purpose. As noted above, I consider intravenous atropine, 0.4 to 1 mg, administered immediately prior to anesthesia induction, to be the anticholinergic method of choice for blocking the vagal effects on heart rate.

Although all the patients described in the studies cited above survived their episodes of prolonged asystole or cardiac arrest, I nevertheless have some difficulty considering the phenomena in question benign. I certainly agree with the recommendation of Zielinski et al. (1993) to administer atropine before treatment whenever stimulus titration is to be performed, but it is clear from some of the cases cited that this precaution may be insufficient.

In summary, the occurrence of subconvulsive responses, the administration of beta-adrenergic blocking agents, and the omission of adequate anticholinergic premedication all increase the risk of bradycardia, prolonged asystole, and cardiac arrest during ECT. The following recommendations should virtually eliminate the risk of such cardiac events, without in any way reducing efficacy.

1. Always administer a vagal-blocking dose of atropine (e.g., at least 0.4 mg) intravenously immediately prior to anesthesia induction in patients who are receiving beta-adrenergic blocking agents, or for whom stimulus titration is planned. Glycopyrrolate should not be considered equivalent to atropine for this purpose.
2. Avoid stimulus titration in patients with clinically significant cardiac disease.

Because no one claims or has demonstrated that the relatively frequent, entirely unpredictable, and occasionally prolonged periods of ECT-induced cardiac asystole are without risk, and until and unless adverse consequences of giving anticholinergic premedication for ECT are demonstrated, a risk-benefit analysis stipulates that an anticholinergic agent should be given before ECT. Moreover, because excessive salivation is not known to complicate ECT, and parenteral administration of anticholinergics 30 to 60 minutes before ECT serves only to cause an uncomfortable dry mouth that may stimulate the patient to drink water, I further recommend that the anticholinergic be given intravenously immediately preceding anesthesia induction. Finally, since glycopyrrolate has no demonstrable advantage over atropine, a drug that has been intensively studied for ECT premedication over several decades, the latter remains, in my view, the anticholinergic agent of choice for ECT.

Sympathetic Cardiovascular Effects

Attenuation or blockade of the acute hemodynamic and myocardial consequences of ECT may be desirable in patients with brain tumors, cardiac conduction defects or ectopy, hypertension, recent myocardial infarction or hemorrhagic stroke, and aortic or cerebral aneurysms.

AGENTS THAT LOWER BLOOD PRESSURE

In the previous edition, I devoted considerable text to the consideration of several potent intravenous agents for lowering blood pressure, such as trimethaphan (no longer available), sodium nitroprusside, and hydralazine. The intervening years have shown less heroic measures to be safer and equally effective for this purpose: nitrates, calcium channel blockers, and beta-adrenergic blocking agents, in order of increasing efficacy.

1. Of the *nitrates*, both nitroglycerine ointment and sublingual spray provide modest to moderate attenuation of the hypertensive response to ECT (Lee et al., 1985; Villalonga et al., 1989; Parab, Chaudhari, and Apte, 1992). A typical regimen of 2 inches of 2% nitroglycerine ointment applied to the anterior chest 45 minutes before ECT achieves a 15% to 20% reduction in the systolic pressure recorded 2 minutes post-ECT (Parab, Chaudhari, and Apte, 1992). However, nitroglycerine can induce substantial heart rate elevations (O'Flaherty et al., 1992), and therefore increase myocardial oxygen consumption, an effect that is likely to be undesirable in many cardiac patients.

2. *Nifedipine* is a calcium channel blocking agent that relaxes the smooth muscle of coronary arteries and peripheral arterioles. Its vasodilating action has been safely and effectively used to manage acute hypertensive crises (Schillinger, 1987), and to prevent or attenuate the ECT-induced hypertensive response. Sublingual administration of the contents of one 10-mg nifedipine capsule 20 minutes before anesthesia induction reduced the maximum ECT-induced systolic blood pressure elevation by almost two thirds (24 mm Hg vs. 62 mm Hg) in a placebo-controlled study of 5 previously hypertensive patients who served as their own controls (Wells et al., 1989). In a single case report (Kalayam and Alexopoulos, 1989), the same method reduced the maximum systolic pressure increase by almost 90%, from 300 mm Hg to 160 mm Hg. Heart rate was unaffected in both studies, and no complications were reported, but tachycardia can occur.

3. The *beta-blockers* are generally the most useful and widely used of the 3 classes of medications described in this section. Although propranolol was the first to be used in association with ECT, subsequent experience with this compound for this purpose has been neither extensive nor particularly favorable (Gaitz and Essa, 1991; Maneksha, 1991), and it has been abandoned.

Labetalol is the most systematically studied beta-blocker for use during ECT. In a single case report of a 74-year-old woman whose

post-ECT hypertension (e.g., 240/140 mm Hg) was resistant to clonidine and hydralazine, Foster and Ries (1988) achieved success with
labetalol, 15 mg intravenously immediately after her seizure, followed
by maintainance oral therapy. In a randomized, double-blind, placebo-
controlled study in elderly depressive patients of the effects of 5 to 10
mg labetalol given intravenously 90 seconds before seizure induction,
Stoudemire et al. (1990) reported significant reductions in ECT-
induced mean arterial blood pressure, tachycardia, and atrial and ventricular ectopy over a 30-minute observation period, without untoward
side effects. In a subsequent dose-response study of similar design,
McCall and coworkers (1991) found that 5-mg and 10-mg doses of
labetalol safely and effectively lowered blood pressure and rate-
pressure product (but not heart rate), without shortening seizure
duration.

It is notable that Holtzman et al. (1986) found that hypertensives
who receive single doses of atenolol, propranolol, and labetalol significantly reduced their cardiac output and heart rate—but not their
blood pressure—with the two former drugs, but exhibited precisely
the reverse pattern with labetalol: It lowered blood pressure without
affecting heart rate or cardiac output—primarily by reducing peripheral vascular resistance. This ability of labetalol to lower blood pressure without reducing cardiac output is of obvious import in the treatment of high-risk or geriatric patients who need to maintain their
cerebral and myocardial perfusion to meet the increased metabolic demands of the induced seizure.

Esmolol, a selective beta-1 receptor blocker and the shortest-
acting of the beta-blockers (distribution half-life, 2 minutes, elimination half-life, 9 minutes), was used by Kovac et al. (1990) to attenuate
the hemodynamic response to ECT in a randomized, within-patient
comparison against no esmolol in 17 subjects. An intravenous bolus
of 80 mg esmolol, followed by a 24-mg/minute infusion, blunted maximal heart rate response by 26%, blood pressure response by 14%, and
RPP by 37%, during the 4 minutes immediately following the stimulus.
Equivalent effects were obtained with a 100- or 200-mg bolus injection
of the drug given 2 minutes before ECT. Compared to the no-esmolol
condition, however, esmolol substantially, but not significantly, shortened seizure duration by 15% to 25%, depending on the dose.

Similar results were obtained by Howie et al. (1990), who used
an analagous design to study 20 patients in a double-blind, randomized, within-subjects study of placebo compared with esmolol. The
authors administered a 10- to 15-minute infusion of either placebo or

esmolol at an intial rate of 500 μg/kg/min, decreasing to 300 μg/kg/min for 3 minutes postictally, before ceasing altogether. Heart rate and blood pressure were monitored every minute during the infusion and every 5 minutes thereafter. Esmolol significantly reduced baseline (prestimulus) heart rate below that achieved with placebo and sustained this reduction over 2 to 15 minutes poststimulus, reducing maximum heart rate by 24% (from 152 to 115 beats/minute). Arterial blood pressure was also significantly lower with esmolol, systolic more than diastolic. Like Kovac et al. (1990), these authors found that esmolol reduced EEG seizure length by about 22% (from a mean of 86 to 67 seconds). In a subsequent dose-response study of 3 dosage levels of esmolol, Howie et al. (1992) found that an initial intravenous bolus of 500 μg/kg followed by an intravenous infusion of 100 μg/kg/min was as effective as higher dosages in controlling the hemodynamic response to ECT, and without significantly reducing seizure duration.

Weinger et al. (1991) compared the relative efficacies of labetalol and esmolol in blocking the hemodynamic response to ECT. In a double-blind, intrapatient, balanced randomized comparison among fixed, single-bolus doses of intravenous esmolol, labetalol, fentanyl, lidocaine and saline placebo conducted in 10 patients, these authors found labetalol (0.3 mg/kg) and esmolol (1 mg/kg) to be similarly effective compared with saline in attenuating the ECT-induced hypertension and tachycardia (e.g., RPP increase was attenuated 46% after labetalol, and 64% after esmolol). Both compounds shortened seizure duration (esmolol by 19%, labetalol by 35%), an effect that reached significance only for the latter drug. Although these authors conclude by expressing a preference for esmolol, it is clear from their study and the others discussed earlier that with proper adjustment of dosage, either drug is capable of safely and effectively attenuating the hemodynamic response to ECT without unduly shortening seizure duration.

Castelli et al. (1995) studied 18 patients with at least one cardiovascular risk factor during 5 ECT sessions in which 5 different pretreatment regimens were administered in a randomized block design: no drug; esmolol, 1.3 or 4.4 mg/kg; labetalol, 0.13 or 0.44 mg/kg, all administered by bolus push within 10 seconds of anesthesia induction. Systolic and diastolic blood pressure, heart rate, and ST-segment deviation were measured at baseline, and 1, 3, 5, and 10 minutes postictally. Compared with no drug, the low-dose beta-blocker conditions significantly reduced, and the high-dose conditions virtually eliminated, the peak heart rate and systolic blood pressure responses. ST-segment deviations were not affected by either compound at either dosage level. The effects of labetalol, but not esmolol, on systolic blood pressure could still be observed 10 minutes postictally.

Labetalol and nifedipine have also been combined to take advantage of the heart rate control achieved with the former, and the blood pressure control with the latter (Figiel et al., 1993). In a sample of 38 patients over the age of 50 years, these authors gave 10 mg of labetalol intravenously at the first ECT treatment and observed 10 patients who nevertheless exhibited sustained systolic blood pressure elevations (two consecutive readings >210 mm Hg) despite adequate control of heart rate. These 10 were then treated with nifedipine, 10 mg sublingually 15 minutes pre-ECT, in combination with the dose of labetalol already described. The addition of nifedipine appeared to achieve substantial control of blood pressure at all measurement intervals without further affecting heart rate; no episodes of hypotension or bradycardia occurred. Unfortunately, the statistical analysis is flawed (multiple paired t-tests rather than repeated-measures ANOVA were used), and the authors failed to describe the response vis-à-vis the criterion for entry in the study—that is, how many of the 10 patients exhibited sustained blood pressure elevations despite the drug combination. The relatively low dose of labetalol used—equivalent to the low-dose condition of the Castelli et al. (1995) study reviewed in the previous paragraph—also raises the question whether simply increasing the labetalol dose would have achieved the same results.

The beneficial effects of beta-blockers on cardiac ectopy, blood pressure, and myocardial oxygen consumption during ECT are, however, entirely safely enjoyed only after treatment with atropine. Based on studies in dogs that had electrically induced seizures in the presence of high spinal anesthesia, Anton et al. (1977) predicted that ECT-induced "activation of the autonomic nervous system in the presence of a sympathetic block would lead to a vagally induced protracted asystole." The aptness of this warning is illustrated by several of the case reports described above (Decina et al., 1984; London and Glass, 1985; Kaufman, 1994; McCall, 1996).

AGENTS THAT REDUCE HEART RATE AND ECTOPY

Prevention and management of the sympathoadrenal cardiac arrhythmias of ECT involve the use of lidocaine or beta-blockers. The most frequent of these extravagal tachyarrhythmias are VPCs occurring late in the seizure or in the immediate postictal phase. Occasional VPCs are of no concern; it is the frequent or multifocal ones that present a risk because of the increased chance that one might coincide with the apex of the T wave of the ECG and precipitate ventricular tachycardia or fibrillation (Lown, 1979).

1. Lidocaine (xylocaine) is a local anesthetic agent that prolongs the refractory period of the cardiac conduction system and increases the myocardial threshold to abnormal stimulation; it has been used successfully for many years to control ECT-induced tachyarrhythmias (Usubiaga et al., 1967; McKenna et al., 1970; Hood and Mecca, 1983; London and Glass, 1985). It is available for intravenous administration in 100-mg ampules. In patients with preexisting multiple ventricular premature contractions, a constant intravenous infusion is administered at a rate of 1 to 5 mg/min, permitting moment-to-moment titration of ventricular ectopic activity. For quick control of multiple ventricular premature contractions that develop for the first time during ECT, a rapid bolus push of 50 to 100 mg of lidocaine (1 to 2 mg/kg body weight) is safe and effective. A significant drawback of intravenous lidocaine, however, is that it shortens (Ottosson, 1960; Usubiaga et al., 1967; Weinger et al., 1991) or even abolishes (Hood and Mecca, 1983; London and Glass, 1985) ECT-induced seizure activity when given at the preceding doses, thus partially or entirely blocking the therapeutic effect as well.

2. Of the beta-blockers, labetalol and esmolol are therefore of particular interest because of their more modest effects on seizure duration (McCall et al., 1991; Weinger et al., 1991).

Treatment of the High-Risk Geriatric Cardiac Patient

Because virtually all cardiac patients referred for ECT are over 50 years of age (Zielinski et al., 1993; Rice et al., 1994), it is reasonable to combine geriatric and cardiac patients for purposes of this discussion.

Burke et al. (1985, 1987) employed a retrospective chart-review method to assess the safety and efficacy of ECT in a total sample of 70 patients over age 60 years, many with cardiovascular disease. In the first study, 5 of 30 patients were described as having "cardiovascular" complications from ECT (including one death); in the second study, 15 of 40 were described as having "cardiorespiratory" complications, for an apparent overall risk of about 30%, which led the authors to warn in the first paper that ECT "should be used with caution, particularly in those over the age of 75 years with cardiovascular disease," and in the second paper that "at particular risk [with ECT] are the very old, those in poor general health, and those taking multiple medications, particularly cardiovascular agents.'' Because they bear the imprimatur of Washington University, these articles are often cited—together with the article by Gerring and Shields (1982), discussed below—in support of withholding ECT in the aged patient with cardiovascular disease.

However, the lack of a control group of elderly, medically ill hospitalized psychiatric patients who did not receive ECT makes it impossible to assess whether all—or even any—of the adverse affects claimed by Burke et al. (1985, 1987) can be attributed to ECT. Moreover, insufficient details of the claimed adverse cardiac effects are presented to allow the reader to judge their severity. For example, in the first article (Burke et al., 1985), one of the 5 adverse effects is described only as ''an episode of hypotension,'' without providing even a blood pressure value in support of this diagnosis. In another instance, a sustained elevated blood pressure of 230/110 is claimed as an adverse effect, without any mention of what the patient's baseline values were or how long the elevation lasted. Worse yet, the death these authors attributed to ECT actually occurred several weeks after treatment, and in a patient who was taking theophylline at the time of ECT, a drug known to have caused severe complications and death when co-administered with ECT (see p. 196, this volume). The second article (Burke et al., 1987) commits the same errors as the first, claiming 2 episodes of ''marked, sustained elevation of blood pressure'' without providing the actual values or comparison with baseline; an episode of ''hypotension following treatment,'' otherwise unspecified; another episode of ''sustained tachycardia following treatment,'' otherwise unspecified; and so forth. In sum, both articles have to be excluded from consideration as lacking even a modicum of objectivity or scientific validity.

In addition to the question of the cardiac risk of subconvulsive stimulation, Zielinski et al. (1993) compared the overall rates of cardiac complications in their samples of patients with and without cardiac disease who received ECT. Cardiac medications were adjusted as necessary, and when the regimens were stable for 7 to 10 days, ECT was administered without specific additional cardiotropic medications. Although the patients with cardiac disease had significantly higher rates of cardiac complication during ECT, no deaths occurred in this group, and only 5% failed to complete the treatment course. This is remarkable in view of the criteria for inclusion in the cardiac group —which required at least one of the following: left ventricular ejection fraction <50% by radionucelide angiography; QRS complex of at least 0.1 second by ECG; at least 10 VPCs per hour by Holter monitoring —and the fact that 15 patients had a history of myocardial infarction. The cardiac complications observed in the cardiac group—many of whom were referred for ECT because of the intolerable cardiovascular side effects of tricyclic antidepressants—included 15 instances of ventricular arrhythmias (2 of ventricular tachycardia), 9 ischemic events (including one episode of myocardial infarction); 6 instances of atrial arrhythmias; and 5 episodes of bradycardia. Eight patients had major complications consisting of persistent ECG changes accompanied by chest pain, asystole, or persistent arrhythmia.

Thus, although the 40 patients with preexisting cardiac disease suffered more, and more severe, cardiac complications during ECT than a matched control group of noncardiac patients, and had received no specific therapy with cardiotropic medications at the time of ECT, intensive medical management of complications once they occurred enabled the vast majority to safely and effectively complete their course of treatment.

Rice et al. (1994) conducted a case-control chart review of consecutively treated patients over age 50 years that yielded a group of 26 at increased risk for cardiac complications, and a group of 21 at standard risk. No specific cardiotropic medications were administered at the time of ECT. Unlike patients in the study of Zielinski et al. (1993), patients in the cardiac risk group were no more likely to experience a major complication during ECT than patients in the no-risk group; minor cardiac complications, however, were twice as frequent in the risk group. Three of 26 risk group patients suffered complications severe enough (e.g., ventricular tachycardia) to necessitate transfer to the medical service; 2 of these (8%) discontinued ECT, and none sustained lasting sequelae. The results of this study stand in striking contrast to the widely cited report of Gerring and Shields (1982), two residents who unaccountably found an extreme and unacceptable risk of cardiac morbidity and mortality in cardiac patients receiving ECT at the same institution as Rice et al. (1994), but 20 years earlier. Gerring and Shields' (1982) findings have never been replicated and must therefore be considered aberrant.

As might be expected, the stress of ECT on the heart is similar to that which might result from vigorous exercise. Messina et al. (1992) assessed left ventricular regional wall motion via echocardiogram in 11 patients (mean age, 54 years) before and immediately after ECT, and found that in 3 patients (2 of whom had coronary risk factors and a family history of heart disease), the stress of ECT on the heart was similar to that typically observed during treadmill exercise testing, producing signs suggestive of reversible myocardial ischemia. No patient experienced myocardial infarction, and all ECGs and echocardiograms returned to normal by the end of the study.

Thus, one may conclude that ECT is generally safe and effective in geriatric patients with or without preexisting cardiac disease; that patients with cardiac disease have a moderately increased risk of untoward cardiac events (and a small risk of death) during ECT; and that these risks are effectively managed with appropriate cardioactive medications administered before, during, or after treatment. Indeed, it is precisely in this group of older cardiac patients referred for ECT that Figiel and Stoudemire (1994) have recommended routine pretreatment with beta-blockers—particularly labetalol—alone or in conjunction with nifedipine. Considering the relatively benign nature of these medications, and the potential severity of some of the adverse cardiac events reported (e.g., ventricular tachycardia, myocardial infarction), this recommendation appears both reasonable and prudent. The initial prophylactic dose of labetalol recommended by these authors for this purpose is 10 mg given intravenously 1 to 2 minutes prior to anesthesia induction, and adjusted at subsequent treatments to maintain peak systolic blood pressure below 210 mm Hg. If increases up to 20 mg of labetalol prove insufficient for this purpose, the contents of one 10 mg capsule of nifedipine can be placed under the patient's tongue 25 minutes before administering the labetalol. Fewer than 5% of patients develop post-ECT orthostatic hypotension on this regimen, which responds to continued bed rest and intravenous fluids.

Cardiac Pacemakers

There are numerous reports of the successful use of ECT in patients with implanted cardiac pacemakers (Youmans et al., 1969; Gibson et al., 1973; Abiuso et al., 1978; Jauhar et al., 1979; Alexopolous and Frances, 1980; Alexopolous et al., 1984a; Tchou et al., 1989). Although the ECT stimulus itself is normally prevented from reaching the heart by the high resistance of the intervening body tissues, and pacemakers are constructed with protective electrical circuitry and shielding to withstand electrical stimuli within the range of those used for ECT, the low-resistance pathway to the myocardium created by an endocardial electrode may allow a large current to pass through the art during ECT if the patient is in contact with ground. Thus, all monitoring equipment must be properly grounded; the stretcher on which the patient is lying must be completely insulated from ground (e.g., by rubber wheels); and the patient must not be held or touched during treatment by anyone who is in contact with ground. (Contact with an improperly grounded monitor is dangerous even if it is turned off at the time.) Pacemaker wires should be checked for breaks or faulty insulation because these also provide ready entry of currents into the heart. Previous editions of this book have suggested using a magnet to convert fixed-mode pacemaker operation to demand mode during ECT to avoid the theoretical occurrence of either bradycardia or tachycardia, depending on the circumstances. Because I am aware of no reports since 1980 in which the feared episodes actually occurred, or in which the magnet technique was used, I have omitted this recommendation in the present edition. External (temporary) cardiac pacemakers must, of course, be grounded; they are, therefore, substantially riskier than implanted ones because they provide a ready conduit through the heart for current flow from improperly grounded monitoring equipment, on or off, even if unattached to the patient and only touched by an assistant who is touching the patient at the same time.

Aortic Aneurysm

Of the many published reports of patients with aortic aneurysms who received ECT (Monke, 1952; Wolford, 1957; Weatherly and Villein, 1958; Moore, 1960; Chapman, 1961; Pomeranze et al., 1968; Abramczuk and Rose, 1979; Alexopolous and Frances, 1980; Rosenfeld, Glassberg and Sherrid, 1988; Devanand et al., 1990), either for untreated aneurysms or after dissection or surgical grafting, no untoward effects occurred in any patient, despite the fact that no particular efforts were made to augment the usual degree of muscle relaxation or to reduce the blood pressure response to treatment. In fact, one patient with multiple aortic homografts (Greenbank, 1958) safely received 10 ECTs without any muscle-relaxant at all. Although these cases suggest that aortic aneurysm is not an important risk with ECT, it seems prudent to recommend that succinylcholine doses in such patients be adequate to provide full relaxation of the abdominal musculature (e.g., 60 to 80 mg), especially in the presence of an untreated abdominal aneurysm.

Cardiac Surgery

There are six reported instances of patients who received ECT at varying intervals after cardiac valvular surgery, two of them after replacement of both aortic and mitral valves (Blachly and Semler, 1967; Weinstein and Fisher, 1967; Hardman and Morse, 1972; Viparelli et al., 1976). Again, no special precautions were taken and no untoward cardiovascular effects of ECT were observed, even in one patient who was treated only 27 days after surgery.

Myocardial Infarction

Ventricular arrhythmias and cardiac rupture constitute the primary fatal risks of ECT in the presence of recent myocardial infarction. Although the risk is greatest during the first 10 days postinfarction (Willerson, 1982), and probably least after 3 months have elapsed (Perrin, 1961), there are no hard data to support the safety (or lack of it) of administering ECT at any given postinfarction interval. Ungerleider (1960) reported the case of a 68-year-old woman who inadvertently received an ECT without any ill effect during an acute myocardial infarction that was documented electrocardiographically, and described another instance personally communicated to him of a patient successfully treated with ECT 3 days postinfarction. Despite these lucky outcomes, the risks of such treatment are substantial and may be reduced by waiting as long as possible after infarction before giving ECT and by the judicious use of antiarrhythmic and antihypertensive agents, and the administration of 100% oxygen by positive pressure before, during, and after the seizure.

Intracardiac Thrombi

Mensah, Schoen, and Devereux (1990) presented two patients with echocardiographically detected left ventricular apical mural thrombi who were safely and successfully treated with courses of 10 and 12 ECT, respectively. Short-acting beta-blockers (otherwise unspecified) were given before each treatment to blunt the sympathetic response, but anticoagulation was not given because neither patient had a history of embolization.

Myocardial Stunning

Myocardial stunning is an ECG diagnosis of doubtful validity that is purported to reflect reversible myocardial dysfunction. I am mentioning it here because of two case reports (Zhu et al., 1992; Eitzman et al., 1994) of alleged myocardial stunning during ECT; neither patient experienced chest pain, and both went on to successfully complete their course of ECT without further episodes, one receiving nifedipine during subsequent ECTs, the other labetalol.

Management of Central Nervous System Risks

Brain Tumor

If one considers the fixed cranium, the noncompressibility of cerebrospinal fluid and blood, and the substantial increases in cerebral blood flow and blood-brain barrier permeability that occur during ECT, it is not surprising that major neurologic deterioration—and death—have been reported when this treatment is administered in the presence of a space-occupying lesion of the brain. The difficulty in interpreting the older literature on the subject, however, derives from the fact that most of the case reports describing the consequences of such a procedure are subject to ascertainment bias, having come to the attention of physicians precisely because of neurologic deterioration that occurred in association with a course of ECT. Thus, Savitsky and Karliner's (1953) patient with occult glioblastoma who developed stupor, papilledema, and hemiparesis after ECT; Shapiro and Goldberg's (1957) six patients with previously undiagnosed brain tumors who deteriorated rapidly after ECT; Gassel's (1960) three patients with occult meningiomas who fared likewise; and Paulson's (1967) three cases of rapid neurologic progression after ECT in the presence of undiagnosed brain metastases or cerebellar sarcoma, are largely responsible for the widely quoted but long-outdated clinical dictum that "brain tumor is an absolute contraindication to ECT." Nevertheless, such case reports are indispensable because they provide a major source of information for assessing the risks and benefits of ECT in the presence of a brain tumor.

Maltbie et al. (1980) conducted an extensive review of 28 cases reported in the literature, adding 7 from their own hospital files. Only 34% of the 35 cases exhibited improvement in their psychiatric symptoms with ECT, whereas 74% exhibited neurologic deterioration, providing a risk about twice as large as the possible benefit. Only 21% improved psychiatrically without showing neurologic morbidity. Four patients died within a week of ECT, and 4 more died within a month; all 8 had major neurologic complications precipitated by ECT. Considering the rarity of ECT-induced mortality, even in the presence of severe cardiovascular disease, it is apparent that brain tumor constitutes a major risk for the administration of ECT. However, theirs was a retrospective review and is subject to the ascertainment bias already noted. At the time of this writing, ten instances of prospective administration of ECT to patients with known brain tumors, mostly meningiomas, demonstrate the relative safety of this procedure (Dressler and Folk, 1975; Hsiao and Evans, 1984; Alexopolous et al., 1984; Greenberg et al., 1988; Fried and Mann, 1988; Goldstein and Richardson, 1988; Malek-Ahmadi and Sedler, 1989; Zwil et al., 1990).

Much of the risk in administering ECT in the presence of a brain tumor has been attributed to aggravation of increased intracranial pressure by the cerebral hemodynamic effects of ECT. Maltbie et al. (1980) do not present data addressing this point, but it is notable that Dressler and Folk's (1975) patient had normal spinal fluid pressure and dynamics and that all of the other prospectively treated patients described previously had meningiomas that were unlikely to have caused increased intracranial pressure. An ECT-induced increase in peri-brain tumor edema may contribute significantly to increased intracranial pressure; although steroids (especially dexamethasone), which effectively reduce such edema, should also reduce the risks of treatment (Carter, 1977; Fried and Mann, 1988; Zwil et al., 1990), they were used in only 2 of the 10 cases described.

In considering whether to give ECT to a patient with a brain tumor, the risks are likely to be least in the presence of small, slow-growing (or calcified) lesions and in the absence of increased intracranial pressure. The administration of dexamethasone in doses sufficient to reduce peri-brain tumor edema seems prudent, although no prospective trials exist to demonstrate the effectiveness of this procedure. Oral dexamethasone, 40 mg/day, for example, was introduced several days before ECT in a patient who had no evidence of increased intracranial pressure (Zwil et al., 1990). Prospective administration of ECT in the presence of a brain tumor accompanied by increased intracranial pressure has not yet been described in the literature. Were ECT to be deemed essential under such circumstances, and after neurosurgical consultation, parenteral administration of steroids beginning 24 to 48 hours before the first treatment might be considered, followed by an oral maintenance dose until the course is completed.

Other Space-occupying Lesions

Cerebral compression by subdural hematoma should increase the risk with ECT in the same fashion as a brain tumor. Paulson (1967) reported a 47-year-old agitated depressed woman who became unresponsive immediately after her first ECT and remained comatose for 2 days. A large subdural hematoma was demonstrated on angiography and evacuated, at which point the patient immediately became responsive and alert. More recently, however, Malek-Ahmadi et al. (1990) successfully used bilateral ECT to relieve a major depressive illness in an elderly woman with a chronic subdural hematoma, without any resultant neurologic deterioration.

Patients with intracranial arachnoid cysts can also present with increased intracranial pressure. Escalona et al. (1991) described their treatment of a depressed man with an asymptomatic intracranial arachnoid cyst in whom 11 right unilateral ECTs relieved the depression without undue cognitive impairment, emergence of neurologic signs or symptoms, or change in any aspect of magnetic resonance images obtained before and after treatment.

Craniotomy and Cerebral Trauma

Years ago, Savitsky and Karliner (1953) reported the successful use of ECT in a patient whose skull fracture was followed by 5 days of coma. Additional successful reports have accumulated in the last decade. Ruedrich et al. (1983) successfully gave ECT to a 21-year-old woman with a depressive psychosis 3 weeks after she had shot herself in the right parietal lobe in a suicide attempt; the wound required debridement of her right motor and sensory cortex and resulted in left hemiparesis. A total of 17 treatments were given with bitemporal treatment electrode placement to avoid the parietal skull defect and with concomitant anticonvulsant therapy to prevent prolonged seizures or status epilepticus. Not only was there no evidence of ECT-induced aggravation of her hemiparesis, but there was steady improvement following the course of ECT until she had regained nearly full use of her left arm and leg.

The patient of Hsiao and Evans (1984) described earlier subsequently underwent elective craniotomy for removal of her meningioma, which left a left parietal calvarial defect. Four months postcraniotomy, a second course of ECT was given for a recurrence of her psychotic depression, using bifrontotemporal treatment electrodes placed well away from the cranial defect; no complications resulted from a course of nine treatments. Levy and Levy (1987) reported the case of a 72-year-old man with a plastic plate covering a skull defect over the entire right cerebral hemisphere resulting from the earlier removal of a meningioma and more recent surgery for a cerebral abscess. A course of nine left unilateral ECTs induced full remission of his depression without any neurologic sequelae. Ries and Bokan (1979) described a 39-year-old woman who received a course of 12 right unilateral ECTs for a depressive psychosis 30 days after undergoing the transsphenoidal-transnasal removal of a basophil adenoma of the pituitary. She enjoyed a full psychiatric recovery without neurologic complications or sequelae. Roccaforte and Burke (1989) reported a dramatic response to a course of 11 ECT (bilateral at first, then right unilateral) in a 26-year-old, right-handed man who developed psychotic depression 2 months after surgical removal of a third ventricle colloid cyst. Notably, the authors continued diphenyl-hydantoin at therapeutic serum levels throughout the treatment course.

Most recently, Hartmann and Saldivia (1990) successfully used ECT to treat a patient who had sustained large neurosurgical defects of the cranium many years earlier secondary to a hand-grenade explosion. Following Gordon's (1982) advice, the authors placed the ECT treatment electrodes well away (and equidistant) from the 6- × 4.5-cm right temporoparietal defect to avoid local intracerebral concentration of the stimulus current through the defect. (The bony flaps temporarily raised during most craniotomies do not require any special precautions in this regard.)

Cerebral Vascular Malformation

Husum et al. (1983) successfully administered a course of 10 ECTs to a severely melancholic 42-year-old woman who 6 months earlier had undergone a craniotomy for surgical clipping of a bleeding sacculate aneurysm of the upper internal carotid artery and muscular wrapping of another located on the right medial cerebral artery. Although the patient was normotensive, these authors elected to block the sympathoadrenal response to ECT with a combination of hydralazine (to relax arteriolar smooth muscle) and propranolol (to prevent hydralazine-induced reflex sympathetic activation and ameliorate the effects of ECT-induced catecholamine release). Under this regimen, no significant blood pressure response to ECT was observed, with the maximum increase being 10 mm Hg. As noted previously, Drop et al.

(1988) successfully treated a depressed patient with multiple intracranial aneurysms whose dramatic hypertensive response to ECT required combined timolol-nitroprusside therapy for its control. Notably, this patient experienced no untoward effects of ECT despite systolic blood pressure levels reaching 340 mm Hg.

Many patients with occult berry aneurysms must have received ECT without any ill effect because they occur in 1% to 2% of the population but have never been implicated in an ECT-related death. Untreated aneurysms that have previously bled presumably constitute a significant risk with ECT because of their inherent tendency to rebleed; however, there are no reported instances of ECT having been administered under such circumstances.

Greenberg et al. (1986) reported a 24-year-old man with a left parietal cerebral venous angioma who received a course of 12 ECTs without incident. Although a nitroprusside drip infusion was available, it was never used (venous angiomas are low-pressure malformations, and the maximum ECT-induced systolic blood pressure levels recorded in this patient rarely exceeded 200 mm Hg). Of special interest is the fact that MRI performed 18 days after the last ECT revealed no change compared with the pre-ECT record.

Stroke

Shapiro and Goldberg (1957) described 6 patients who were given ECT for severe depressive states occurring 4 weeks to 2 years after a cerebrovascular accident (CVA). Four of these patients, including two who were treated 4 and 9 weeks poststroke, had remission of their depression without neurologic complications. Two patients died during treatment: A 55-year-old woman with severe diabetes whose right-sided CVA preceded ECT by 6 weeks failed to recover consciousness after her sixth ECT, and a 48-year-old man with hypertensive cardio-vascular disease whose right-sided CVA preceded ECT by 2 years suffered cardiorespiratory standstill during his first ECT.

Murray et al. (1986) reported more favorable results in 14 patients, age 46 to 86 years, who received ECT for poststroke depression, a sample selected from the records of 193 patients with stroke and depression who were treated at Massachusetts General Hospital from 1969 to 1981. All strokes had been completed and none were evolving at the time ECT was given. Twelve of the 14 patients improved markedly with ECT, and none developed new neurologic findings or exhibited worsening of old ones, despite the fact that 4 patients were included whose stroke preceded ECT by less than 1 month. Of great clinical importance is the observation that of 6 patients who exhibited cognitive impairment before ECT, 5 experienced improvement in this impairment (and in depression) as a result of ECT. Kwentus et al. (1984) reported the case of a depressed, catatonic 52-year-old woman with a history of a left-hemisphere CVA 2 years before who was successfully treated with a course of 9 right-unilateral ECTs without neurologic complications. In fact, a coexisting neuroleptic-induced tardive dystonia also remitted with ECT and remained so at examination 7 months later. The shortest interval between stroke and ECT was reported by Alexopolous et al. (1984a), who briefly mentioned the uneventful treatment of a patient 4 days after a cerebral infarction documented by CT scanning.

Allman and Hawton (1987) used a combination of two beta-blockers—practolol and atenolol—given intravenously to inhibit completely the ECT-induced surge in blood pressure in a 60-year-old normotensive woman who had suffered a cerebral hemorrhage 3 years previously. Her depression responded to 9 ECTs, without associated complications. DeQuardo and Tandon (1988a) reported equally favorable results in a 48-year-old depressed man who had suffered a large right parietotemporal stroke—secondary to atrial fibrillation—15 months earlier. Eight right unilateral ECTs induced a full remission of his depressive syndrome without any change in his neurologic or neuropsychological status when he was examined 2 days post-ECT, despite the fact that he continued oral anticoagulation therapy with coumadin throughout.

The only instance of a specific neurologic complication (Todd's palsy) secondary to ECT in a patient with a history of stroke was reported by Strain and Bidder (1971), who gave four closely spaced seizures during a single treatment session of multiple-monitored ECT (MMECT) to a 62-year-old woman who, unknown to the authors, had had a CVA 7 years earlier. Status epilepticus lasting 28 minutes occurred after the fourth seizure, from which the patient awakened with a left hemiparesis that partially remitted over the following week. The fact that this patient had received two previous courses of six to eight conventional ECTs since her CVA without neurologic sequelae illustrates the increased neurotoxicity of MMECT.

Although it usually takes about 3 months for radioimaging evidence of cerebral damage to resolve (Jeffries et al., 1980), the data of Murray et al. (1986) suggest that ECT given even as soon as 1 month after a CVA does not present a major risk to the patient. Indeed, the well-documented increases in cerebral blood flow and oxygenation following induced seizures described in Chapter 5 have been used as therapy for experimental strokes in dogs (Reed et al., 1971) and in monkeys (Roberts et al., 1972). In the latter study, bilateral ECTs enhanced by pentylenetetrazol induced mean intracerebral pO_2 increases of 74% lasting 40 minutes or more in monkeys rendered hemiparetic by middle cerebral artery occlusion an hour earlier. Although both experimental and no-ECT control monkeys had substantial and equivalent recovery of neurologic function 3 months poststroke, the authors noted that only one session of induced seizures had been used and that seizures would have had to have been repeated frequently to maintain elevated pO_2 levels. This study is cited not so much as a plea for controlled trials of ECT in human stroke, which would indeed be a rational approach, but as a demonstration of the apparent safety of induced seizures in the presence of acute or recent ischemic stroke.

Anticoagulation Therapy

Loo, Cuche, and Benkelfat (1985) reviewed the safety of administering ECT to patients on anticoagulant therapy and reported 4 patients who successfully received this combination: 3 on heparin, one on a warfarin derivative. Tancer, Pedersen, and Evans (1987) found additional successful cases in their literature review, adding the example of their own patient who received two full courses of ECT while on oral warfarin therapy (prothrombin times, 1.4 to 2.1 times control). Subsequently, Tancer and Evans (1989) and Hay (1989) reported the uneventful administration of ECT in 4 additional geriatric patients on oral warfarin, bringing to 13 the total number of patients reported in the literature to have safely received ECT while receiving anticoagulants.

Lupus Cerebritis

Guze (1967) described the successful use of ECT in three patients with affective episodes—including catatonia—secondary to lupus cerebritis, but did not mention whether any adverse effects occurred as a result. Since then, several additional patients have been described (Allen and Pitts, 1978; Douglas and Schwartz, 1982; Mac and Pardo, 1983; Kurokawa et al., 1989; Fricchione et al., 1990) whose lupus-induced organic affective syndromes with catatonia responded fully to ECT without exacerbating the underlying disorder. The two most recent reports document the generally dramatic responses that have been obtained in patients unresponsive to high-dose corticosteroids and neuroleptic agents. Kurosawa et al. (1989) described a 30-year-old lupus patient with recurrent manic-depressive attacks whose 13-month history of mutism, incontinence, and clouded consciousness was abruptly terminated by ECT. Fricchione et al. (1990) gave ECT to a 25-year-old woman with a 3-year history of lupus who exhibited facial grimacing, mutism, rigidity, and an elevated temperature. An intial course of ECT was aborted because of a high seizure threshold, but a second course—given in conjunction with cyclophosphamide—resulted in full remission of her psychiatric syndrome.

Dementia

Because of the transient, but occasionally pronounced, cognitive side effects of bilateral ECT, psychiatrists have been understandably cautious in administering any form of ECT to patients with preexisting cognitive impairment. In a study of acute organic mental syndrome after bilateral ECT, Summers et al. (1979) reported that the only two instances of markedly prolonged confusional states (lasting 45 and 65 days post-ECT) occurred in the only two patients with preexisting mild chronic dementia. Tsuang et al. (1979) reported the development of profound disorientation and urinary and fecal incontinence after six ECTs (electrode placement unstated) in a 70-year-old woman with normal pressure hydrocephalus (NPH) and a right ventriculojugular shunt. (She had been stuporous, disoriented, and occasionally incontinent of urine just before starting ECT, but had become fully oriented and continent by the fourth treatment.) Her cognitive functioning gradually improved over 3 weeks post-ECT, and she was fully oriented at discharge.

Subsequent reports have been more sanguine. Demuth and Rand (1980) gave eight unilateral ECTs to a depressed 80-year-old man with documented severe primary degenerative dementia who achieved a full remission without any increase in confusion. Snow and Wells (1981) treated a woman with probable Alzheimer's disease who also improved significantly with ECT without evidence of any worsening of her organic state—in fact, her incontinence cleared during the course of treatment. McAllister and Price (1982) described two depressed patients with dementia (one with NPH, one with Creuzfeldt-Jakob disease) who improved substantially with ECT without any exacerbation of their cognitive deficits. Unilateral ECT was used for one patient, but the other's treatment was not described. Perry (1983) reported the case of a demented man in his 50s whose muteness and catatonia responded dramatically to ECT without any worsening of his dementia; Dubovsky et al. (1985) successfully treated a 53-year-old depressed man with dementia and increased intracranial pressure with a course of nine ECTs (four unilateral and five bilateral) that resulted in marked improvement in his memory as well as in his depression. Not every depressive patient improves with ECT, of course, and Young et al. (1985) reported the case of a depressed 73-year-old woman with Parkinson's disease and dementia who exhibited no relief from depression, but also no persistent worsening of her dementia, after 7 unilateral ECTs (there was, however, long-term improvement in some of her parkinsonian symptoms).

Benbow (1987) described five patients in his ECT practice who had received ECT for depressive illness complicated by dementia: Two recovered fully, one improved, and two did not respond—four of the five were discharged after ECT to live in their own homes in the community. Liang et al. (1988) observed substantial improvement in affective and vegetative features in two elderly demented women but neither improvement nor worsening of their cognitive dysfunction. In their extensive literature review of the results of ECT in 113 cases of depression occurring in the presence of organic dementia (mean age, 67 years), Price and McAllister (1989) found an 83% overall positive therapeutic response to ECT, with 20% of patients experiencing significant cognitive or memory side effects, virtually all transient and reversible, and 15% showing improved cognition or memory consequent to ECT. In general, patients with subcortical dementias (e.g., Huntington's or Parkinson's disease) showed more improvement in depression than those with cortical dementias (e.g., Alzheimer's or Pick's)—93% compared with 73%, respectively—while exhibiting no cognitive improvement, compared with 30% cognitive improvement for patients with cortical dementia.

In the largest study to date, Nelson and Rosenberg (1991) retrospectively analyzed a 4-year sample of 21 elderly demented patients who had received primarily right unilateral ECT for major depression. The method was safe and effective despite transitory increased confusion in some patients, and the antidepressant efficacy of ECT was similar to that found in a group of nondemented elderly depressives previously studied in the same setting.

When one is prescribing ECT for patients with dementia, the general recommendation for starting with a brief-pulse stimulus delivered through right-unilateral treatment electrodes is virtually obligatory. Only if improvement fails to occur after six ECTs—or the severity of the patient's condition dictates an earlier change—should the switch be made to bilateral electrodes. Twice-weekly treatments are also less likely to induce cognitive dysfunction than those given three times a week, yet they are ultimately no less effective—they just take longer. The improvement in the dementia syndrome noted after ECT by Price and McAllister (1989) does not suggest any ameliorative effect of the treatment on the primary syndrome. Rather, the cognitive deficits of melancholia (depressive pseudodementia) that have been superimposed on the existing features of dementia remit with successful ECT just as they do in nondemented patients.

Mental Retardation

In his review and case studies of affective disorders among mentally retarded patients, Reid (1972) noted in passing that "tricyclic antidepressants and ECT appeared to be effective in most of the cases where they were prescribed." There are several case reports that specifically address this use of ECT. Bates and Smeltzer (1982) reported the case of a 25-year-old, severely mentally retarded man (full scale IQ range 21 to 25) whose persistent self-injurious, head-banging behavior resulted in a wide-based staggering gait, loss of manual fine motor control, a Babinski sign, and other symptoms of upper motor neuron damage. Insomnia, agitation, and weight loss were prominent. A course of 12 bilateral ECTs induced a dramatic improvement in all areas of behavior, without any adverse consequences. Guze et al. (1987) reported a 21-year-old bipolar man with spastic diplegia and mild mental retardation (IQ 65) whose depressive symptoms were rapidly and fully relieved by a course of 8 unilateral ECTs. Kearns (1987) successfully used ECT to treat nihilistic delusional psychosis (Cotard's syndrome) in a severely mentally retarded man (IQ 35) who had not responded to antidepressant drugs, and Goldstein and Jensvold (1989) reported full recovery without adverse effect (described by his internist as "a miracle") in a 68-year-old mildly retarded (IQ 65) man whose relentlessly progressive mental and physical decline had begun following orchiectomy several years earlier. Warren, Holroyd, and Folstein (1989) described an excellent response to ECT in three patients with trisomy 21 (Down's syndrome) who were referred for evaluation of apparent dementia but were instead found to have major depression. In each instance, ECT was dramatically effective in restoring the patient to normal functioning despite failure to respond to antidepressant drugs (one patient returned to school, one to work in the family business, and one remained well on lithium maintenance over a 2-year follow-up interval).

Epilepsy

The anticonvulsant effects of ECT described elsewhere in this volume were well known to older clinicians who used them to good effect in the treatment of epileptic patients with and without psychiatric symptoms (Kalinowsky and Kennedy, 1943; Caplan, 1946; Kalinowsky et al., 1982, p. 267). Sackeim et al. (1983) reported using the seizure threshold-raising effect of ECT to successfully treat a 19-year-old patient with lifelong, intractable, idiopathic secondary generalized seizures. More recently, Viparelli and Viparelli (1992) successfully used bilateral ECT to treat a 19-year-old woman with grand mal epilepsy who suffered from as many as 46 partial seizures over a 12-hour period, and who was unresponsive to diphenylhydantoin and diazepam. After the second ECT, all seizures ceased and she remained seizure-free over a 7-year follow-up interval, on very low doses of carbamazepine (plasma levels of 2.2 μg/ml). Thus, ECT is more likely to ameliorate than aggravate an epileptic disorder, at least temporarily, and can be especially useful in patients with the psychiatric manifestations of complex partial seizures (usually temporal lobe epilepsy). Epileptic patients already receiving anticonvulsants should continue to do so during the course of ECT because abrupt discontinuation increases the risk of status epilepticus (Hauser, 1983). If one considers the potent anticonvulsant properties of ECT, there seems little rationale for initiating anticonvulsants before ECT in epileptic patients not already receiving them. In any case, although higher-than-usual electrical doses may be required, seizures of adequate length and therapeutic potency can be obtained despite concomitant therapy with anticonvulsants (Weiner, 1981; Sackeim et al., 1986a; Kaufman et al., 1986; Cantor, 1986), although some manipulation of their dose may be required, and an occasional patient may not develop a seizure at all (Roberts and Attah, 1988). Although Kaufman et al. (1986) found it easier to obtain seizures in the presence of blood levels of carbamazepine than of diphenylhydantoin, Roberts and Attah (1988) could not obtain a seizure in their patient on carbamazepine despite several double bilateral applications of 4 and 5 seconds of "stimulating current" (no further stimulus details were provided).

Hydrocephalus

In addition to the cases of NPH described previously (Tsuang et al., 1979; McAllister and Price, 1982), Karliner (1978) and Mansheim (1983) reported the successful administration of ECT to a hydrocephalic patient. Mansheim's (1983) patient is particularly interesting because ECT not only relieved his depression but also markedly improved some long-standing functional deficits despite the presence of meningomyelocele, a ventriculogastric shunt, and epilepsy. Most recently, Cardno and Simpson (1991) safely and successfully used ECT to relieve depressive illness in a 54-year-old woman with a ventriculoperitoneal shunt in place for hydrocephalus secondary to Paget's disease of the skull.

It is unclear whether shunting reduces the likelihood of severe cognitive side effects of ECT in patients with NPH. Improvement in depression but with marked post-ECT confusion and memory loss occurred in a patient with NPH (Price and Tucker, 1977) who received ECT before shunting, but Tsuang et al. (1979) and Levy and Levy (1987) had patients who received ECT after shunting who also developed severe disorientation (as well as incontinence in the former instance), both transient. Another NPH patient treated with a shunt in place (McAllister and Price, 1982) recovered fully from depression without any unusual cognitive side effects, as did the patient of Cardno and Simpson (1991) described above.

Tardive Dyskinesia

Considering the clinical evidence presented below that ECT increases postsynaptic dopamine receptor responsivity and, in particular, that ECT-emergent dyskinesias regularly occur in Parkinson's disease patients receiving this treatment for depression (Rasmussen and Abrams, 1991), it might be expected that ECT would aggravate tardive dyskinesia. It is puzzling that the opposite is often the case, although published case reports are equally divided on whether ECT ameliorates or aggravates this disorder.

Asnis and Leopold (1978) found that the frequency of oral movements in 3 of 4 women with neuroleptic-induced, orofacial dyskinesia fell below baseline during ECT and remained so after the course in two of the women; the other two showed increased abnormal movements after ECT. Price and Levin (1978) described a 49-year-old woman whose pronounced buccolingual dyskinesia improved suddenly and dramatically after her third ECT seizure, and Chacko and Root (1983) reported two women, aged 62 and 63 years, whose prominent orofacial and buccolingual dyskinesias also improved markedly after their third and fourth ECT seizures. One patient had no return of tardive dyskinesia (TD) over the following 2 years; the other showed only an occasional dyskinetic tongue movement 1 year later. Malek-Ahmadi and Weddige (1988) gave ECT to an elderly depressed woman whose persistent tardive dyskinesia improved significantly with remission of her depressive symptoms, and Gosek and Weller (1988) reported even more favorable results: The dyskinetic movements in their 54-year-old woman improved dramatically with ECT and remained so over a 14-month follow-up interval. In the only prospective study of ECT for tardive dyskinesia conducted to date, however, Yassa, Hoffman, and Canakis (1990) reported that only one patient of nine showed dramatic improvement.

Tardive dystonia, an entity less well known than tardive dyskinesia, is diagnosed in the presence of chronic torticollis or other dystonia in a patient exposed to neuroleptic drugs and without other known cause or family history of dystonia. Kwentus et al. (1984) described a 52-year-old woman whose severely dystonic gait and posture completely remitted by her fourth ECT and remained so at a 7-month follow-up examination. A similarly favorable, although temporary, response to ECT was reported by Adityanjee et al. (1990), whose 30-year-old male patient enjoyed almost full remission of pronounced sternocleidomastoid dystonia (anterocollis) for about 1 month after completing a course of 11 ECTs for a severe, chronic hallucinatory psychosis.

There are some negative reports, however. Holcomb et al. (1983) reported a 72-year-old woman with Parkinson's disease and buccolingual dyskinesia whose formal ratings of tardive dyskinesia worsened substantially during and after a course of ECT despite remission of her depressive state and improvement in her parkinsonian symptoms. Roth, Mukherjee, and Sackeim (1988) described a manic patient whose preexisting parkinsonian-athetoid complex remitted with ECT, only to be replaced by an emergent marked orofacial dyskinesia. Liberzon et al. (1991) described three depressed patients who developed transient dyskinesias after right unilateral ECT, but responded well to ECT for their affective syndromes and were free from ECT-induced dyskinetic movements at the time of discharge.

Leukoencephalopathy

The advent of MRI has brought with it the radiologic diagnosis of subcortical leukoencephalopathy (Coffey et al., 1988b, 1990a, 1991; Price and McAllister, 1989; Pande et al., 1990), which is characterized by small areas of increased signal intensity in the subcortical white matter. Although this finding is reported in about two thirds of elderly depressed patients referred for ECT, it neither predicts an unfavorable outcome nor is aggravated by ECT (Coffey et al., 1988b; Pande et al., 1990).

Neuromuscular-Neurodegenerative Disorders

Affective symptoms (depression or euphoria) occur frequently in patients with multiple sclerosis and are occasionally severe enough to require ECT. Savitsky and Karliner (1951) successfully treated two such patients diagnosed as having manic-depressive psychosis, without any significant worsening in neurologic status (indeed, one bedridden and incontinent woman regained bladder control and the ability to walk with a cane after treatment). In later papers, Savitsky and Karliner (1953) and Karliner (1978) reported several additional cases, although it is unclear whether any were reported twice. Most patients showed improvement in psychiatric status with no change or modest improvement in neurologic symptoms. Savitsky and Karliner (1953), however, cite an additional case from the German literature of a catatonic woman with multiple sclerosis who improved after a single, unmodified ECT but developed paraparesis with bilateral pyramidal tract signs and right upper extremity weakness and hyper-reflexia that took 3 months to resolve. In general, however, a pattern of psychiatic improvement with at least no neurologic worsening has been consistently observed by subsequent clinicians treating patients with multiple sclerosis (Gallinek and Kalinowsky, 1958; Hollender and Steckler, 1972; Kwentus et al., 1986; Coffey et al., 1987), with the exception being a 38-year-old manic-depressive man with multiple sclerosis in remission who developed a gait disturbance and dyscalculia requiring cessation of treatment after 8 ECTs, with only minor improvements in mental state (Regestein and Reich, 1985). A patient examined with brain MRI by Coffey et al. (1987) before and after the ECT showed no change in the preexisting white matter lesions.

ECT has also been used successfully to treat psychiatric patients suffering from cerebral palsy (Lowinger and Huston, 1953; Guze et al., 1987), myasthenia gravis (Martin and Flegenheimer, 1971), muscular dystrophy (Zeidenberg et al., 1976), and Friedrich's ataxia (Casey, 1991), all without any complications.

ANESTHESIA CONSIDERATIONS

Although many patients with multiple sclerosis have received ECT with succinylcholine-induced muscle relaxation without ill effect, Marco and Randels (1979) warned that the potassium-releasing and muscle-depolarizing action of succinylcholine might adversely affect patients with neuromuscular disorders. For this reason, Hicks (1987) recommended using atracurium, the curariform nondepolarizing muscle-blocker, as a muscle-relaxant instead of succinylcholine when giving ECT to a patient with multiple sclerosis.

Because of the overlapping symptoms of neuroleptic malignant syndrome and malignant hyperthermia, a familial syndrome induced by general anesthesia and succinylcholine, concern has also been raised that using this muscle-relaxant when giving ECT to patients with neuroleptic malignant syndrome might reactivate their symptoms (Liskow, 1985). This author also chose atracurium instead of succinylcholine in treating a patient with neuroleptic malignant syndrome. However, Addonizio and Susman (1986) found no instances of malignant hyperthermia in any of 13 patients with neuroleptic malignant syndrome who received ECT with succinylcholine muscle relaxation, and Hermesh et al. (1988) reported no symptoms or past or family history of malignant hyperthermia in 12 patients who had both a history of neuroleptic malignant syndrome and treatment with a total of 20 courses of ECT (146 exposures to succinylcholine). In any case, the protective value of substituting a nondepolarizing muscle-blocker for succinylcholine was questioned by Grigg (1988), who reported a patient, apparently recovering from neuroleptic malignant syndrome with coma that had occurred 2 days earlier, who again developed fever, tachycardia, and marked elevation in serum creatine phosphokinase several hours after receiving ECT administered with pancuronium hydrochloride for muscle relaxation.

Other Risk Factors

Pregnancy

Several early reviews of the effects of ECT during pregnancy (Boyd et al., 1948; Charatan and Oldham, 1954; Laird, 1955; Forssman, 1955;

Smith, 1956; Sobel, 1960) failed to demonstrate any increased risk of complications of labor and delivery, fetal damage, or growth and development that could be attributed to the treatment. More recently, the Collaborative Perinatal Project did not find an excess of malformations in fetuses exposed to methohexital, succinylcholine, and atropine (Walker and Swartz, 1994). Doppler ultrasonography, external uterine tocodynamometry, ultrasonography, and continuous fetal heart electric monitoring have revealed no significant alterations of fetal heart rate, fetal movement, or uterine tone during ECT (Wise et al., 1984; Repke and Berger, 1984); both infants that were studied were normal at delivery and at follow-up examination. In the light of these facts, there seems little justification to monitor routinely mother and fetus during ECT (Remick and Maurice, 1978; Wise et al., 1984; Repke and Berger, 1984); rather, these procedures should be reserved for patients with high-risk pregnancies. The call for performing ECT in pregnant women only under endotracheal intubation (Wise et al., 1984) seems particularly unwise, because this procedure requires substantially higher doses of barbiturate and muscle-relaxant drugs and stimulates tracheal-laryngeal reflexes that can increase pressor responses and the incidence of cardiac arrhythmias (Pitts, 1982).

Because of the release of oxytocin by ECT-induced seizures— and potential resultant stimulation of uterine contractions and induction of labor—Walker and Swartz (1994) have suggested the potential usefulness of tocolytic therapy with ritodrine or magnesium in patients who develop persistent uterine contractions accompanied by cervical changes during or shortly after ECT, or in case vaginal bleeding occurs.

Osteoporosis

With unmodified ECT, the presence of osteoporosis approximately doubles the incidence of vertebral compression fracture (Lingley and Robbins, 1947; Dewald et al., 1954). The modern use of muscle-relaxant drugs, however, has eliminated the risk of any type of fracture during ECT, along with the influence of osteoporosis on that risk, so long as the cuffed-limb method is avoided.

Glaucoma

A transient rise in intraocular pressure during ECT is reported to occur in some patients, whereas others experience a reduction (Manning et al., 1954; Epstein et al., 1975). Edwards et al. (1990) recently carefully defined the time-course of intraocular pressure changes in 10 nonglaucomatous patients undergoing ECT. Applanation tonometry performed at baseline and every 15 seconds poststimulus until return to baseline revealed that succinylcholine significantly increased intraocular pressure, which was then further significantly increased during the induced seizure by 60%; all values returned to baseline within 90 seconds of seizure termination. The authors characterized these changes as benign in all nonglaucomatous and many actively glaucomatous patients and of potential importance only in those with severe or end-stage glaucoma, for whom they recommended ophthalmologic consultation before administration of ECT.

Old Age

Increased age does not of itself increase the risk with ECT, and, as described in Chapter 2, some of the most rewarding results with convulsive therapy are obtained in elderly, debilitated patients whose primary affective disorder masquerades as senile dementia.

6

The Electroconvulsive Therapy Stimulus

A few basic electrical concepts are required to understand the properties of the ECT stimulus. Although most ECT devices utilize alternating current, some of the principles involved are more readily presented through the simpler situation that obtains for direct current. The primary variables of direct current electricity are voltage, current, and resistance, which are measured in units of volts, amperes, and ohms, respectively. Voltage is an electromotive force that drives a current of electrons through a conductor just as hydraulic pressure drives water through a pipe. The greater the resistance to the flow of current, the greater is the voltage required to maintain the same current. Therefore, the flow of current through a conductor varies directly with the voltage and inversely with the resistance, a relationship known as Ohm's law and expressed by the following equation:

$$\text{Current} = \text{voltage/resistance}$$

Energy

Energy (expressed in joules) is the work required to overcome resistance. It is the time-integral of power, which is simply the product of voltage and current:

$$\text{Power} = \text{voltage} \times \text{current}$$

Energy is therefore expressed as the product of voltage, current, and time (the duration of electron flow):

$$\text{Energy (in joules, J)} = \text{voltage} \times \text{current} \times \text{time}$$

Because voltage = current $\times$ resistance (by Ohm's law), the equation for determining the energy of a stimulus becomes:

$$\text{Energy} = \text{current}^2 \times \text{resistance} \times \text{time}$$

Charge

Charge is the total quantity of electrons flowing through a conductor during a given period of time: It is the time integral of current. For a constant current, the charge is equal to the product of the current and its duration:

$$\text{Charge (coulombs)} = \text{current (amperes)} \times \text{time (seconds)}$$

and, therefore:

$$\text{Energy} = \text{voltage} \times \text{charge}$$

The main difference compared with direct current in the principles governing the behavior of the alternating currents used to generate the ECT stimulus lies in the concept of impedance, which is analogous to direct current resistance. Impedance is a measure that combines resistance with capacitance (the property of being able to accumulate a charge) and inductance (the property of being able to induce an electromotive force, e.g., an electromagnetic field). Inductance does not occur during ECT because the brain contains no ferrous material. Although neural membranes exhibit the capacity to store current, the magnitude of this effect is quite small compared to the impedance of the electrode-skin interface, which can be substantial (Sackeim et al., 1994). Until further data become available on the nature of capacitance during ECT, however, it is safe for practical purposes to assume that the impedance during ECT is primarily attributable to resistance, and therefore subject to Ohm's law as expressed above:

$$\text{Current} = \text{voltage/impedance}$$

The seizure of ECT is generated when a quantity (charge) of electrons flows through the brain with sufficient voltage to depolarize cell membranes synchronously. The charge passing through the brain is related to the impedance of the head in a complex fashion. Most of the impedance is across the skull, estimated at 18,000 ohms/cm, compared with about 200 ohms/cm across the skin or brain (Weaver et al., 1976). Although the charge with a constant current device does not vary with impedance, its distribution among the three compartments of scalp, skull, and brain does vary with the voltage. At low voltages there is insufficient electromotive force to drive enough current through the high-impedance skull to induce a seizure; most of it is shunted (short-circuited) between the electrodes via the low-impedance scalp. As voltage increases, more and more current penetrates the skull to pass through the brain, increasing the likelihood of depolarizing enough neurons to exceed the threshold for a grand mal seizure.

An inverse relation for constant-current devices between seizure threshold (the charge required to induce a seizure of specified duration) and dynamic impedance was documented by Sackeim et al. (1987a), and replicated by Coffey et al. (1995a). It results in the counterintuitive observation that the high-threshold patients in whom seizures are the most difficult to elicit are actually those with the lowest impedances. This is probably due to greater shunting of the stimulating current through extracranial tissues, resulting in a lower dynamic impedance and less current entering the brain (Sackeim et al., 1994). The finding of McCall et al. (1993a) that higher thresholds were associated with larger (and presumably, thicker) skulls is consistent with this view.

Brief-pulse devices deliver a constant current, so the voltage varies directly with the dynamic impedance of the patient. Because extremely high impedances would draw correspondingly high voltages to maintain the same current across the electrodes—thus markedly increasing the energy generated—brief-pulse devices also limit the maximum voltage that can be applied to about 500 volts (the point is moot, however, because in clinical practice a patient with 500 ohms' dynamic impedance is never encountered).

Stimulus Waveform

The electrical stimulus can be delivered in an infinite variety of forms, of which the two most common are the sine wave and brief-pulse square wave. Sine-wave currents are characterized by a continuously changing stream of electrons, flowing alternately in opposite directions, at a frequency of 50 to 60 wave pairs (one negative, one positive) per second (Hertz, or Hz). This is the current waveform that is universally supplied by wall outlets and was the first type to be used for ECT (Cerletti and Bini, 1938). The alternating rise and fall of the sine wave current delivers substantial amounts of electrical stimulation below seizure threshold. Such below-threshold stimulation contributes little to seizure intensity or generalization and, therefore, to the therapeutic effect, but adversely affects memory functions (Ottosson, 1960).

The brief-pulse square wave current, with its sharp leading edge, was recognized early to be a more efficient and physiological stimulus for inducing seizures (Merritt and Putnam, 1938). It rises and falls almost vertically, delivering all of its charge above the seizure threshold in about 1/1000 of a second. The current is off during most of the time that the stimulus is administered (e.g., current flows for only 0.14 second during a typical 1-second brief pulse stimulus of 140 pulses of 0.001 second each). It therefore induces seizures with substantially less charge and energy than do sine-wave currents, achieving the same therapeutic effects with significantly less memory loss and EEG abnormality (Weiner et al., 1986a,b).

Attempts to reduce the neurotoxicity of the sine-wave stimulus by chopping or clipping a portion of it (e.g., Siemens Konvulsator, Ectron Duopulse) are only partially effective (McClelland and McAllister, 1988). Because sine-wave stimuli exhibit no therapeutic advantage over brief-pulse stimuli (Weiner et al., 1986a,b), they have long been considered obsolete for ECT (Weaver and Williams, 1982; Royal College of Psychiatrists, 1989, 1995). In 1982 the British government replaced sine-wave devices in its National Health Service hospitals with brief-pulse instruments (Department of Health and Social Security, 1982), and the Ontario Psychiatric Association (Position Paper, 1985) and Danish Psychiatric Association (Bolwig, 1987) have made similar recommendations. The Siemens Konvulsator, arguably the most widely used ECT device in the world at one time, was discontinued by its manufacturer during the late 1980s.

Nevertheless, a few old-timers continue to maintain that they obtained better results with sine-wave than with brief-pulse ECT. In a double-blind, controlled prospective comparison of sine-wave and brief-pulse stimuli for bilateral ECT in patients with endogenous depression, Andrade et al. (1988a) reported that 93% of the sine-wave group compared with 60% of the brief-pulse group exhibited depression rating scale reductions of 75% or better after an average course of about 6 ECTs. However, mean seizure durations were borderline— 27 seconds in each group—and patients in the sine-wave group received more than a threefold higher mean stimulus charge: 317 mC compared with only 97 mC for the brief-pulse patients, suggesting that the latter group received suboptimal treatment (Weiner and Coffey, 1989). The 97 mC mean dose for unilateral ECT is, in fact, substantially lower than the mean dose that Sackeim et al. (1987a) found to be without therapeutic effect for unilateral ECT.

In an open retrospective comparison of the records of 197 patients who received sine-wave ECT with those of 144 who received brief-pulse ECT, Fox, Rosen, and Campbell (1989) found that the mean number of ECTs received by each group was about 7.5 and that both groups were equally improved at time of discharge, according to the treating physician's global impression.

Brief-Pulse Stimulus Parameters

The brief-pulse, square-wave stimulus can be described in terms of frequency, pulse width, and number of pulses. The standard stimulus is a train of bidirectional square waves, with each cycle consisting of one negative and one positive pulse. Thus, for this type of stimulus, a frequency of 70 Hz delivers 140 pulses per second. For a pulse width of 1/1000 of a second (1 millisecond, msec), for example, one second of stimulation will deliver 140 pulses of 1 msec each, or a total of 140 msec (0.14 seconds) of stimulation. The charge of this stimulus delivered by an instrument with a constant current of 0.9 amps is calculated as follows:

$$
\begin{aligned}
\text{charge} &= \text{current} \times \text{time} \\
&= 0.9 \text{ amps} \times 0.14 \text{ seconds} \\
&= 0.126 \text{ ampere-seconds} \\
&= 126 \text{ milliampere-seconds (mC)}
\end{aligned}
$$

(Ampere-seconds are known as coulombs, C, and milliampere-seconds as millicoulombs, mC.)

The energy (in joules, J) of the same stimulus can be calculated only if the impedance is known or assumed, e.g., 220 ohms. The equation is:

$$
\begin{aligned}
\text{Energy} &= (\text{current})^2 \times \text{impedance} \times \text{time} \\
&= 0.81 \text{ amps} \times 220 \text{ ohms} \times 0.14 \text{ seconds} \\
&= 24.95 \text{ J}
\end{aligned}
$$

Should the patient's impedance double for the next treatment because the skin was not cleaned properly, the total stimulus energy would also double, suggesting to the unsophisticated operator that a greater stimulus had been delivered to the brain. Almost twice as much variance in the seizure threshold can be accounted for in units of charge as units of joules (Sackeim et al., 1987b, 1994; Coffey et al., 1995a). Moreover, units of joules were insensitive in detecting a rather strong sex difference in the seizure threshold that was demonstrated with the unit of charge (men had a higher threshold than women), and the authors concluded, with others (Gordon, 1982; Gangadhar et al., 1985), that for brief-pulse, constant-current ECT, the unit of charge was superior to joules as a measure of electrical dose.

Ultrabrief Stimuli

The term ultrabrief describes pulsed square wave stimuli of less than 0.1 msec duration. Ultrabrief pulses require extremely high peak current levels to generate seizures, which are often difficult to elicit or incomplete as a result (Weiner, 1988). Cronholm and Ottosson (1963b) administered ultrabrief stimuli with the Elther ES apparatus and obtained a smaller therapeutic effect in depression than with the higher energy Siemens Konvulsator III, which employed a modified sine wave. Moreover, it was harder to get seizures with the Elther, suggesting that incompleteness of seizure generalization may have played a role. A similar analysis applies to a later study (Robin and De Tissera, 1982) that found a reduced therapeutic effect for ultrabrief pulsed spike stimulation (Ectonus Duopulse) compared with pulsed square waves (Theratronic Transpsycon). Hyrman et al. (1985) were able to induce seizures in rabbits and a pig with 40- to 50-microsecond (0.04–0.05 msec) pulses, at frequencies of 100 to 300 Hz, generating only a fraction of the energy that would be expected from standard brief-pulse instruments, but these investigators subsequently abandoned such ultrabrief pulses for clinical purposes.

Constant Current, Constant Voltage, or Constant Energy?

An ECT stimulus can have a constant voltage or a constant current, but Ohm's law enjoins it from having both. Constant current stimulation is the more physiological method of the two for inducing neuronal depolarization and is more likely to induce a seizure in the presence of a high impedance—for example, in the elderly—because of insufficient current delivery with constant voltage or constant energy devices (Weiner, 1980a; Weiner and Coffey, 1986, 1988; Sackeim et al., 1994).

Railton et al. (1987)—as corrected by Railton (1987) and McClelland and McAllister (1988)—found that much more energy was delivered by constant-voltage than by constant-current devices, which were more consistent in stimulus delivery. A constant current ensures stable delivery of the stimulus over a wide range of impedances, in contrast to constant voltage or energy, which more readily induce brief or missed seizures when administered close to the patient's threshold (McClelland and McAllister, 1988; Sackeim et al., 1994). In its report, cited above, the British Department of Health and Social Security (1982) also recommended constant-current instruments for ECT.

Impedance Measurements

Impedance to the electrical stimulus during ECT is primarily attributable to the patient, although corrosion may cause substantial impedances to develop in the stimulus leads delivering the current, their connectors, and the electrode discs themselves. During a given treatment, the high impedance of the skull relative to the skin and subcutaneous tissues causes 40% to more than 60% of the stimulus current to be shunted through the scalp (Weaver et al., 1976; Gordon, 1981); the closer the treatment electrodes are placed to each other (e.g., as for anterior bifrontal or unilateral ECT), the greater this shunt will be. The charge entering the brain is then distributed along the paths of least impedance. With bilateral ECT, current densities are greatest in the frontal poles, diminishing in more remote areas in proportion to the square root of the distance traversed; with unilateral ECT, current density is greatest in the pathway between the electrodes, across the surface of the brain (Weaver et al., 1976).

Measurement of the patient's skin (static) impedance before administering the electrical stimulus for ECT provides important information on the quality of the skin-to-electrode contact: If the skin is oily, or if the electrodes are applied loosely or with inadequate conductive gel, a high impedance will be registered, informing the physician that his technique requires improvement. Such impedance testing is performed with a high frequency, very low milliamperage current that is undetectable by the patient. The static impedance is much higher than the dynamic impedance that is recorded during the actual passage of the treatment stimulus; the dynamic impedance is function of the summed electrical properties of the skin, hair, scalp, subcutaneous tissues, periosteum, bone, dura and pia mater, brain, blood vessels, blood, and cerebrospinal fluid (Weaver et al., 1976), and falls dramatically during the passage of the treatment stimulus (Maxwell, 1968).

Umlauf et al. (1951) measured the static and dynamic impedances of the human head during ECT while systematically varying voltage. They found no correlation between static and dynamic impedance but observed the latter to vary inversely with the voltage applied (200 to 300 ohms over a range of 60 to 160 volts, with a mean impedance of about 200 ohms above 160 volts), a result later confirmed by other investigators (Maxwell, 1968; Gordon, 1981; Gangadhar et al., 1985; Railton et al., 1987; Sackeim et al., 1987b), although often with great variability.

Seizure Threshold, Dosage, Stimulus Duration, and Treatment Response

At least a dozen studies (Weaver et al., 1976; Weiner, 1980a; Sackeim et al., 1987b, 1993; Letemendia et al., 1993; McCall et al., 1993a, 1995; Rasmussen et al., 1994; Beale et al., 1994; Enns and Karvelas, 1995; Coffey et al., 1995a; Isenberg et al., 1996) have now systematically employed an iterative stimulus titration procedure to determine, through incrementally repeated subconvulsive stimulations, the smallest electrical dosage for brief-pulse ECT to evoke a grand mal seizure of specified minimum duration. The resultant 600% to 4,000% individual variability obtained (McCall et al., 1993a) reflects differences in peak current, age, sex, treatment electrode placement, seizure duration criteria and measurement method, electrical stimulus parameters, and the strength of the initial and incremental dosages of the titration schedule. Across patient samples, there is at least a threefold variability in the mean threshold dosages obtained—ranging from 49 mC (Rasmussen, Zorumski, and Jarvis, 1994) to 164 mC (Letemendia et al., 1993).

Estimates of the seizure threshold obtained by varying one of the parameters determining stimulus dosage (e.g., the stimulus frequency) are not inherently more valid than estimates obtained by varying another parameter (e.g., stimulus train duration). Thus, Swartz and Larson (1989) found that a 144 mC brief-pulse stimulus charge for bilateral ECT was more effective in producing seizures of at least 20 seconds' duration when administered with a 2-second stimulus train than with a 1-second stimulus train, voltage and energy remaining constant. Their study nicely demonstrates the dependence of seizure threshold estimates on the stimulus parameters selected, focusing on stimulus-train length.

Swartz and Larson's (1989) finding has been confirmed and extended in two clinical studies using stimulus titration. Rasmussen et al. (1994) performed stimulus titration for right unilateral ECT using 3 iterative dosage levels of 25.2 mC, 50.4 mC, and 75.6 mC, delivered via a 0.5-msec pulse width, 30-Hz frequency, and stimulus-train durations of 0.93 second, 1.9 seconds, and 2.8 seconds, respectively (mean = 1.8 seconds). However, no minimum seizure duration criterion was specified. The mean seizure threshold for their sample was 48.9 mC, significantly lower than the mean threshold of 73.5 mC reported by Sackeim et al. (1993), using a 1-second stimulus train duration. Even more to the point, the mean threshold of Rasmussen et al. (1994) was significantly lower than the 73.5-mC threshold found by McCall et al. (1993a), who used the identical dosage and increments for the first 3 stimuli as Rasmussen et al. (1994), but administered via a 30-Hz, 1-msec stimulus, and therefore with stimulus trains that were only half as long. It is, of course, unclear whether halving the pulse width or doubling the stimulus train duration is the key to the observed differences between the two studies; however, in clinical practice the two cannot be separated: Halving the pulse width at a given charge setting doubles the stimulus duration.

However, a recently-completed study (Swartz and Manly, 1997) sheds some light on the relative importance of stimulus pulsewidth and stimulus frequency for seizure induction. In this study, 24 patients receiving asymmetric anterior bilateral ECT (Swartz, 1994a) at a stimulus charge 2.5 times age were randomly assigned to a sequence of four treatments with stimuli of pulsewidth either 0.5 msec or 1.0 msec, and frequency of either 30 Hz or 60 Hz, in a balanced, repeated measures design: all subjects received all stimuli. Of seven subjects with at least one failed motor seizure, 71% failed with both 1 msec stimuli, and none failed with both 0.5 msec stimuli (p = 0.005). Differences between 30 Hz and 60 Hz stimulus frequencies were negligible, suggesting that a 0.5 msec pulsewidth is more efficient at inducing seizures than wider pulsewidths, and that frequency hardly affects efficiency as long as it is below 70 Hz.

Isenberg et al. (1996) included by far the largest sample of patients treated (N=403) and used the identical titration dosages and increments as McCall et al. (1993a) and Rasmussen et al. (1994), for patients receiving either unilateral or bilateral ECT given under two different conditions: long vs. short stimulus train duration. The long stimulus train was administered via a 30-Hz, 0.5-msec stimulus at the lowest possible frequency, and the short stimulus train via 1- to 2-msec pulse widths at varying frequencies. With the 0.5 msec pulsewidth, long stimulus train, 80% of patients receiving unilateral ECT had seizures at 50 mC or less, compared with only 37% of patients receiving 1 to 2 msec pulsewidth, short-duration stimuli. For bilateral ECT, 100% of patients receiving short pulsewidth, long-duration stimuli exhibited seizures at stimuli of 100 mC or less, compared with only 29% of those receiving long pulsewidth, short-duration stimuli. Seizure duration was not different among the 4 groups; age and seizure threshold were positively correlated ($r = 0.32$).

This study provided the additional opportunity to compare the seizure-inducing efficacy at matched charge dosages of two different brief pulse ECT devices during stimulus titration for unilateral ECT: one with a maximum stimulus duration of 2 sec and a minimum pulsewidth of 1 msec, the other with a maximum stimulus duration of 8 seconds and a minimum pulsewidth of 0.5 msec. At increasing stimulus titration dosages across the study range of approximately 25 mC to 100 mC, the seizure-inducing advantage of the shorter pulsewidth, longer stimulus train device became apparent, approaching 100% successful seizure induction at the 75 mC to 100 mC charge settings, compared with only 60% to 70% for the longer pulsewidth, shorter stimulus train device.

At the present state of knowledge, therefore, the seizure threshold cannot be viewed as a fixed or absolute quantity, but rather as infinitely variable across an endless range of stimulus combinations—in fact, more of a metaphor than a measure. The best that can be said is that under the right circumstances, every human being is capable of experiencing a grand mal seizure, and that it is the study of those circumstances that informs our knowledge of the mechanisms through which ECT exerts its diverse influences.

Seizure Threshold, Seizure Duration, and Therapeutic Impact

Seizure duration typically decreases across a course of ECT (Sackeim et al., 1987b, 1993; Shapira et al., 1996)—an exception being the study of DiMichele et al. (1992)—often, but by no means always, with a concurrent increase in the seizure threshold. Although several studies have reported an inverse relation between seizure threshold and duration (Sackeim et al., 1987b, 1993; Krueger et al., 1993; Coffey et al., 1995a), evidence for a dissociation also exists (Sackeim, Devanand, and Prudic, 1991; McCall et al., 1993a; Shapira et al., 1996), and even where such a relation obtains across a sample, almost half the subjects fail to show it (Coffey et al., 1995b).

Stimulus Parameters in Relation to Efficacy

To begin with, I should stress that high-dose stimulation is recommended primarily for unilateral ECT, because just-above- or moderately-above-threshold dosing is highly effective for bilateral ECT (Sackeim et al., 1987a, 1993).

A study by Sackeim and associates (Sackeim et al., 1992, 1993) is instructive because it shows that even 2.5-times-threshold dosing for unilateral ECT may be only partially effective if (a) the stimulus charge is relatively small and (b) it is delivered over too short a period of time. Thus, these authors obtained a 51% reduction in Hamilton depression scale scores after 6 right unilateral ECTs administered via a 1-second, 175-mC stimulus. In comparison, my colleagues and I achieved a 68% reduction in Hamilton depression scale scores with 6 right unilateral ECTs administered via a 3-second, 378-mC stimulus (Abrams, Swartz, and Vedak, 1991). Moreover, our right unilateral ECT patients exhibited 13% more improvement after 6 ECTs than even the high-dose bilateral ECT patients of Sackeim et al. (1992, 1993).

Table 6-1 includes all studies I could find of brief-pulse unilateral ECT that provided the mean dosages used and percent improvement obtained, or the raw data from which they could be calculated. To facilitate comparison among the studies I have generally displayed the percent improvement obtained after 6 ECTs. Exceptions are the studies of McCall et al. (1995), who examined patients after a mean of 5.7 treatments, and Lamy et al. (1994), who gave a mean of 7.7 treatments.

Table 6-1 Studies of brief-pulse unilateral ECT

Author	Mean dose	Improvement (percent)	Duration (seconds)
Letemendia et al. (1993)	107 mC	45	1–2
Sackeim et al. (1987a)	154 mC	34	1
Sackeim et al. (1993)	175 mC	51	1
Abrams et al. (1991)	378 mC	68	3
Lamy et al. (1994)	394 mC	60*	6 (4–10)
McCall et al. (1995)	403 mC	69	2
Pettinati et al. (1990)	476 mC	89	2–3

*As tabulated in d'Elia, 1992.

Where reported, stimulus-train durations are also listed. Without claiming all-inclusiveness, I found the articles listed in Table 6-1, which I have arranged in order of increasing mean stimulus dose.

Interestingly, only the first three studies employed stimulus titration to set the initial dose. Because several of the higher-dose studies also employed longer-stimulus train durations, it is impossible to separate the effect of dosage from duration in this table (although I suspect dosage plays the more important role). Nevertheless, it is apparent that brief-pulse unilateral ECT given via high-dose, long-duration stimuli is a highly effective treatment irrespective of the seizure threshold.

Excluded from the table because of the large number of ECTs administered is the study of Bean et al. (1991), who used an age-based, fixed-dose method, assigning patients below 50 years of age to receive unilateral ECT with an initial stimulus dose of 60 to 64 mC (depending on the treatment device used), and the remainder to a dose three times as large: 180 to 192 mC. Stimulus dosages were adjusted at subsequent treatments to ensure adequate seizures; the total number of treatments given was determined on clinical grounds by the treating physician. Using the same criteria for recovery as Sackeim et al. (1987a), 82% of the high-dose patients recovered after a mean of 10 ECTS, compared with 40% of the low-dose patients, after a mean of 11 ECTs. Depression scale scores fell 53% in the low-dose group, and 77% in the high-dose group. Mean stimulus dosages across the treatment course were 105 mC for the low-dose group and 245 mC for the high-dose group.

Also excluded from the table was the study of Coffey et al. (1995b), because the percent improvement in depression scores could not be calculated separately for patients receiving unilateral ECT, and because of the long treatment courses administered (mean = 9 ECTs).

In addition to their greater absolute efficacy, higher stimulus intensities also accelerate the therapeutic response to ECT (Ottosson, 1960; Robin and de Tissera, 1982; Sackeim, Devanand and Prudic, 1991; Abrams, Swartz, and Vedak, 1991; Pettinati et al., 1994; McCall et al., 1995).

Although Sackeim et al. (1987a, 1993) have repeatedly tested their data for the relative clinical impact of dosage substantially exceeding threshold versus absolute dosage—and found only the former related to improvement—such a comparison is not intended to assess the efficacy of fixed, high-dose unilateral ECT, nor could it. This is because the dosages used by Sackeim et al. (1987a, 1993) were substantially lower than those in the high-dose studies cited, and because the efficacy of fixed, high-dose unilateral ECT is purely empirical— independent of whether or not there is a direct therapeutic component of the electrical stimulus that is separate from the induced seizure.

Another concern raised by Sackeim's group (Prudic et al., 1994) is that with fixed, high-dose stimulation some patients receiving unilateral ECT will receive dosages that are barely suprathreshold, thereby undermining the therapeutic effect. This argument overlooks the fact that the fixed, high-dose studies reported to date have achieved therapeutic results that are substantially better than those using the titration method (Abrams et al., 1991; Pettinati, 1994; Lamy et al., 1994; McCall et al., 1995).

To date, the study of McCall et al. (1995) shown in the table is the only prospective comparison of the clinical efficacy of unilateral ECT given with dosages derived from stimulus titration versus a fixed, high-dose protocol. In their sample of elderly patients (mean age 76), those receiving ECT with a fixed 403-mC dose responded faster and required fewer treatments than those receiving titrated, moderate-dose ECT (mean dose = 151 mC). They also exhibited shorter seizures and greater regularity of EEG morphology (McCall and Farah, 1995). Strikingly, despite the almost threefold higher dosage received by the fixed-dose group, memory self-ratings after ECT were not different for the two groups.

Cognitive Effects of High-Dose ECT

The fear has often been expressed that because fixed high–dose unilateral ECT without titration—especially the 378-mC dose my associates and I employed (Abrams et al., 1991)—is potentially many multiples of the seizure threshold in some patients, excessive cognitive dysfunction might result (Sackeim, 1994a; Beale et al., 1994; Enns and Karvelas, 1995):

> ... the practice of using electrical intensities far in excess of that needed to produce seizures undoubtedly contributes to adverse cognitive side effects. (Sackeim, Devanand, and Prudic, 1991)

However, the fact is that many studies that demonstrated dramatically less memory loss with right unilateral than with bilateral ECT used a sine-wave stimulus that delivered stimulus dosages for unilateral ECT that were substantially larger than the 378 mC used by Abrams et al. (1991).

The failure of McCall et al. (1995) to find excessive dysmnesia with fixed, high-dose (403 mC) unilateral ECT is in accord with other studies. Squire and Zouzounis (1986) found that brief-pulse right unilateral ECT administered with a fixed 336-mC stimulus caused no more verbal memory disturbance than observed in controls who received no ECT, and Pettinati et al. (1989) reported no change in verbal memory performance after a course of right unilateral ECT administered at a mean dose of 476 mC, which Pettinati et al. (1994) later estimated to be 4.5 to 7 times the seizure threshold.

It is further notable that Sackeim et al. (1993), although reporting significantly greater effects of high-dose than low-dose unilateral ECT on 2 highly sensitive right hemisphere-specific neuropsychological measures (nonsense shape recall and memory for facial emotional expression), nevertheless found no deleterious effect of high dosage on the more clinically relevant measure of autobiographical retrograde amnesia, the phenomenon that is most troubling to patients and their families. Moreover, despite the hemisphere-specific memory decrements found for high-dose unilateral ECT, this group (as well as all others) actually rated their memory as substantially improved on the self-rating scale of Squire et al. (1979) for post-ECT memory complaints.

Perhaps the most practical finding relative to the putative cognitive risks of high-dose unilateral ECT is the fact that both of the high-dose versus low-dose neuropsychological differences found by Sackeim et al. (1993) immediately after a course of treatment were no longer detectable a week later. Thus, fears of undue cognitive consequences of high-dose right unilateral ECT are unwarranted.

Cognitive Effects of Long Stimulus-Train Duration

Many of the high-dose studies cited also employed longer stimulus trains, and Sackeim (1994a) has raised the theoretical possibility that such long-duration stimuli might cause excessive dysmnesia by stimulating the brain after it was already in a hyperactive state—that is, while it was in seizure. In support of this view, he introduced the concept, derived from animal data, that the seizure threshold might act as a "filter" for the cognitive side effects of ECT.

Reification of a metaphor aside, this view does not take into account the fact that a 1 second stimulus dose that crosses the seizure threshold by the end of that second is unlikely to do so when its rate of administration is cut by 90% (e.g., by decreasing the frequency to spread the same dose over 8 seconds). Indeed, it is more likely that reducing the rate of administration of the ECT dose will substantially retard seizure onset, thus reducing, rather than accentuating, cognitive side effects (analogous to the relation between the steepness of the increase in plasma concentrations of a drug and the occurrence and severity of side effects). Moreover, long stimulus trains of up to 10 seconds have for many years been used routinely for unilateral ECT in Scandinavia (d'Elia et al., 1983) without incurring excess cognitive dysfunction, either on clinical observation or as measured by standardized test batteries of learning and retention (d'Elia, 1970; Fromholt et al., 1973; Strömgren et al., 1976; Lamy et al., 1994).

Relation of Stimulus Parameters to Seizure Quality and Efficacy

It has only been quite recently that investigators have turned their attention to defining the specific parameters of the brief-pulse, square-wave (pulsed) stimulus necessary for optimal induction of neuronal depolarization and the quality of the induced seizure (Abrams, 1996).

The variable features of the pulsed stimulus are pulse width, frequency, current, and stimulus train duration. From these, two others can be calculated: the charge and the charge rate. Optimizing the parameters of the pulsed stimulus requires an analysis of the characteristics of neuronal depolarization, as in the single-neuron action potential model. The validity of generalizing from a single neuron to the entire brain is supported by depth-electrode and scalp-recorded EEGs obtained during ECT-induced seizures. These uniformly show generalized, repetitive, bilaterally symmetrical high-voltage spikes, followed by spike and slow-wave complexes, often taking the form of rhythmic burst activity. Such patterns and sequences are typical of the simultaneous firing of massive numbers of neurons by a central pacemaker, suggesting that during an ECT-induced seizure the brain indeed acts as a virtual neuron.

Two other parameters of this model are (1) the smallest electrical dose that will initiate depolarization (this is the threshold, or rheobasic, dose) and (2) the minimum duration that a dose of twice this strength must be applied in order to initiate depolarization (the twice-threshold duration, or the chronaxie). This duration is entirely arbitrary, of course, as a higher or lower than twice-neuronal threshold dose might equally well have been chosen. In fact, had a 2.5- to 5-times-threshold dose originally been chosen (similar to what is now recommended for the clinical administration of unilateral ECT), the chronaxie would be much shorter.

Recent discussions on optimizing the parameters of the pulsed stimulus have addressed several interrelated topics: stimulus crowding, the relation of stimulus pulse width to cerebral neuron chronaxie, stimulus charge rate, and stimulus-train duration.

Stimulus Crowding

Sackeim et al. (1992) observed that "packing in more pulses during the same time frame . . . may be less efficient . . . because stimulation is given while neurons are refractory due to insufficient recovery from prior depolarization." Because the cycle of neuronal stimulation, depolarization, and repolarization—including absolute and relative refractory periods—takes about 6 msec, stimulus pulses should not be applied more frequently than about once every 6 msec (Abrams, 1994).

As noted earlier, the standard brief-pulse stimulus is bipolar, so a 70 Hz stimulus delivers 140 pulses per second, or 1 pulse every 7 msec. If the pulse width is 1 msec, for example, the first pulse depolarizes the neuron, after which the next stimulus follows in 6 msec, leaving just enough time for completion of the neuronal cycle. This suggests that the 70-Hz stimulus is the maximum that ought to be used, and that lower stimulus frequencies—which provide more time between stimuli, thus lengthening the stimulus-train duration proportionately—should be even more effective.

Pulse Width in Relation to Cerebral Neuron Chronaxie

Excessively wide pulse widths also stimulate neurons while they are unresponsive (Sackeim et al., 1994), and Sackeim (1994a) further refined this observation by considering the effect of pulse width from the physiologic vantage point of the chronaxie of cerebral neurons:

> Once the neuron has depolarized, there is a refractory period (reverse depolarization) and continued stimulation will not yield a response. Consequently, phase or pulse durations that markedly exceed the chronaxie of cerebral neurons are inefficient. Yet, the pulse durations commonly used in ECT are in the range of 1 to 2 msec.

The most recent estimate of the chronaxie of human alpha fibers (Malmivuo and Plonsey, 1995) is 0.2 msec, with a range in the earlier literature generally reported as up to 0.5 msec (H. Sackeim, personal communication). This means that pulse widths for ECT that substantially exceed the 0.2- to 0.5-msec range are also inefficient, because they exceed the minimum duration needed to initiate neuronal depolarization at the twice-threshold dose. Thus, based on the single-neuron model, for the pulsed stimulus to be optimally effective its frequency should be below 70 Hz and its pulse width in the 0.2- to 0.5-msec range.

Stimulus Charge Rate

Swartz (1994b, 1995) has approached the problem pragmatically by focusing on the rate of administration of the stimulus charge in relation to the efficiency of seizure induction. He observed that lower charge rates were consistent with greater efficacy in seizure induction and better quality seizures, and recommended a charge rate of about 25 to 50 mC per second.

Of course, because current is fixed in modern brief-pulse ECT devices, the charge rate is a function of pulse width and frequency: reducing either will reduce the charge rate proportionately (other things being equal, reducing the pulse width and/or pulse frequency lowers charge rate by spreading the dose over a longer interval).

Swartz makes the additional important point that it is essential for efficiently low charge rates to be available at the highest total stimulus charge settings for ECT devices. This is because it is the older— usually male—patients that have the greatest difficulty in obtaining good quality seizures, sometimes failing to develop any seizure activity at maximum device capacity. Whereas inefficient stimuli can readily induce seizures in low-threshold patients, they often cannot do so in high-threshold patients.

Stimulus-Train Duration

According to Sackeim et al. (1994), "manipulating the stimulus train duration may be a particularly efficient means of adjusting stimulus dosage relative to increasing pulse width, pulse frequency, or current intensity." As noted earlier, experimental data suggesting that increasing the pulse train duration—while keeping the charge constant—lowers the seizure threshold initially came from the study of Swartz and Larson (1989), with subsequent confirmation by Rasmussen et al. (1994) and Isenberg et al. (1996).

EEG Seizure Quality

At least a dozen studies in the modern era have failed to demonstrate a positive correlation between seizure duration and therapeutic outcome—there are no contrary data—and the subject must be considered closed. Moreover, several recent studies have consistently reported that an inverse relation actually exists (Nobler et al., 1993; Krystal et al., 1995; McCall et al., 1995; Shapira et al., 1996)—the shorter the seizure, the better the treatment response—an association that may have an important interaction with dosage. Thus, several investigators (Robin et al., 1985; Sackeim et al., 1991; Krystal et al., 1993; Shapira et al., 1996) have also reported an inverse relation between stimulus dose and seizure duration—the higher the dose, the shorter the seizure—sharply contrasting with the frequently offered advice to increase the stimulus dose if seizures are too short, and vice versa.

Swartz (1993a,b) has reviewed the available data and concluded that it is time to look beyond seizure duration for clinical and laboratory measures of seizure quality, focusing particularly on the tachycardia response to ECT (Swartz, 1996). Krystal and Weiner (1994) further suggest that several attributes of the ictal EEG other than its duration are candidates for markers of relative stimulus intensity, namely amplitude, symmetry, coherence, and postictal suppression.

These views reflect a consensus of expert opinion that effective

stimulation (e.g., stimulation at higher dosages) results in morpho-
logically well-developed, symmetrical, coherent, synchronous, high-
voltage seizure activity that is followed by marked postictal suppression and accompanied by substantial prolactin release and a
prominent tachycardia response—phenomena that all reflect increased
intracerebral seizure intensity or generalization (e.g., more rapid development and spread) and therefore shorter, more effective, seizures
(Robin et al., 1985; Krystal et al., 1992, 1993; Abrams, 1992, 1996;
Swartz, 1993a,b, 1996; Nobler et al., 1993; Krystal and Weiner, 1994;
McCall and Farah, 1995; Krystal, Weiner, and Coffey, 1995).

    Nobler et al. (1993) found that, compared to just-above-threshold
ECT, ECT given at 2.5 times threshold induced seizures that exhibited
greater midictal slow-wave amplitude and greater postictal suppression, and that the magnitude of this latter variable was positively associated with clinical improvement in depression.

    Krystal et al. (1993) confirmed this work, finding that 2.25-times-
threshold ECT was associated with significantly greater immediate
EEG post-stimulus and midictal spectral amplitude, greater immediate
post-stimulus interhemispheric coherence, and lower postictal spectral
amplitude (greater postical suppression) than observed with just-above-
threshold ECT.

    In a later study using a global scale to score severity of illness,
Krystal, Weiner, and Coffey (1995) employed a computer program to
select the EEG segment with maximum amplitude in each of 3 frequency bands for the early, middle, and postictal portions of the record.
These segments were then subjected to spectral amplitude and interhemispheric coherence analysis.

    All the EEG measures significantly differentiated threshold ECT
from that given at 2.25 times threshold, with greater ictal amplitude
and postictal suppression, and a more rapid onset and synchronous
(coherent) onset of slowing, characterizing the larger stimulus.

    The authors stated that their results confirmed that more highly
suprathreshold ECT was associated with ictal EEG evidence of more
intense seizure activity, greater early and midictal amplitude, and more
extensive postical suppression. The earlier onset of slow-wave activity
and greater coherence of ictal slowing suggest that such seizures may
be more rapidly generalized and neuronally synchronous.

    McCall and Farah (1995) examined the ictal EEG regularity ob-
tained with fixed-high-dose (403 mC) versus 2.25-times-threshold dosing in 17 elderly patients receiving right unilateral ECT. The fixed-
high-dose group exhibited greater EEG regularity, shorter seizures, and

a more rapid antidepressant effect than the moderately suprathreshold group.

Krystal et al. (1996) re-analyzed earlier data (Krystal et al., 1993, 1995) for spectral amplitude and interhemispheric coherence in 3 frequency bands and 3 seizure phases. They also obtained depression rating scale scores at baseline and after the fifth ECT, and found that improvement in scores correlated most highly with the EEG measures of low-frequency postictal coherence (the less coherence, the better the response) and high-frequency postictal spectral amplitude (the lower the amplitude—that is, the greater the postictal suppression—the better the response).

Recommendations

The trick, of course, is to be able to administer the optimal stimulus dose for a particular patient and treatment method, using stimulus parameters that maximize seizure generalization. Sadly, this is not possible for many patients, for two reasons.

First, there is an arbitrary energy limitation imposed on modern ECT devices by the International Electrotechnical Commission (IEC) and the Food and Drug Administration (FDA) of 100 joules at 220 ohms impedance, or about 500 to 600 mC of charge, which simply does not permit giving the doses of 2.5 to 5.5 times threshold that are required to treat many patients when administering unilateral ECT. Especially in older patients, some of whom will have seizure thresholds as high as 896 mC, dosages approaching 2,000 mC will therefore be required in order to reach the therapeutic range (Sackeim et al., 1992; Lisanby et al., 1996).

Second, delivering the present maximum allowable dose, using pulse widths no greater than 0.5 msec and frequencies no greater than 70 Hz, already requires a stimulus train duration of about 8 seconds; and the potentially more desirable (because closer to the chronaxie of human neurons) 0.25-msec pulse width, combined with, say, a more physiological 50-Hz stimulus, would require a stimulus-train duration for unilateral ECT of over 22 seconds!

In recent years, I have suggested that investigations into the clinical efficacy of ECT in depression should focus on further refinements of the technique of unilateral ECT, using higher doses and more efficient stimuli, because of the substantial cognitive advantage of this form of therapy over traditional bilateral ECT.

In fact, one could make the cogent argument to give every patient who is to receive brief-pulse unilateral ECT stimulation at full device capacity—period. Therapeutic response will be maximized for all; whatever memory disturbances result will be far less than previously obtained with bilateral sine-wave ECT—and no different a week or so later from those consequent to the frequently lower dosages determined via stimulus titration—and the patient will experience a subjective improvement in memory.

The neurophysiological considerations detailed above, however, suggest that the dose-sensitivity of unilateral ECT presents a limit that may already have been reached (at today's present maximum allowable dosages) in terms of maximizing the efficacy of this therapy. Because bilateral ECT is not dose-sensitive (it is effective when given with just-above- or moderately-above-threshold dosing), and because the range of impedances encountered in clinical practice is about 90 to 350 ohms (Sackeim et al., 1993)—permitting a stimulus charge well below the presently-set maximum—it is possible to give bilateral ECT to virtually all patients using stimuli that lie within the physiological range: pulse widths no larger than 0.5 msec and frequencies no greater than 70 Hz. In fact, if the finding of Isenberg et al. (1996) is confirmed—that the seizure threshold to bilateral ECT using long-duration stimuli doesn't usually exceed 100 mC—it will be possible to routinely administer this therapy using a pulse width of 0.25 msec and a frequency of 30 Hz without exceeding an 8-second stimulus train.

Moreover, the cognitive side effects of bilateral ECT can be reduced without altering its therapeutic impact by simply lowering its frequency of administration to the British standard of twice each week from the present U.S. standard of 3 times each week (Lerer et al., 1995).

Thus, until and unless the FDA and the IEC change their view on the maximum allowable stimulus dose of ECT devices, twice-weekly bilateral ECT given with these more physiological stimulus parameters should be the most effective treatment for a substantial number of patients. It also seems likely that such stimuli will further reduce the cognitive side effects of bilateral ECT, thus possibly rendering marginal any cognitive advantage for unilateral ECT.

My recommendation, therefore, is that all patients should routinely receive an initial trial of thrice-weekly brief-pulse unilateral ECT at maximum device capacity (e.g., at least 500 mC), and without stimulus titration. If several such treatments do not produce the anticipated result, I recommend a switch to biweekly conventional or anterior bilateral ECT at a dosage expected to be substantially suprathreshold (as determined by stimulus titration or the age-based method), administered via a pulse width of 0.25 to 0.5 msec, a stimulus frequency of 30 to 70 Hz, and a stimulus-train duration of 4 to 8 seconds.

7

Unilateral Electroconvulsive Therapy

Unilateral ECT—especially when administered with a brief-pulse square-wave stimulus—represents the most important technical advance in the field of convulsive therapy since Cerletti and Bini (1938) invented ECT. More clinical research has been conducted since 1960 on the cognitive and therapeutic effects of this modality than on any other single topic in the ECT literature; much of this research has been directed primarily at resolving the controversy concerning the precise clinical role of this method in relation to the older bilateral ECT (Fink, 1979; Welch, 1982; Abrams and Fink, 1984; Abrams, 1986; Mathisen and Pettinati, 1987; Overall and Rhoades, 1986, 1987). This chapter will review the history and development of unilateral ECT, concentrating on studies of therapeutic efficacy in comparison with bilateral ECT; the many cognitive studies will be considered in Chapter 10.

The early history of ECT research was largely characterized by attempts to reduce the side effects of seizures induced by the original sinusoidal currents delivered via bifrontotemporal electrodes. Only a year after the first English-language papers on ECT appeared (Kalinowsky, 1939; Fleming et al., 1939; Shepley and McGregor, 1939), Douglas Goldman demonstrated the new treatment at the annual American Psychiatric Association meeting, using a device built to his specifications by Offner (Fink, 1987). In view of the fact that Offner subsequently marketed the first commercial brief-pulse device 6 years later (Weiner, 1988), it is likely that Goldman used such a device in his demonstration. Friedman (1942) and Friedman and Wilcox (1942) were the first to publish data on the use of modified sine-wave currents—chopped portions of half-waves—which they administered via a left-sided unilateral electrode placement. These authors' primary interest was technical—to investigate the amount of electric current delivered—and they made no mention of therapeutic effects, memory loss, or confusion. These studies were continued and expanded by Proctor and Goodwin (1943), Liberson (1944)—who introduced the term "brief-stimulus" to describe the 0.16- to 0.33-msec spikes employed and was also the first to report right-sided unilateral ECT placement—Liberson and Wilcox (1945), Moriarty and Siemens (1947), and Liberson (1948). A variety of electrode placements were used (most of them right unilateral), but they were not applied systematically, and these authors all reported reduced cognitive side effects with their new techniques.

Goldman (1949) invented unilateral ECT as we know it: He was the first to specify that unilateral treatment electrodes should be placed over the right hemisphere in order to avoid the speech areas. In 112 patients, he observed clinical improvement equal to that produced by bilateral ECT but with a "marked diminution and, at times, absence of confusion associated with the electric shock therapy." His attribution of the beneficial effect thus obtained to the brief-pulse, square-wave stimulus he used was only partly correct—right unilateral electrode placement probably played the more important role. Bayles et al. (1950) confirmed these results with brief-stimulus right unilateral ECT and also reported reduced EEG effects compared with sine-wave ECT. Workers into the mid-1950s (Blaurock et al., 1950; Impastato et al., 1953; Liberson, 1953; Liberson et al., 1956) continued to report reduced memory loss and confusion with unilateral placements, particularly right-sided ones, but they never attempted to separate the effects of stimulus type from electrode placement, or to further characterize the specific benefits accruing from right unilateral placement.

The Argentine psychiatrist Thenon (1956) was the first to demonstrate the specific link between right unilateral electrode placement and reduced memory loss and confusion; he also observed an accentuation of post-ECT slow-wave EEG activity over the treated hemisphere. He called his method monolateral electroshock. Two years later, Lancaster, Steinert, and Frost (1958), apparently entirely unaware of the work of Goldman or Thenon, published the first English-language paper devoted to this technique, giving it its present name of unilateral ECT. Their study was also notable for employing random assignment to treatment and blind assessment of depression and orientation using rating scales. In 21 patients receiving unilateral ECT, orientation and recall returned significantly faster than in 15 controls who received bilateral ECT. Moreover, these authors observed automatic behavior, dazed expression, and restlessness to be less prominent after unilateral ECT. They reported that four bilateral ECTs reduced depression scores by 71%, compared with 54% for unilateral ECT, noted "slightly better and more complete remission" with bilateral ECT, and therefore recommended that it be preferentially given to involutional depressives, patients who were actively suicidal, depressed patients who failed to show substantial improvement after six unilateral ECTs, and to catatonic schizophrenics who were "dangerously impulsive" (these latter patients might well receive a diagnosis of acute mania today). This report of Lancaster, Steinert, and Frost (1958) already contained each of the elements of what later was to become "the unilateral ECT controversy": (1) sharply reduced memory loss and confusion with unilateral ECT; (2) a formal equivalence for right unilateral and bilateral ECT on objective outcome measures; and (3) the authors' clinical impression that bilateral ECT was nonetheless more therapeutically potent than right unilateral ECT.

By 1972 there were 15 published comparisons of unilateral and bilateral ECT, of which only 5 unequivocally reported the two methods to be equally therapeutic (Abrams, 1972). Most workers, although finding the methods equally effective on the objective measures of rating scale scores or the total number of ECT prescribed by a "blind" psychiatrist, nevertheless added their clinical impressions to the effect that unilateral ECT was less rapidly effective, had to be given more frequently or required more total treatments (Cannicott, 1962; Halliday et al., 1968; Cronin et al., 1970; d'Elia, 1970), and that bilateral ECT was globally more effective or was to be preferred in patients who were more severely ill, endogenously depressed, suicidal, catatonic or dangerous (Lancaster, Steinert, and Frost, 1958; Levy, 1968; Halliday et al., 1968; Small et al., 1970; Fleminger et al., 1970a; Cronin et al., 1970).

By 1975 d'Elia and Raotma could find 24 published comparisons of unilateral and bilateral ECT, which they tabulated for research findings and clinical impressions: 12 studies reported equal efficacy, 11 reported an advantage for bilateral ECT, and one an advantage for unilateral ECT ($\chi^2 = 9.25$, $p < 0.001$).

Even among the studies finding approximate global equivalence for the two methods using objective measures, large differences favored bilateral ECT in certain clinically important subgroups. Thus, Cronin et al. (1970) found that six bilateral ECTs reduced depression scale scores in endogenous depressives by 72% compared with 35% for unilateral ECT, and Strömgren (1973) found a statistically significant advantage for bilateral ECT in relieving depression in patients over age 44.

Considering its marked cognitive advantages over bilateral ECT, right unilateral ECT has been used far less widely than might be expected. A 1976 survey of its members conducted by the American Psychiatric Association Task Force on ECT (1978) revealed that 75% used bilateral ECT exclusively and that fewer than 10% of all patients received unilateral ECT. In a 1975 to 1976 survey of ECT usage in New York City, Asnis et al. (1978) reported that 83% of the respondents used bilateral ECT exclusively. Similar observations were recorded in single-hospital surveys of patterns of ECT usage in the 1980s compared with the 1970s (Tancer et al., 1989). In Great Britain, Gill and Lamborn (1979) found that 50% of the senior psychiatric consultants preferred bilateral ECT, and Pippard and Ellam's (1981) survey 2 years later found that 80% of all clinicians "rarely or never" used unilateral ECT. Unilateral ECT is probably most widely used in the Scandinavian countries, but even there only 25% of the Danish centers (Heshe and Roeder, 1976) and 50% of the Swedish centers (Fredericksen and d'Elia, 1979) used unilateral ECT exclusively at the time they were surveyed. In a nationwide survey of ECT practice in the United States, Farah and McCall (1993) reported that 52% of ECT providers initiated treatment with bilateral ECT, and 48% with unilateral ECT—a substantial increase in usage of the latter method since the previous U.S. survey by Asnis (1978)—virtually always administered with a brief-pulse device.

The many studies demonstrating therapeutic equivalence for unilateral and bilateral ECT have been reviewed by d'Elia and Raotma (1975) and Fink (1979). Contrary data have been less well publicized (Abrams, 1986), however, and the following selective review describes in more detail studies—most of which used a random-assignment, double-blind, controlled methodology—that have reported an advantage for bilateral over unilateral ECT.

Strain et al. (1968) assigned 96 hospitalized depressives to right unilateral or bilateral ECT and assessed the outcome under double-blind conditions. Forty percent of the right unilateral ECT group required 10 or more treatments, compared with 17% of the bilateral group. The bilateral ECT group improved substantially more on the two Clyde mood scale factors found to be the most valid indicators of depression: *unhappy* and *dizzy*, and the right unilateral ECT group required an average of one extra treatment and a stay of 2 days longer in the hospital.

Abrams and Taylor (1974) treated 30 melancholics with either one bilateral ECT, two right-sided unilateral ECTs, or one right- followed by one left-sided unilateral ECT each treatment session. On assessment by Hamilton rating scale, four bilaterally-induced seizures produced the same therapeutic effect as eight seizures induced by either of the two unilateral methods over the same period of time.

In a different sample of patients, Abrams and Taylor (1976b) assigned 20 melancholics to receive six seizures either with bilateral placement or two sets of unilateral electrodes separately and simultaneously applied to both sides of the head. After 6 treatments, the bilateral ECT group exhibited significantly lower depression scale scores, and 91% of the patients in the left–right unilateral group went on to receive additional treatments, compared with only one third of the bilateral group.

Reichert et al. (1976a,b) assigned 50 patients with varied diagnoses to unilateral or bilateral ECT and found a significant advantage for the latter method at several points during the treatment course on a self-rated mood scale. Significantly more patients in the unilateral group also required an additional course of ECT within 6 months after terminating treatment.

Heshe et al. (1978) treated 51 endogenous depressives with either right unilateral or bilateral ECT and rated their global outcome 1 week and 3 months after the treatment course. At the 1-week rating, more than one third of the patients who received right unilateral ECT were scored "unimproved" compared with none in the bilateral group (exact $p = 0.01$). No differences were found at 3 months. For patients over age 60, more than 50% of those given unilateral ECT were rated "unimproved" at 1 week, compared with none in the bilateral group (exact $p = 0.003$), and at 3 months 75% of the unilateral ECT patients were rated "unimproved" compared with 30% of the bilateral ECT group (exact $p = 0.003$).

Abrams et al. (1983) assigned 51 melancholics to right unilateral or bilateral ECT and monitored all treatments by EEG. Hamilton depression scale scores after 6 ECTs were reduced by 81% in the bilateral group compared with only 56% in the right unilateral group. Moreover, patients receiving right unilateral ECT required an average of three more treatments, more often required 10 or more ECTs, and were more frequently switched to the alternate form of treatment by a psychiatrist who was blind to treatment assignment.

Sackeim et al. (1987a) assigned 52 primary major depressives to right unilateral or bilateral ECT, both administered with just-above-threshold stimulation. Hamilton Depression Scale scores obtained before treatment and after the sixth and the final ECT showed much greater improvement with bilateral than with right unilateral ECT (70% improvement for bilateral ECT after the full course, compared with only 37% with right unilateral ECT), a result also confirmed when global outcome ratings were used to divide patients into treatment responders and nonresponders (right unilateral ECT was associated with a strikingly high nonresponse rate of 34%). Despite the low-dose electrical stimulation, EEG seizure duration was the same in both groups and similar to that usually reported for conventional bilateral ECT.

Gregory et al. (1985) treated 60 depressives with either bilateral, right unilateral, or sham ECT. Both genuine methods were superior to sham ECT, an advantage that appeared after the second bilateral ECT but not until after the fourth unilateral ECT. Moreover, patients receiving unilateral ECT required significantly more treatments after their sixth compared with those in the bilateral group.

Tandon et al. (1988) prospectively studied 46 medication-resistant depressives who had received bilateral (the first 30 patients) or right unilateral (the next 16 patients) ECT with blind weekly evaluations performed on the Hamilton scale during the treatment course. After five treatments, bilateral ECT induced a 57% improvement compared with only 19% in the right unilateral group. Global assessments after the full course of ECT showed 72% of the bilateral group to be fully recovered, compared with 32% of the unilateral group. This advantage for bilateral ECT was also observed when seizure length was equivalent for the two methods.

Thus, numerous investigators report a statistically significant therapeutic advantage for bilateral over various forms of unilateral ECT in depression. Of 18 controlled trials in depression completed since d'Elia and Raotma's (1975) paper (Abrams and Taylor, 1974; Abrams and Taylor, 1976b; Reichert et al., 1976a,b; Heshe et al., 1978; Weeks et al., 1980; Fraser and Glass, 1980; Abrams et al., 1983; Horne et al., 1985; Gregory et al., 1985; Weiner et al., 1986b; Malitz et al., 1986; Welch et al., 1982; Tandon et al., 1988; Abrams, Swartz, and Vedak, 1991; Letemendia et al., 1993; Sackeim et al., 1993; Lamy et al., 1994), 10 favor bilateral ECT.

The results of sham ECT studies are also instructive: of 12 comparisons of the efficacy of genuine versus sham ECT in the treatment of depression (Ulett et al., 1956; Harris and Robin, 1960; Robin and Harris, 1962; Wilson et al., 1963; McDonald et al., 1966; Lambourn and Gill, 1978; Freeman et al., 1978; Johnstone et al., 1980; West, 1981; Ghangadar et al., 1982; Brandon et al., 1984; Gregory et al., 1985), 11 used bilateral placement as the active treatment and found an advantage for genuine ECT; the single study that compared right unilateral ECT with sham ECT (Lambourn and Gill, 1978) found no such advantage. Finally, meta-analysis, a statistical method for integrating the results from diverse studies on a single topic, has been used to review the unilateral versus bilateral ECT literature. Although Janicak et al. (1985) and Pettinati et al. (1986) both used meta-analytic procedures to arrive at the conclusion that the two electrode placements were equally effective in treating depressed patients, Overall and Rhoades (1986, 1987) reanalyzed both studies using three different meta-analytic techniques, each of which revealed statistical significance in favor of bilateral ECT in the relief of depression.

Thus, although right unilateral and bilateral ECT are often reported to be therapeutically equal in depressed patients, right unilateral ECT frequently yields less improvement or requires more treatments to achieve the same outcome. Moreover, some patients who do not respond to even substantial numbers of unilateral ECTs (e.g., 10 to 20 treatments) nevertheless achieve a remission when switched to bilateral ECT (Price, 1981; Abrams et al., 1983). The most striking example of this phenomenon was reported by Pettinati et al. (1990), who found that 9 of 11 patients who did not respond to high-dose (391 mC) right unilateral ECT did respond when switched to bilateral ECT, enjoying a remarkable 80% total reduction in depression scale score after achieving only 16% improvement in response to the initial 5 or 6 unilateral ECTs. This report is all the more convincing for having come from the same research group that only a few years earlier had claimed therapeutic equivalence for the two methods (Horne et al., 1985).

The following considerations may help to explain the discrepant findings among the various studies reviewed (Abrams, 1986a,b).

1. *Diagnosis.* Endogenous depression (melancholia) constitutes the prime indication for ECT; it is the patients in this diagnostic group that are most likely to show between-group differences in any treatment comparisons. For example, as cited earlier, Cronin et al. (1970) found bilateral ECT to induce substantially more improvement than right unilateral ECT in melancholics but not in reactive depressives. Unfortunately, many comparisons of unilateral and bilateral ECT fail to specify the proportion of melancholics in their

samples, or report the treatment results separately for this diagnostic group.

2. *Age.* As previously noted, Strömgren (1973) reported a statistically significant advantage for bilateral over unilateral ECT in patients over 44 years of age, a result later confirmed by Heshe et al. (1978) for patients over age 60. In the recent meta-analytic review cited earlier, Pettinati et al. (1986) noted that older patients tended to show a larger bilateral compared with right unilateral ECT advantage.

3. *Sex.* The same meta-analytic review found an even stronger trend for men to exhibit larger bilateral compared with right unilateral ECT differences than women. Sackeim et al. (1987b) reported that the seizure threshold is about 50% higher in men than in women.

4. *Electrical dosage.* Stimulus dosing is considered elsewhere in this volume (p. 124), but suffice it to say here that the most important discovery about unilateral ECT in the past decade is that it is far more dosage-sensitive than bilateral ECT (Sackeim et al., 1987a, 1993). Thus, those studies employing the smallest stimulus doses (Sackeim et al., 1987a, 1993) report the largest clinical advantage for bilateral ECT, and vice versa (Pettinati et al., 1990; Abrams, Swartz, and Vedak, 1991; Lamy et al., 1994; McCall et al., 1994). Moreover, the only study failing to find an advantage of genuine over sham ECT (Lambourn and Gill, 1978) gave unilateral ECT with the smallest fixed stimulus ever reported: just 10 joules.

5. *Interelectrode distance for unilateral ECT.* The original hypothesis of d'Elia and Raotma (1975) that smaller interelectrode distances for unilateral placements resulted in a smaller therapeutic effect was confirmed in the meta-analytic study of Pettinati et al. (1986): A larger bilateral compared with unilateral ECT advantage occurred in studies using smaller interelectrode distances for unilateral ECT.

6. *Relevance of technique.* Is the therapeutic advantage frequently reported for bilateral ECT simply a result of poor technique in administering unilateral ECT, so that inadequate seizures and a reduced therapeutic effect are obtained? That is, would monitoring of seizures in those studies reporting an advantage for bilateral ECT have revealed shorter, incomplete, or abortive seizures in the unilateral ECT groups and thus a reduced effect? This is a plausible but untenable argument because it applies primarily to earlier studies reviewed by Abrams (1972) and d'Elia and Raotma (1975) that were performed before seizure monitoring had become a routine

part of ECT; virtually all of these reported equal therapeutic effects of bilateral and unilateral ECT.

In an earlier hypothesis (Abrams, 1986a), I attempted to explain how age, gender, electrical dosage, and unilateral ECT interelectrode distances might interact to influence the likelihood of finding a therapeutic advantage for bilateral ECT. Seizure threshold and intracerebral current density both vary with changes in each of these factors and are themselves related because a sufficient quantity of electricity, or charge, must enter the brain to exceed the seizure threshold (reducing electrical dosage has the same effect on obtaining seizures as increasing the threshold). Seizure threshold increases with age and is higher in men than in women (Sackeim et al., 1987b). Intracerebral current densities are reduced with smaller interelectrode distances (Weaver et al., 1976) and, of course, with low-dose stimulation. Relevant in this context are the reports that seizure threshold is higher with bilateral than unilateral ECT (Weaver et al., 1978; Weiner, 1980; Sackeim et al., 1987b), requiring a larger electrical charge to be introduced into the brain to elicit seizures with the former method.

What effect might the intensity of the electrical stimulus have on the seizure and the therapeutic effect of ECT in depression? Evidence for a therapeutic effect of the stimulus was found by Ottosson (1960) in a comparison of the clinical efficacy of moderately and markedly suprathreshold stimuli. On all measures of improvement the markedly suprathreshold group fared better, a difference that was statistically significant for the improvement in depression score per second of seizure discharge in patients who received four or fewer treatments. Abrams and Taylor (1976b) found that conventional bilateral ECT was significantly more effective in relieving depression than simultaneously administered left- and right-sided unilateral ECT. We interpreted our findings in terms of differential intracerebral distribution of the stimulating currents and resultant seizure activity and proposed that the therapeutic differences observed were due to greater diencephalic (specifically, hypothalamic) stimulation with bilateral ECT.

Robin and De Tissera (1982) compared high- and low-energy, brief-pulse ECT and found a significantly greater therapeutic effect for high-energy stimulation at every post-ECT assessment interval. Evidence for greater cerebral stimulation with bilateral than unilateral ECT comes from Swartz and Abrams (1984) who demonstrated that bilateral ECT induces more prolactin release into the bloodstream than unilateral ECT (Figure 7-1), a finding confirmed by Papakostas et al. (1984) and by Swartz (1985) in a sample of women.

Observations (Abrams and Swartz, 1985b) that the electrical stimulus can induce prolactin release in the absence of an observable motor or EEG seizure (Figure 7-2), and that multiple electrical stimuli tend to induce more prolactin release than single ones, provide further evidence for a physiologic effect of the stimulus current. In a comparison of ECT devices with different energy outputs, Robin et al. (1985) found that ECT-induced prolactin release varied directly with stimulus energy, although this correlation was not statistically significant and there were some methodological problems as well. Nevertheless, subsequent studies of high- versus low-dose stimulation in patients receiving unilateral or bilateral ECT have confirmed a strong effect of stimulus dosage on ECT-induced prolactin release that is independent of the induced seizure (Zis et al., 1993; Lisanby et al., 1996).

The electrical stimulus might contribute directly to the therapeutic effect of ECT either by influencing the intensity or the generalization of the induced seizure activity, or both. Ottosson's (1960) finding of a greater therapeutic effect per seizure second with markedly compared with moderately suprathreshold stimulation, albeit only in patients who

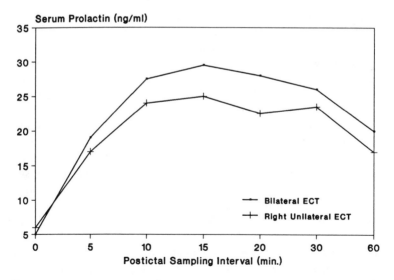

Figure 7-1 Prolactin release with bilateral and right unilateral ECT. (Adapted from Swartz and Abrams, 1984.)

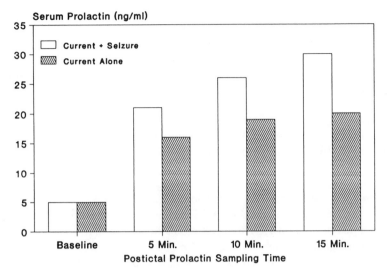

Figure 7-2   Stimulus-induced release of prolactin in one patient. (Adapted from Abrams and Swartz, 1985.)

received small numbers of treatments, suggests that the larger electrical stimulus acted by affecting the intensity or generalization of the induced seizure activity. More intense or completely generalized seizures are followed by greater immediate post-ictal EEG suppression: Ottosson's (1960) comparison of seizures with and without lidocaine modification showed that lidocaine-modified seizures often failed to terminate in the usual EEG phase of electrical silence (postictal suppression). Postictal EEG suppression is greater with bilateral than with unilateral ECT (Small et al., 1970; Abrams et al., 1973; Weiner, 1986), presumably because the larger charge of electricity bilateral ECT introduces into the brain results in more intense or generalized seizures. Greater seizure generalization with bilateral ECT is also suggested by the finding of Swartz and Larson (1986) that the correlations between each pair of four separate estimates of seizure duration (motor activity, heart rate, and two EEG measures) were significantly greater with bilateral compared with unilateral ECT; by the report of fewer missed or abortive seizures with bilateral compared with unilateral ECT (Pettinati and Nilsen, 1985); by the 83% greater increase in MRI spin-lattice relaxation times after bilateral compared with unilateral ECT (Mander et al., 1987); by the greater cardiac response to bilateral compared with unilateral ECT (Lane et al., 1989); and by the fact that bilateral ECT induces more prolactin release than does unilateral ECT (Swartz and Abrams, 1984; Papakostas et al., 1984, 1986; Abrams and Swartz, 1985a; Swartz, 1985; Zis et al., 1993; Lisanby et al., 1996).

Sackeim et al. (1987a, 1993) have suggested that the degree to which the electrical stimulus exceeds the seizure threshold is critical for the fully developed therapeutic effect of a given treatment, and that differential stimulation of specific anatomic brain sites determines the differential efficacies of high- versus low-dose unilateral or bilateral ECT (Sackeim, 1994a,b). In this view, triggering seizures from prefrontal brain areas—which occurs most effectively with high-dose bilateral ECT—is considered fundamental to the efficacy of ECT.

I have suggested (Abrams, 1986b) that the seizure and the electrical stimulus both contribute to the therapeutic activity of ECT in depression. Once a seizure with well-developed polyspike (tonic) and polyspike-and-slow-wave (clonic) phases occurs, its therapeutic effect does not depend on its duration, but on how intense, complete, or well-generalized throughout the brain the seizure activity is. At substantially suprathreshold levels of stimulation, the therapeutic effect attributable to the electrical stimulus is dwarfed by the effects of the fully generalized seizure. With reduced electrical dosage or elevated seizure threshold, however, therapeutic effects of the stimulus emerge. Under these circumstances bilateral ECT introduces more electrical charge into a larger volume of brain than unilateral ECT, resulting in more efficient seizure generalization, greater diencephalic stimulation, and more rapid or complete relief of depression. Common to both views of the therapeutic role of the electrical stimulus, however, is the notion that increasing the stimulus charge with unilateral ECT should result in an increased therapeutic effect.

A study by my colleagues and me (Abrams, Swartz and Vedak, 1991) supports the validity of this prediction. We conducted a random-assignment, double-blind, controlled comparison of the antidepressant effects of 6 bilateral or right unilateral ECT in 38 melancholic men, employing a brief-pulse stimulus, a wide inter-electrode unilateral placement, and a fixed, high-dose (378 mC) stimulus that should have been about 2.5 times threshold according to the population data collected by Sackeim et al. (1987b). No significant differences between bilateral and right unilateral ECT were found for depression rating scale improvement (79% vs. 68%, respectively), the proportion of patients categorized as responders (77.8% vs. 65.0%, respectively), or the total number of ECTs prescribed (7.5 in each group), although there was a trend ($p = 0.06$) for faster improvement with bilateral ECT (Figure 7-3).

Because we found a significant clinical advantage for bilateral ECT in an earlier study that was conducted in the same clinical setting and used the same rating scale (Abrams et al., 1983)—but employed a sine-wave stimulus and a narrow interelectrode unilateral ECT placement—we concluded that changing the unilateral ECT stimulus and application site had substantially augmented its therapeutic impact. (The mean depression scale score reduction of 81% in response to bilateral ECT in the new study was virtually identical to the 79% reduction obtained earlier, but the reduction in response to unilateral ECT was much larger: 68% vs. 55%.)

No definitive comparison of the charges administered in the two studies is possible, because the first employed a fixed-voltage, sine-wave stimulus and the second, a fixed-current, brief-pulse stimulus, but the sine-wave stimulus of 170 volts for 1 second is likely to have been greatly above threshold for virtually all patients. Indeed, at the average patient impedance of 220 ohms, this stimulus would have had a charge of 773 mC, more than double the dosage recently used. The fact that the much smaller, but nonetheless markedly suprathreshold,

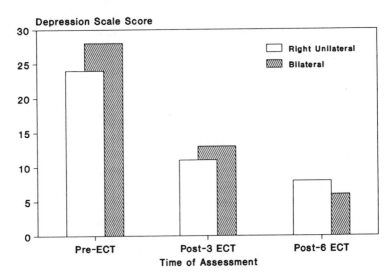

Figure 7-3   Antidepressant effects of high-dose brief-pulse ECT. (Adapted from Abrams, Swartz, and Vedak, 1991.)

brief-pulse stimulus augmented the therapeutic potency of unilateral ECT suggests that brief-pulse stimuli—especially when delivered through unilateral electrodes—are more therapeutically efficient than sine-wave stimuli.

Whether, and to what extent, the high-stimulus dosing we used might have attenuated the widely reported and clinically important cognitive advantage of right unilateral compared with bilateral ECT is discussed elsewhere in this volume (p. 126).

Sackeim et al. (1993) confirmed the greater efficacy of an increased stimulus dose for unilateral ECT in a prospective comparison of titrated high- versus low-dose unilateral or bilateral ECT. In this study, 2.5-times-threshold dosing for unilateral ECT was substantially more effective than just-above-threshold dosing, although still less effective than bilateral ECT given at low or high dosage. Moreover, the effect of stimulus intensity on clinical response was not associated with the absolute electrical dose administered, but rather with whether the dosage substantially exceeded the seizure threshold.

Although the authors interpreted this latter observation as falsifying the theory that the electrical charge itself may be inherently therapeutic, the dosages used in their studies have not generally been nearly as large as those in several of the high-dose, high-efficacy studies reported (Pettinati et al., 1990; Abrams, Swartz, and Vedak, 1991; Lamy et al., 1994; McCall et al., 1995), and they may easily have missed a dosage threshold effect similar to that observed for the relation between seizure duration and therapeutic outcome.

Seizure intensity or generalization and differences in intracerebral current densities are reflected in the interictal as well as in the immediate postictal EEG. There are several reports of accentuation of sine wave unilateral ECT-induced EEG slowing ipsilateral to the treated hemisphere (Martin et al., 1965; Zamora and Kaelbling, 1965; Sutherland et al., 1969; Abrams et al., 1970; Volavka et al., 1972; Sackeim et al., 1996); less well-known is the documented tendency for left-hemispheric accentuation of EEG slowing after bilateral sine-wave ECT (Green, 1957; Marjerrison et al., 1975; Abrams et al., 1970, 1987; Volavka et al., 1972; Sackeim et al., 1996). This differential lateralization of EEG slowing with unilateral and bilateral ECT is age-related, with increasing age associated with a relative reduction of left versus right hemisphere frequencies (Volavka et al., 1972).

As detailed previously, however, our initial demonstration (Abrams et al., 1987) of a significant correlation between the side of hemispheric lateralization of ECT-induced EEG change and antidepressant response was not confirmed in a subsequent study employing a modified methodology (Abrams, Volavka, and Schrift, 1992). Just as changing from a sine-wave to a brief-pulse stimulus and from a narrow to a wide temporoparietal unilateral placement abolished the previously detected therapeutic difference between bilateral and right unilateral ECT (Abrams, Swartz, and Vedak, 1991), so the same change in the attempted replication of the EEG data abolished the differential lateralization of EEG slowing we had previously detected for the two methods. Compared with the earlier study, in which all patients with left-sided slowing had received bilateral ECT and all patients with right-sided slowing had received right unilateral ECT (Abrams et al., 1987)—the study that assigned patients to right, left, or bilateral ECT simply found no ECT-induced left-sided slowing. Moreover, the 6 instances of right-sided slowing were evenly divided among treatment groups. A comparison of the two studies (Table 7-1) shows that the brief-pulse stimulus induced less global EEG abnormality, equivalent reduction in depression score, and more relief of depression per unit of induced EEG abnormality than the sine-wave stimulus—that is, the same improvement with less EEG slowing, consistent with the report of Weiner et al. (1986a).

Using EEG computer analysis, Sackeim et al. (1996) confirmed the differential lateralizing effects of right unilateral and bilateral ECT on interictal EEG slow activity previously reported by Abrams et al. (1987) but were unable to find a correlation between such lateralized slowing and therapeutic response in depression. The ability of Sackeim et al. (1996) to detect such lateralized differences with brief-pulse stimulation—when Abrams, Volavka, and Schrift (1992) could not— is probably due to the greater sensitivity of computer, compared to visual, EEG analysis.

Table 7-1 Comparison of results reported in Abrams et al. (1987) and Abrams, Volavka, and Schrift (1992)

Abrams et al.	(1987)	(1992)
Global EEG abnormality after 6 ECTs	3.66 (SD 1.1)	3.12 (SD 1.2)
Percent reduction in HRS	72.4 (SD 24.5)	68.1 (SD 36.0)
HRS improvement per unit of global EEG abnormality	20.2 (SD 15.5)	29.5 (SD 22.3)

Left Unilateral Electroconvulsive Therapy

Left unilateral ECT has suffered from an undeservedly bad reputation, due largely to a selective reading of the handful of studies on the subject. A claimed antidepressant advantage of right over left unilateral ECT has been mustered to support a general theory of cerebral hemispheric asymmetry in the expression of emotions—specifically, depression—and to explain the antidepressant effects of ECT as well. Thus, Galin (1974) states that "... examination of the literature on unilateral ECT for depression suggests that the two hemispheres differ in the response to treatment, and that it may be useful to consider the effect of this treatment in terms of changing the balance or interaction between the two hemispheres." Sackeim et al. (1982) draw similar conclusions: "Studies of the therapeutic efficacy of unilateral electroconvulsive therapy generally have found that administration on the right side produces a greater decrease in depressed affect, and therefore, better therapeutic response than left-sided administration." Sackeim (1986) again states, "It is noteworthy that, of six comparative clinical trials in depression of left unilateral and right unilateral ECT, when differences were observed they were all in the direction of superior results with right unilateral ECT."

Flor-Henry (1986) concurs that "a number of studies in fact find unilateral nondominant ECT superior to bilateral ECT," and affirms, authoritatively, that "the neuropsychological, neurological, and acoustic evidence then is quite consistent and indicates that the beneficial effects of induced seizures in depression, be they bilaterally symmetrical or asymmetrical nondominant, are mediated through the repercussions of the seizure discharge in critical neural networks in the right hemisphere which are thereby normalized."

A careful examination of the relevant controlled studies, however, reveals that they provide scant support for the advantage claimed for right unilateral ECT; indeed, only two of six controlled comparisons of the antidepressant effects of right unilateral ECT compared with left unilateral ECT show an advantage of right unilateral ECT. The studies, all conducted before 1974, employed random assignment to treatments and blind outcome measures; they are summarized briefly as follows.

Halliday et al. (1968) assessed patients before and 2 to 4 days after 4 ECTs administered with a sine-wave device through temporomastoid treatment electrodes. Mean Hamilton rating scale scores fell 48.5% in the left unilateral ECT group compared with 47.5% in the right unilateral ECT group (n.s.); 81% of patients treated with left unilateral ECT were rated recovered or improved, compared with 72% of patients treated with right unilateral ECT (n.s.). In a re-analysis of their data, Galin (1974) claimed to have detected a therapeutic advantage for right unilateral ECT 3 months after completion of the treatment course. The data presented, however, were seriously contaminated by nonsystematic and unequal administration of additional ECTs and maintenance antidepressant drugs during the follow-up interval and therefore cannot provide any useful information. Moreover, one third of the patients treated with unilateral ECT had predominantly focal contralateral seizures, a technical idiosyncrasy that disqualifies the study from serious consideration, because such partial seizures have sharply attenuated therapeutic efficacy.

Sutherland et al. (1969) administered sine-wave treatments via the placement described by Lancaster et al. (1958). The mean total number of ECTs prescribed on clinical grounds by a psychiatrist who was blind to group assignment were 5.7 and 5.5 for the right unilateral ECT and left unilateral ECT groups, respectively (n.s.). No depression ratings were obtained in this study, which was aimed primarily at assessing the cognitive effects of treatment.

Fleminger et al. (1970a) assigned 12 patients to each treatment, administered with brief-pulse stimulation via the Lancaster placement, and found that self-rated Beck Depression Inventory (BDI) scores fell 70.0% 3 days after 6 left unilateral ECTs, compared with 75.5% after right unilateral ECT (n.s.).

Costello et al. (1970) gave sine-wave ECT via the Lancaster placement and reported that BDI scores shortly after 4 treatments fell 42% with left unilateral ECT compared with a fall of 32% with right unilateral ECT (n.s.).

Cronin et al. (1970) delivered a partial sine-wave stimulus via the Lancaster placement to a mixed group of endogenous and reactive depressives. Eight right unilateral ECTs were significantly more effective in lowering BDI scores than an equal number of left unilateral ECTs ($p = 0.05$). Means and standard deviations were not given, but their graph shows that the group receiving right unilateral ECT improved slightly more than twice as much as the group receiving left unilateral ECT.

Cohen et al. (1968) examined patients after 2 sine-wave ECT administered via the Lancaster placement. Zung self-rating depression scores fell 23% in the group receiving right unilateral ECT compared with 8.8% in the group receiving left unilateral ECT ($p < 0.01$). The atypically low number of ECT given in this study, however, renders its interpretation problematic.

Thus, out of six controlled trials, only one—that of Cronin et al. (1970)—provides unequivocal support for a therapeutic advantage of right unilateral ECT versus left unilateral ECT. Moreover, the studies were all conducted with techniques that are no longer considered optimal for unilateral ECT. All but one used a sine-wave stimulus; all but one used the now-abandoned Lancaster unilateral placement; and, where rating scales were used, all but one employed self-rating scales (BDI, Zung) that have been criticized for their questionable sensitivity and validity (Carroll et al., 1981; Bailey and Coppen, 1976).

The observation of a striking instance of recovery from melancholia after 6 left unilateral ECTs in a fully dextral man (Leechuy and Abrams, 1987) suggested that it was premature to attribute the beneficial effects of ECT in melancholia primarily to right hemisphere mechanisms and led us to undertake a random-assignment, double-blind, controlled comparison of the antidepressant potencies of right and left unilateral ECT in 30 melancholic male veterans, of whom 19 received right-sided and 11, left-sided, ECT (Abrams, Swartz, and Vedak, 1989).

Hamilton depression scale scores obtained blindly after the 3rd and 6th ECTs exhibited equivalent antidepressant effects across the treatment course, but with a significantly faster rate of improvement with left unilateral ECT (Figure 7-4). Two patients who were incidentally readmitted for second courses of ECT more than 6 months after the end of their initial participation in the study were again randomly assigned to treatment but were excluded from further analyses. One received his first treatment course with right unilateral and his second with left unilateral ECT, improving 97% and 96%, respectively, and the other received left unilateral ECT the first time with a 64% improvement, and right unilateral ECT the second time with a 27% improvement.

Again, differences in stimulus administration technique may account for the superior clinical results we obtained with left unilateral ECT, because we used a brief-pulse stimulus administered via a wide temporoparietal unilateral placement, whereas all but one of the earlier studies used a sine-wave stimulus, and all used a narrow temporoparietal unilateral placement. We did not compare the cognitive or memory effects of the two methods, but no striking or untoward effects of left unilateral ECT were observed.

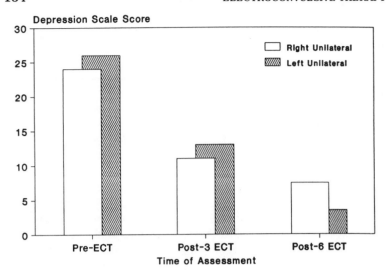

Figure 7-4 Antidepressant effects of left vs. right unilateral
ECT. (Adapted from Abrams et al., 1989.)

Cerebral Locus of Action of
Electroconvulsive Therapy

So far, I have considered primarily evidence for the ways in which
differences in ECT technique might result in differential cerebral stimulation because of the current used or the seizure it induces. Equally
important is the related question of where in the brain this stimulation
acts to relieve depression. On the basis of the investigations of his
group into the differential efficacies of titrated unilateral and bilateral
ECT given at low or high dosages, Sackeim (1994a,b) has proposed
that the efficacy of ECT is related to the spatial intracerebral distribution of charge density, with unilateral ECT producing an even distribution across the anterior two thirds of the stimulated hemisphere,
and bilateral ECT concentrating its effects in the prefrontal regions. In
this view, increasing the stimulus intensity with unilateral ECT results
in its becoming more like bilateral ECT in the spatial distribution of
its charge density, thus enhancing participation of the prefrontal
regions in seizure initiation, which is theorized to be central to the
antidepressant efficacy of ECT.

My own view is somewhat different, and proposes that increasing the stimulus intensity of unilateral ECT leads to greater intracerebral (including diencephalic) generalization of the induced seizure activity via more efficient triggering of a central pacemaker.

The notion that convulsive therapies reduced the vegetative changes in depression by providing "massage of diencephalic centers" was already clearly expressed by 1939 (King and Liston, 1990). Pollitt (1965) subsequently detailed the way in which the diencephalon directly controls a variety of biological functions that are frequently altered in depression through its hypothalamic releasing factors and pituitary and autonomic connections, pointing out that melancholia is frequently associated with disturbances in appetite, gastrointestinal functions, sleep, temperature regulation, secretory patterns, diurnal rhythms, menstrual cycle, libido, and cardiovascular function, all more or less regulated by diencephalic centers and virtually always restored toward normal by a course of ECT.

Beginning around 1971, Dr. Michal Taylor and I undertook what was to be a series of three studies attempting to understand what we had both observed to be a clear therapeutic advantage of bilateral over right unilateral ECT in the treatment of melancholia. In the first study (Abrams and Taylor, 1973), we tested the hypothesis that bilateral electrical cerebral stimulation was central to the fully developed, antidepressant effect of ECT by applying bilateral treatment electrodes forward over the anterior forehead (anterior bifrontal ECT) and away from the temporal lobes as described previously.

Our findings, presented in Figure 7-5, that this method produced an antidepressant effect intermediate between that produced by bilateral and right unilateral ECT, as observed in an earlier clinical comparison (Abrams et al., 1972), led us to to reject the hypothesis that the therapeutic advantage for bilateral over right unilateral ECT lay solely in the bilateral electrical cerebral stimulation of the former method and to consider that bilateral temporal lobe stimulation might play the critical role. We then tested this hypothesis (Abrams and Taylor, 1974) by comparing the effects of three different electrode placements for ECT that stimulated one or both temporal lobes in a systematic fashion, using the same stimulus parameters for each. We randomly assigned 30 melancholic patients to receive four treatment sessions with one of the following methods: 2 right-unilateral ECTs per session; one right- followed by one left-unilateral ECT each session, or one bilateral ECT per session, all admininstered with a fixed high-dose sine-wave stimulus of 170 V for 1 second. Our finding (Figure 7-6) of no clinical difference among the three methods in reducing

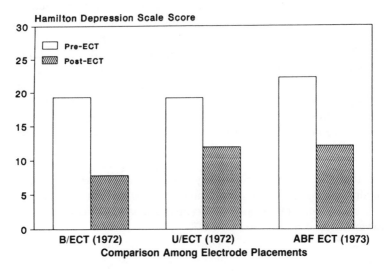

Figure 7-5 Clinical efficacy of anterior bifrontal ECT. (Adapted from Abrams and Taylor, 1973.)

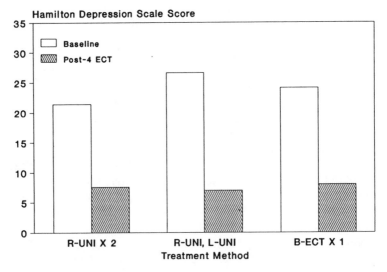

Figure 7-6 Antidepressant effects of right, then left, unilateral ECT. (Adapted from Abrams and Taylor, 1974.)

Hamilton depression scale scores led us to reject bilateral temporal-lobe stimulation as critical to the antidepressant effects of ECT and to investigate the proposition expressed by Carney and Sheffield (1973) that ECT worked through a specific effect on diencephalic structures.

In a third study (Abrams and Taylor, 1976b), we compared two treatment methods: Conventional bilateral ECT and simultaneously administered left and right unilateral ECT given through two separate sine-wave ECT devices and treatment electrode assemblies (at the time of treatment, the stimulus buttons of both devices were simultaneously activated). Each patient received a single ECT per session with an identical, fixed stimulus dose, for a total of 6 treatments. All patients satisfied research criteria for endogenous depression and were randomly assigned to treatment methods. Hamilton depression scores were obtained blindly at baseline and the afternoon of the 6th ECT, after which additional conventional bilateral ECTs were given as needed, until maximum benefit had been obtained (this decision was also made blind to treatment assignment).

Nine patients receiving bilateral ECT and 11 receiving right–left ECT had similar depression scores at baseline (20.6 versus 20.0, respectively), and the bilateral group had significantly lower mean post-ECT depression scores than the right–left unilateral group (Figure 7-7). The mean reduction in depression scores for the right–left group was only 7.3 points (n.s.); for the bilateral group it was 15 points ($p < 0.001$). Following the first 6 study ECTs, 10 of 11 patients in the right–left group went on to receive additional ECTs, compared with 3 of 9 bilaterally treated patients ($p < 0.05$).

With all stimulus parameters held constant and with both groups receiving simultaneous bitemporal stimulation, the marked therapeutic advantage for the bilateral group could only have derived from differences in the intracerebral distribution of the stimulating current or the induced seizure activity—specifically through the greater expected diencephalic stimulation with bilateral ECT.

Specific evidence that bilateral ECT stimulates the diencephalon more than unilateral ECT comes from our comparisons of the effects of bilateral, left, and right unilateral ECT on heart rate (Lane et al., 1989; Swartz et al., 1994) described previously. Although we initially interpreted our finding of a greater duration of ECT-induced tachycardia with bilateral ECT as an indication of greater catecholamine release, the recent report of a full hemodynamic response to ECT in a bilaterally adrenalectomized woman (Liston and Salk, 1990) suggests that differential neural—presumably diencephalic—activation was re-

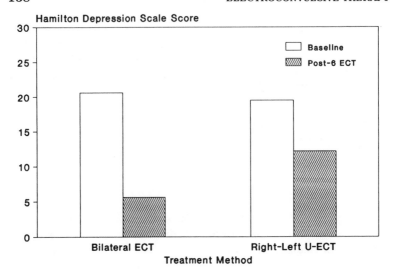

Figure 7-7 Comparison of simultaneous right-and-left unilateral ECT with bilateral ECT. (Adapted from Abrams and Taylor, 1976.)

sponsible for our finding. Our subsequent demonstration of a greater ECT-induced tachycardia with right than left unilateral ECT supports this interpretation, because only hypothalamic driving of brain-stem cardioacceleratory centers could explain such a result.

Lisanby et al. (1996) found no evidence that the ECT-induced prolactin surge was associated with the therapeutic efficacy of ECT, and therefore concluded that their data did not support the view that diencephalic seizure propagation—at least as measured by pituitary prolactin release—was central to the antidepressant potency of ECT. However, these authors were the first to report a significant inverse correlation between the ECT-induced prolactin surge and the clinical response, with treatment responders demonstrating a fall in peak prolactin levels across their treatment course. Such a fall in peak prolactin levels across a treatment course has been reported by many other investigators (this volume, p. 257), and is consistent with a sustained increase in pituitary postsynaptic dopamine receptor sensitivity, a phenomenon that might itself be central to the therapeutic effects of ECT in depression, just as it surely must be central to the therapeutic effects of ECT in Parkinson's disease.

Discussion

It is a cornerstone of scientific psychiatry that an intimate relationship exists between brain function and behavior. In many ways, modern psychiatry can be viewed as the study of the abnormal aspects of this relationship, which is also subsumed under the rubric of behavioral neurology. In this context it would certainly be unexpected if treatment methods such as bilateral and unilateral ECT, which exert such different effects on various parameters of cerebral activity, nevertheless had identical effects on the melancholic syndrome, which is surely another manifestation of brain (dys)function.

In their influential review, d'Elia and Raotma (1975) concluded that right unilateral ECT was "the treatment of choice in endogenous depression," a sentiment subsequently echoed in various ways by other reviewers and investigators (American Psychiatric Association, 1978; Squire, 1982; Strömgren, 1984). The Royal College of Psychiatrists—on the basis of the same information—has asserted exactly the opposite: ". . . it is our opinion that the balance of evidence points to bilateral electrode placement being preferable in terms of speed of action and overall effectiveness . . ." (Royal College of Psychiatrists, 1989). The present review suggests that such assertions are premature because they do not consider all of the available data. A more appropriate focus would attempt to elucidate the precise clinical differences among the methods so that a fuller understanding might be provided of their relative risks and benefits. Reports of persistent amnesia with bilateral ECT (Squire, 1986; Weiner et al., 1986a,b) make such an assessment critical. An accurate understanding of the relative therapeutic effects of the two methods is no less important than that for their amnesic effects, for when a patient who might have recovered with bilateral ECT commits suicide after receiving unilateral ECT (Gambill and McLean, 1983), any cognitive advantages of the latter method are rendered moot.

Clinical Recommendations

The pronounced cognitive advantages of brief pulse right unilateral compared with bilateral ECT—including in particular the evidence presented by Weiner et al. (1986b) that patients receiving brief-pulse right unilateral ECT improve just as much as those receiving bilateral ECT, but with no more memory loss than controls who do not receive

ECT—mandate using the former method in preference to bilateral ECT wherever possible. This is what I wrote in the previous edition and still believe to be generally true. However, as my comments at the end of Chapter 6 suggest, the dosage sensitivity of unilateral ECT, combined with the FDA limitation on maximum device output, and the high stimulus intensities generally required to make it a fully effective method, mitigate against being able to administer unilateral ECT at fully therapeutic dosages with what now appears to be an optimal configuration of stimulus parameters (i.e., pulse width no greater than 0.5 msec, frequency no greater than 70 Hz).

Nevertheless, because many patients—especially in the younger age range—can be successfully treated with high-dose, brief-pulse, unilateral ECT (e.g., a fixed dose in the 375 mC to 500 mC range, or a titrated dose of 3 to 5 times threshold), I continue to recommend such therapy for at least the first few treatments, to determine whether a suitable response will be obtained. If such a response is not forthcoming, a switch to bilateral ECT (with conventional or anterior placement) is indicated, administered at a substantial (e.g., not just-above-threshold) dose, and via the physiological stimulus parameters set forth in Chapter 6.

8

Technique of Electroconvulsive Therapy: Theory

ECT is not a trifling or inconsequential procedure to be delegated to a junior resident or casually administered, unassisted, in the office. It is unique among psychiatric treatments: a significant medical intervention requiring general anesthesia and entailing risks, however, small, of morbidity and mortality. The psychiatrist administering ECT adopts a role most like that of his medical and surgical colleagues; to perform it well requires an intimate knowledge of the physiology and biochemistry of induced seizures, an understanding of the pharmacology of anesthetic agents, familiarity with the physical properties of the electrical stimulus used, and the confidence and skill to lead a treatment team in the event of a medical emergency.

Training

No requirements yet exist for the training of psychiatrists in giving ECT (Fink, 1986b); indeed, neither the American Committee on Graduate Medical Education and its Residency Review Committees nor the American Board of Psychiatry and Neurology provide any guidelines in this regard. It is clear, however, that training in ECT has been sadly neglected by many institutions here and abroad—the surveys of Pippard and Ellam (1981) in Great Britain and Latey and Fahy (1985) in Ireland amply demonstrated how little attention has been paid to this subject in the British Isles; the Consensus Development Conference Statement (1985) from the United States likewise calls for the increased training of medical students and residents in the use of ECT.

A reasonable training program for psychiatric residents should provide didactic course-work on ECT early in the first year of training (usually the inpatient year), including at least 3 hours of lecture and discussion on history, clinical indications, treatment response, side effects, precautions and contraindications, medical physiology, cognitive effects, EEG effects, the physical properties of the electrical stimulus, and the comparative and combined effects of psychotropic drugs. To gain practical experience, the psychiatric resident should personally administer at least 30 to 40 treatments under the direct supervision of a faculty member; this will usually require a 1- or 2-month rotation on an ECT service. The resident's responsibilities should include both the performance of ECT consultations and assistance with the administration of ECT. After an initial week of observing all aspects of the treatment procedure with full discussion by his supervisor, the resident in training should be responsible for treating patients under direct supervision. He should learn to insert an intravenous line, prepare and administer the anesthetic agents, apply the treatment electrodes for unilateral and bilateral ECT, deliver the electrical stimulus, and monitor the induced seizure. He should observe patients in the recovery room awakening from their treatments and learn to manage emergence delirium. He must become thoroughly familiar with the requirements for informed consent for ECT and participate in obtaining such consent from new patients.

For residents enrolled in programs at facilities where ECT is underutilized, educational videotapes can be used to augment their training (Fink, 1986b). Such tapes are available (Frankel, 1986; Ries, 1987; Grunhaus, 1991; Alger, 1991) and should be used in conjunction with assigned readings and attendance at the training courses conducted for credit during the year at various medical centers and at the American Psychiatric Association's annual meeting.

The Electroconvulsive Therapy Unit

The ECT unit is an integral functioning part of the psychiatric inpatient service and ought to be located nearby, not set apart in a surgical suite or other remote area of the hospital.

Physical Requirements

ECT should be given in pleasant, well-lit surroundings, air-conditioned in summer and heated in winter, with ample room for staff and equipment and with waiting and recovery areas designed to maximize privacy and minimize the apprehension engendered in patients by seeing or hearing others receiving or recovering from treatment. These points may seem self-evident, but the Pippard and Ellam report (1981) revealed them, sadly, not to be so.

The treatment room should be large enough to comfortably accommodate a patient on a stretcher, all of the equipment in the following list, and from four to eight people, depending on whether any observers are present. (The ECT unit appropriately serves as a training site for nursing and medical students and should have adequate space for this important function.) This will require from 225 to 400 square feet of space with at least four grounded hospital grade outlets. A telephone is needed for calling the patients' units and in the event that emergency assistance is required. The room should have two doors: One for patient entry, the other leading to a recovery area. Recommended equipment is as follows:

ECT instrument and cart, preferably with integral EEG and ECG monitor
Six rolling stretchers, operating room type, with wheel locks and intravenous pole holders
EEG monitor (if not integral to ECT instrument)
Defibrillator and cart
ECG machine (if not integral to ECT instrument or defibrillator)
Oxygen tank with valve, flow meter, and positive pressure bag
Tracheal suction pump and cart
Refrigerator with lock
Wheeled intravenous pole and stand
Lockable cabinet for medication and supplies
Medication cart
Emergency medication tray (not lockable) containing
    atropine (20-mL vial, 0.4 mg/mL)
    diazepam (2-mL ampules, 5 mg/mL)
    diphenhydramine (30-mL vial, 50 mg/mL)
    epinephrine (1-mL ampules, 1 mg/mL)
    levarterenol (4-mL ampules, 1 mg/mL)
    lidocaine (50-mL vial, 20 mg/mL)
    methylprednisolone (125-mg vial, 62.5 mg/mL)
    esmolol (10-mL vial, 10 mg/mL)
Laryngoscope with three sizes of blades and assorted cuffed endotracheal tubes
Rubber mouthguards (autoclavable)

The recovery area should be large enough to hold at least three stretchers, separated from each other by curtains or screens, and have its own tracheal suction apparatus, portable positive pressure ventilation device (e.g., Ambu bag), and intravenous pole.

Staffing Requirements

To maximize safety and efficiency, ECT should be given by a team consisting of a psychiatrist, a registered nurse, an anesthetic specialist, and a licensed practical nurse or nursing assistant. In hospitals with residency training programs, a resident should be assigned to assist, as well as any additional nursing staff who accompany their patients to the ECT unit and remain to observe them in the recovery room until they are ready to return to their wards.

The psychiatrist directs the treatment; his overall medical responsibility for the procedure is analagous to the surgeon's role in the operating suite. He must ascertain how clinically appropriate ECT is for each patient referred, weigh the treatment risks against the potential benefits, monitor the patient's treatment response, and decide (in consultation with the primary physician) when maximum benefit has been obtained. He selects the anesthetic agents and their dosage, determines the treatment electrode placement, sets and subsequently adjusts the treatment stimulus parameters, administers the electrical stimulus, and observes the patient throughout the treatment course for the occurrence of side effects.

The ECT charge nurse has a large administrative responsibility in coordinating the unit, as well as substantial traditional nursing functions. These responsibilities include the verification that patients have been appropriately prepared for ECT and that all necessary paperwork and laboratory examinations are complete, including consent forms. Medical supplies for the unit must be ordered and maintained; records must be kept of the controlled substances used; and intravenous solutions and injectable medications must be prepared freshly each treatment day. Patient flow from the waiting area to the treatment room to the recovery room must be facilitated; vital signs must be recorded before, during, and after treatment; and nursing personnel must be supervised in the treatment and recovery rooms.

The anesthetic specialist induces the anesthesia with the assistance of the psychiatrist, maintains the airway, ventilates the patient, determines when it is safe to move the patient to the recovery area, and initiates any required resuscitative or corrective procedures (e.g., intubation, treatment of cardiac arrhythmias). To be sure, the 1990 APA ECT task force waffled carefully in its definition of who should give anesthesia during ECT so as not to offend those psychiatrists who prefer to save time or collect a larger fee by administering anesthesia themselves (American Psychiatric Association, 1990). Moreover, the treatment is so inherently safe that thousands of consecutive seizures are routinely induced without fatality, regardless of who is standing at the head of the stretcher (Pearlman, Loper, and Tillery, 1990). However, the increasing age and concurrent medical morbidity of patients who receive ECT, coupled with the progressively complex pharmacologic manipulations of hemodynamic status these patients frequently require (Regestein and Reich, 1985; Hay, 1989; Drop and Welch, 1989), should, in compliance with Gresham's law, inexorably drive psychiatrists out of the practice of administering anesthesia during ECT. I would personally rather undergo brief anesthesia administered by a qualified anesthetic specialist than by a psychiatrist and advise my patients accordingly.

It is noteworthy that in Slawson's (1985) review of ECT malpractice claims against the American Psychiatric Association's insurance program from 1972 to 1983, one of only two claims of wrongful death occurred in a patient who developed laryngospasm and apnea during ECT; the psychiatrist, who was administering the anesthesia himself, had difficulty resuscitating the patient and the case was settled out of court for $270,000, the largest settlement during the 11-year period studied.

The nursing assistant ensures that patients have voided their bladder and are properly attired, that they do not smoke before or chew gum during treatment, and that dentures, jewelry, and eyeglasses have been removed to a safe place. Other duties include wheeling patients to and from the treatment room, applying the ECG monitoring electrodes, and maintaining the unit in clean and orderly condition (by check-list) for the next treatment day.

The Pretherapy Workup

As for any procedure conducted under general anesthesia, a medical history and physical (including neurologic) examination are prerequisite. No laboratory tests are specific to ECT; the purpose of requesting routine examinations of the blood and urine (CBC,

SMA-6, SMA-12, urinalysis), a chest film, and an ECG is simply to screen for medical conditions that may complicate the procedure so that they may be remedied or controlled beforehand. Some examinations that traditionally have been obtained before ECT or suggested by some authorities are not recommended here for the following reasons.

1. *X-ray examination of the spine.* Before the introduction in the mid-1950s of succinylcholine muscle relaxation for ECT, up to 40% of the patients receiving this treatment experienced compression fractures of the dorsal spine (DeWald et al., 1954). It was *de rigueur* to obtain spinal films before treatment for medical-legal purposes. Although the need for such x-rays no longer exists, some facilities continue to require them, which adds not at all to the patient's security, but very considerably to his bill.

2. *Skull roentgenograms.* Skull films are occasionally requested to "rule out brain tumor" before one gives ECT. Such films, however, are insensitive to intracerebral lesions, regardless of cause, and together with spine films needlessly increase the cost of treatment and add to the patient's lifetime radiation exposure. Brain tumors large enough to cause psychiatric symptoms are likely to manifest themselves during a careful behavioral neurologic examination—any clinical suspicion of such a neoplasm should then be investigated with one of the newer imaging techniques (CT scan, MRI).

3. *Electroencephalograms.* Conversely, the high sensitivity and low specificity of the EEG render it a poor screening tool before ECT. One quarter to one third of melancholics exhibit EEG abnormalities (Abrams et al., 1970; Abrams and Taylor, 1979) that are usually in the form of nonspecific slowing, which is not infrequently asymmetrical. Such slowing does not predict a poor outcome with ECT (Abrams et al., 1970) and may even disappear after the acute EEG effects of ECT have passed.

4. *Pseudocholinesterase testing.* Pseudocholinesterase is the enzyme responsible for degrading succinylcholine, the muscle relaxant used in ECT. Absence of this enzyme is transmitted as a rare genetic abnormality affecting fewer than 1 in 3000 (Lehmann and Liddell, 1969) and is responsible, along with liver disease, polyphosphate insecticide poisoning, anemia, malnutrition, or the administration of anticholinesterases, for the complication of prolonged apnea after ECT (Matthew and Constan, 1964; Packman et al., 1978). Concomitant therapy with lithium, certain antibiotics, aminoglycosides,

magnesium salts, procainamide, and quinidine (Hill, Wong, and Hodges, 1976; Packman et al., 1978) may also prolong post-ECT apnea by enhancing the neuromuscular blockade induced by succinylcholine. A rapid screening test for pseudocholinesterase deficiency is available (Swift and LaDu, 1966), but when a sensitive test is used to screen for a rare disorder, virtually all positive responses are false and therefore unhelpful (Galen and Gambino, 1975).

Medical Consultation

The mean age of patients receiving ECT has increased in recent years, probably as a combined result of increased longevity, the greater risk for depressive illness in later life, and insurance coverage under Medicare. More high-risk patients are thus receiving ECT, and medical consultation in their management will often be sought. The consultation process should not be viewed simply as "clearance for ECT"; no such clearance is really possible. Rather, what the referring psychiatrist needs is the consultant's opinion on the nature and severity of the medical disorder in question, its amenability to medical management, and the degree of risk imposed by a grand mal seizure induced under controlled conditions of anesthesia, muscle relaxation, and oxygenation. For the consultant to provide a valid opinion on these matters, he must have an understanding of the medical physiology of ECT, the risks of alternate therapies (e.g., tricyclic antidepressants), and the deleterious effects of the untreated psychiatric illness itself. Because such considerations are not routinely taught in most medical residencies, psychiatrists should seek out consultants with some experience in ECT or provide the requisite information themselves through personal discussions and citations from the literature. (Some internists, not fully aware of the very brief duration of ECT anesthesia or the precise physiological effects of a medically controlled seizure, overestimate the stress of the procedure and reject some patients as inappropriate risks for whom ECT is actually a more conservative treatment than pharmacotherapy.)

Consent

Except for rare instances of judicially ordered treatment or treatment given in a genuine emergency to "preserve life or limb," patients may not receive involuntary ECT any more than they may receive involuntary surgery. The topic is treated in greater detail in Chapter 11, but the essential elements of informed consent always include:

1. A full explanation of the procedure in layman's terms
2. A presentation of the risks and potential benefits of the treatment offered, as well as those of alternative available therapies
3. A statement that the patient may withdraw his consent at any time and for any reason

An educational videotape is useful both to orient patients and their families to the procedures for ECT and to unambiguously document the information that has been presented to the patient when obtaining informed consent (Barbour and Blumenkrantz, 1978). Such videotape aids are available commercially (Baxter and Liston, 1986; Ries, 1987).

Seizure Monitoring

Before the introduction of succinylcholine muscle relaxation for ECT, there was seldom any doubt as to whether or not a patient had a seizure. With succinylcholine-induced attenuation of the motor convulsion, however, it may be difficult or impossible to verify the occurrence and duration of the induced seizure through observation of muscle activity alone. The importance of such verification derives from studies suggesting that it is the induced cerebral seizure, more than any other aspect of the treatment, that is responsible for the fully developed therapeutic effect of ECT (Ottosson, 1960), and from the risks of undetected, prolonged seizures (Scott and Riddle, 1989). Although direct electrical stimulation of the brain may itself play a therapeutic role during ECT (Abrams and Taylor, 1976b; Robin and deTissera, 1982; Robin et al., 1985; Sackeim et al., 1987a), no one doubts that the cerebral seizure is central to the therapeutic process.

An arbitrary minimum of 25 seconds for motor seizure duration (and 30 seconds for EEG seizure duration) has somewhat mysteriously materialized during the last decade; fortunately, this recommendation has received post hoc support in the observation that seizures of shorter duration do not release thyrotropin (Dykes et al., 1987; Scott et al., 1989b) and therefore presumably lack the expected physiologic impact. Seizure monitoring is particularly important during unilateral ECT. In a study employing EEG monitoring, Pettinati and Nilsen (1985) reported significantly more missed seizures with unilateral than with bilateral ECT (63% compared with 29%). Because such missed seizures are not always detected clinically, the authors suggest that without EEG monitoring, patients receiving unilateral ECT may inadvertently receive an inadequate treatment course.

Several manifestations of the seizure may be monitored during ECT: The motor convulsion, the electromyogram (EMG), the EEG, and the induced tachycardia. The motor convulsion can simply be observed and timed but is occasionally obscured by the effect of the succinylcholine. To circumvent this phenomenon, Addersley and Hamilton (1953) applied a blood pressure cuff to one limb and inflated it to 10 mm Hg above systolic pressure before administration of succinylcholine in order to occlude this drug from the muscles distal to the cuff and allow direct observation of unmodified muscle activity. Motor seizure duration estimates thus obtained are reliable and correlate highly with those obtained by EEG (Fink and Johnson, 1982; Larson, Swartz, and Abrams, 1984). The EMG can be monitored during ECT despite the presence of neuromuscular blockade (Abrams, Volavka, and Fink, 1973; Ives et al., 1976; Sørensen et al., 1981; Couture et al., 1988a,b), although the duration of the EMG response varies among muscle groups (Sørenson et al., 1981) in a pattern reflecting the rostral to caudal spread and subsequent abatement of succinylcholine-induced muscle depolarization. Moreover, there is not necessarily a close correspondence between EMG estimates of motor seizure duration in a partially depolarized muscle and an unaffected one: In one study, an estimate of motor seizure duration obtained from a forehead EMG was 37% greater than a visual estimate in the cuffed arm (Couture et al., 1988b). A microprocessor-controlled technique has recently been invented for incorporation into an ECT device to automatically measure and display the duration and end point of the EMG manifestations of the ECT-induced seizure (Swartz and Abrams, 1991a). Swartz et al. (1994a) demonstrated the validity of this method in 114 randomly selected recordings from treatments of 52 patients at two different university-affiliated hospitals, reporting an interrater reliability coefficient (intraclass r) of 0.86 between the computer-determined EMG seizure duration and the independently rated cuffed-arm motor seizure duration. Not included in that article were the interrater correlations between the EMG end-point ratings of the two clinicians and the computer, which were 0.83 and 0.97.

Krystal et al. (1995) confirmed the high reliability of Abrams and Swartz's (1989) computer algorithm for automatically determining

EMG seizure duration, with two clinician-raters achieving 0.89 and 0.90 agreement (by intraclass r), respectively, with the computer-determined durations.

Because the EEG directly measures the brain's electrical activity, it remains the standard against which other techniques must be measured. Two methods are presently incorporated in ECT instruments for amplifying and presenting unprocessed EEG activity during ECT. One uses a chart-drive and penwriter to record the EEG signal on paper; the resulting record is then read by the clinician as it is generated to determine the occurrence, duration, and end-point of the induced seizure. The second method provides an auditory representation of the EEG signal in the form of a tone that fluctuates with the frequency of the seizure activity and becomes constant when the seizure ends. This method is as reliable as the first and correlates highly with it (Swartz and Abrams, 1986); it has been used sucessfully to detect prolonged seizures requiring termination with benzodiazepines (Chen et al., 1990).

Great—and sometimes unacceptable—variability has been reported by some investigators in assessing seizure length during ECT using the unprocessed single-channel EEG (Fink and Johnson, 1982; Brumback, 1983; Greenberg, 1985; Rich and Black, 1985; Zorumski et al., 1986; Ries, 1985; Guze et al., 1989). Others, however, report excellent interrater reliability (Larson et al., 1984; Pettinati and Nilsen, 1985; Swartz and Abrams, 1986; Warmflash et al., 1987; Couture et al., 1988b; Kramer et al., 1989; Gilmore et al., 1991). The experience of the investigators and the uniformity of their recording techniques doubtless contribute more to this variability than do any deficiencies of a particular ECT device.

Electroencephalographic seizure duration derived from graphic displays of mean integrated EEG amplitude (averaged EEG), or power spectral analysis generated by commercially available microprocessor-based EEG analyzers, correlate highly with visual estimates of the unprocessed EEG (Couture et al., 1988a,b; Gilmore et al., 1991). A microprocessor-controlled seizure-monitoring technique for incorporation in an ECT device has recently been invented that automatically detects and prints on the EEG strip the occurrence, duration, and end point of the EEG manifestations of the ECT-induced seizure (Abrams and Swartz, 1989). In the study by Swartz et al. (1994a) cited above, computer-determined EEG seizure endpoint ratings were also obtained and compared with the visual ratings made by the two clinicians from the paper records. The two clinicians achieved a high degree of interrater reliability (intraclass $r = 0.98$) in their visual ratings of the EEG seizure end point, and their equally high correlations with the computer-determined EEG end point (intraclass $r = 0.98$ and 0.99) amply demonstrated the validity of this method.

Krystal et al. (1995) likewise reported a high degree of agreement for EEG seizure duration between the two clinician-raters and Abrams and Swartz's (1989) computer algorithm: intraclass r values of 0.83 and 0.86, respectively. It was further notable that inability of the computer to determine the seizure end point occurred only once despite the fact that the majority of the seizures were rated as having a gradual end point.

Krystal et al. (1995) reported that the presence of artifact, poor postictal suppression, and a gradual seizure end point all reduced the agreement between clinician and computer, although it is impossible to determine from their study whether the computer or the clinician exhibited greater accuracy in judging the end point. In the absence of these confounding variables, however, agreement between clinician and computer was nearly perfect: 0.99 for both raters versus the computer. Moreover, regardless of other considerations, agreement between clinician and computer was also nearly perfect (98%) in the important determination of whether a seizure lasted longer than 24 seconds.

Heart rate may also be used to estimate ECT-induced cerebral seizure duration because the point of maximal decrease in the rate of the ECT-induced tachycardia—which occurs about 10 seconds before the EEG seizure ends—is highly correlated with both EEG and motor measures of the induced seizure (Larson, Swartz, and Abrams, 1984; Swartz and Larson, 1986). Moreover, the heart rate is a sensitive enough reflection of intracerebral seizure generalization to differentiate right unilateral from both bilateral ECT (Lane et al., 1989) and left unilateral ECT (Swartz et al., 1994b). Electroencephalographic seizure duration can be predicted from the durations of the ECT-induced tachycardia and the motor seizure according to a formula derived by linear regression analysis (Larson, Swartz, and Abrams, 1984):

$$\text{EEG duration} = 0.62 \text{ tachycardia duration}$$
$$+ \ 0.60 \text{ motor seizure duration}$$
$$+ \ 3.3 \text{ seconds}$$

indicating that the durations of the ECT-induced tachycardia and motor seizure are equally predictive of EEG seizure duration. This formula provides an objective estimate of cerebral seizure duration that may be useful in the 10% of seizures that are characterized by an indeterminate visual or auditory EEG end point.

The particular characteristics of seizures monitored with motor, visual, and auditory techniques are as follows: The motor seizure is observed in the limb distal to the blood-pressure cuff and consists of an initial sudden contraction of the muscles during the passage of the electrical stimulus and an equally abrupt relaxation as the stimulus terminates. The tonic phase is then ushered in by a gradually increasing, sustained, tetanic contraction of the muscles (arms flexed, legs extended), lasting from 10 to 15 seconds and characterized by rigidity and a fine tremor. This is gradually replaced by the increasingly rhythmical jerking movements of the clonic phase, starting at a frequency of 10 to 12 per second and gradually slowing over the next 20 to 45 seconds to 3 to 4 per second at seizure termination, which always occurs abruptly in the muscles. It is always advisable to monitor the motor seizure as well as the EEG because termination of clonus occasionally provides the only estimate of seizure duration—that is, when the EEG end point is indeterminate or if EEG paper runs out during the seizure (Weiner et al., 1980a).

Electroencephalographic monitoring consistently reveals a progression through a series of characteristic patterns: Build-up, hypersynchronous polyspikes during tonus, and polyspike-and-slow-wave complexes during clonus that terminate in suppression. The approaching end of the seizure is indicated by progressive slowing of the spike-and-wave bursts of clonus. A classical seizure end point occurs when these are abruptly replaced by electrical silence. A distinct end point is also signaled by sudden replacement of paroxysmal clonic activity with lower amplitude, mixed frequencies. The auditory EEG signal fluctuates intensely and rapidly during tonus and becomes increasingly irregular during clonus, with staccato tones that accompany each muscular contraction; seizure termination is typically marked by a distinct change to a nearly steady tone.

Abrams, Volavka, and Fink (1973) were the first to report that ECT-induced paroxysmal EEG activity typically persisted after cessation of clonus, an observation subsequently confirmed by numerous investigators (Weiner, 1980b; Fink and Johnson, 1982; Miller et al., 1985; Warmflash et al., 1987; Liston et al., 1988; Couture et al., 1988b; Gilmore et al., 1991). Liston et al. (1988) measured the duration of EEG and motor seizure activity in 24 patients receiving right unilateral ECT. In each patient, EEG seizure duration continued after cessation of motor activity in a cuffed limb by a mean of 12.4 seconds, a figure close to that of 13 seconds reported earlier by Warmflash et al. (1987), but substantially shorter than those of 25 seconds reported by Couture et al. (1988b) and 22.5 seconds reported by Gilmore et al. (1991). On average, motor seizures were only 76% as long as EEG seizures, a figure that is about 65% for all published studies comparing both monitoring methods. Because cerebral seizure activity sometimes continues for many minutes after the motor component ends (Greenberg, 1985; Scott and Riddle, 1989; Chen et al., 1990) and may require termination by intravenous diazepam to prevent neuronal damage, routine EEG monitoring of the induced seizure is mandatory in addition to observing the motor seizure duration.

The discrepancy between EEG and motor estimates of seizure duration is not always large, however, and the two measures are often coterminous. Because the motor convulsion reflects spike discharges primarily in the motor strip, while the EEG seizure reflects more widespread cortical spike activity, the degree of correspondence between the two measures may be viewed as an index of intracerebral seizure generalization (Swartz and Larson, 1986; Abrams and Swartz, 1989): The smaller the discrepancy, the greater the generalization. Adding the duration of ECT-induced tachycardia to this equation should provide an important dimension of brain-stem seizure activity (Lane et al., 1989; Swartz et al., 1994b) and forms the basis for a new computer-automated method of assessing the degree of intracerebral seizure generalization based on an algorithm incorporating EEG, EMG, and ECG estimates of seizure duration (Swartz and Abrams, 1993; Abrams and Swartz, 1996).

Because the standard bifrontal EEG cannot distinguish generalized seizures from the partial or focal seizures that occasionally occur with unilateral ECT (Welch, 1982), it is advisable to record from contralateral fronto-mastoid leads when administering this form of treatment. However, Brumback's (1987) assertion that single-channel bifrontal EEG recordings during ECT are incapable of differentiating muscle artifact from cortical potentials is wrong because it ignores the close correlations observed between such EEG recordings and the duration of the ECT-induced tachycardia and the fact that bifrontal EEG activity typically continues for many seconds after all muscle activity ceases.

The British, with their commonsense practicality and reluctance to invest time, money, and energy in newfangled ideas from the colonies, have vacillated for some time over the value of EEG monitoring during ECT. A spate of articles in the *British Journal of Psychiatry* has not resolved the issue. In a paper entitled "Is electroencephalo-graphic monitoring of electroconvulsive therapy clinically useful?", McCreadie et al. (1989) found only modest disagreement (2.5% for bilateral, and 8% for unilateral ECTs) between clinical and EEG assessments of whether a seizure had occurred; when the requirement was to state whether a seizure greater than 25 seconds had occurred, the disagreement rose to 7% and 28%, respectively. The authors concluded that EEG monitoring might be worthwhile for unilateral ECT but that the case for this would be strengthened by the demonstration that seizure length was therapeutically crucial. Later that year, Scott et al. (1989a) asked "Would monitoring by electroencephalogram improve the practice of electroconvulsive therapy?" and found that EEG monitoring revealed short seizures in almost one third of 100 ECTs monitored, although this was usually detected by the treating doctor. Nevertheless, the authors suggested that EEG monitoring might be worthwhile in patients observed to have short seizures. Later yet that year, however, Scott and Riddle (1989) reported a patient whose ECT-induced status epilepticus was observed on EEG monitoring for more than 10 minutes after all visible muscle activity had ceased. Despite the authors' acknowledgment that status epilepticus is best terminated without delay and that its diagnosis and treatment would have been delayed without EEG monitoring, they unaccountably omit the corollary recommendation for routine EEG monitoring of ECT. Similarly, The Royal College of Psychiatrists (1989), after candidly admitting that "there are certain patients where it is very difficult to tell whether the fit has occurred and the facility for ECT monitoring may be worthwhile," nevertheless obtusely conclude that ". . . the routine monitoring of EEG during ECT cannot at this stage be recommended"—a recommendation that sadly remains unchanged in the 1995 report of this august body (Royal College of Psychiatrists, 1995).

Electrocardiographic Monitoring

Although ECT is one of the safest procedures that is carried out under general anesthesia, whatever risk the treatment does entail falls primarily on the cardiovascular system and specifically on the heart (see Chapter 5). This risk primarily takes the form of cardiac arrhythmias engendered by the abrupt and massive autonomic stimulation resulting from both the electrical current and the induced seizure. Although such arrhythmias rarely require treatment, an awareness of their presence increases the likelihood of an efficient medical response should corrective measures be required. For this reason, and because of the increased numbers of high-risk patients receiving ECT, ECG monitoring of the procedure is now standard. Most modern ECT devices provide ECG monitoring capability, although any oscilloscope monitor or electrocardiograph is suitable for this purpose—all that is generally required is a determination of the rhythm and a display of the QRS complex. Should evidence of myocardial damage appear, however, it would also be useful to have full limb and chest lead capability.

Benign neglect is a successful strategy for handling the majority of transient ECT-induced cardiac arrhythmias. ECT was given for tens of thousands of consecutive treatments without cardiac arrest long before ECG monitoring or beta-adrenergic blockade was ever dreamed of (Kolb and Vogel, 1942; Impastato and Almansi, 1942; Barker and Baker, 1959) and is remarkably benign even in the presence of cardiac disease (Pitts, 1982). It would be ironic if the routine introduction of sophisticated monitoring techniques and cardioactive agents into the procedure ultimately served to increase, rather than reduce, its risk.

Protection of Teeth and Tongue

The direct electrical stimulation of the temporalis muscles during ECT causes the teeth to clamp shut powerfully, stressing them and risking a severe tongue bite. For this reason, a rubber mouthguard is always inserted between the teeth just before delivery of the electrical stimulus, cushioning the force of contraction and preventing the tongue from protruding between the teeth. The mouthguard should be designed to direct much of the force of the bite to the molars and away from the more fragile incisors (Durrant, 1966). It should have a rim in the front to separate the teeth from the lips as well as a channel to permit the flow of oxygen and the insertion of a suction catheter tip if needed. The rubber portion that fits between the teeth should be thick enough to substantially open the jaws, thus more efficiently diverting the biting strain rearward. Under no circumstances should a Guedel-type plastic airway be in place when the stimulus is administered to a patient with teeth because this exposes the incisors to the full force of the bite on an unyielding surface, possibly fracturing them (Pollard and O'Leary, 1981; Faber, 1983), or dislocating the jaw (M. Fink, personal communication). Of course, edentulous patients require no mouthguard.

Treatment Electrode Placement

The skin, with its oily secretions, presents the main impediment, other than the skull, to the flow of current during ECT (Weaver et al., 1976), and special care should be taken to cleanse it thoroughly with an organic solvent before applying the electrode jelly. Alcohol is generally sufficient for this purpose, but some patients with particulary oily or sebaceous skin may require ethyl acetate (available as nail-polish remover) to bring their skin impedance down to an acceptable level.

For bilateral ECT, bifrontotemporal placement is standard. One flat metal disc electrode is positioned on each side of the head approximately 1 inch above the midpoint of an imaginary line connecting the external auditory meatus and the outer canthus of the eye. This part of the temporal area is usually flat but may be concave in older patients due to temporalis muscle wasting, leading to skin burns where the stimulus concentrates in the small contact area around the electrode edge. In such patients, self-adherent, flexible, disposable stimulus electrodes conform to the surface of the skin and transmit the stimulus more efficiently.

Following a suggestion of Inglis (1970), Abrams and Taylor (1973) introduced a modification of the standard bilateral placement by spacing the electrodes 2 inches apart over the anterior forehead, as described in Chapter 7. In an open clinical trial, we treated 17 depressed patients with 8 high-dose, sine-wave anterior bifrontal ECTs administered daily and found clinical improvement to be intermediate between that previously obtained with 4 bilateral and right unilateral ECTs using the same modification of the Hamilton depression scale (Abrams et al., 1972), and a slight improvement in Wechsler Memory Scale scores during the treatment course, which was virtually identical to that reported earlier for 20 right unilateral ECT treatments, also administered daily (Abrams, 1967). Because there seemed little advantage of this method compared with right unilateral ECT and because the close interelectrode distance used often caused skin burns over the forehead due to shunting of the stimulating current through the skin, we abandoned it.

The method did not die, however, for 20 years later Letemendia et al. (1993)—with Inglis as co-author—revived it in a prospective, random-assignment, double-blind controlled comparison with both right unilateral ECT and bitemporal (conventional bilateral) ECT in 59 patients with major depression. Both bilateral placements were therapeutically superior to unilateral ECT, and—unexpectedly—bifrontal was more effective than bilateral ECT. Because an earlier paper from this group (Lawson et al., 1990) in a subsample of 40 major depressives had found that anterior bifrontal ECT caused the least cognitive disturbance, these authors concluded that this was the method of choice for ECT. Their recommendation must be taken with a grain of salt, however, as their treatment method was inherently biased against unilateral ECT in that just-above-threshold dosing was employed (mean stimulus charge = 107 mC), a method demonstrated to be therapeutically ineffective with unilateral ECT (Sackeim et al., 1987a, 1993). Indeed, their unilateral group showed only a 45% improvement in depression scores after 6 ECTs, the second lowest outcome reported in the literature for this form of ECT. Subsequently, Manly and Swartz (1994) and Swartz (1994a) administered high-dose asymmetrical anterior bifrontal ECT in two uncontrolled open clinical trials in small samples, reporting that all patients recovered completely without any memory disturbance and remained well, observations that await confirmation under random-assignment, controlled, double-blind conditions.

Unilateral ECT has always been preferentially administered to the hemisphere presumed to be nondominant for language, based on the recommendations of Goldman (1949) and Lancaster, Steinert, and Frost (1958), who believed that the reduced cognitive side effects of this treatment method derived from avoiding the direct electrical stimulation of the speech and verbal memory centers of the dominant temporal lobe. Although it is apparent that these reduced cognitive effects (especially on short-term retentive memory) derive mainly from the fact that only one temporal lobe (rather than both) is stimulated, regardless of which side, right unilateral placements remain standard. However, because our recent study (Abrams, Swartz, and Vedak, 1989) demonstrates that left unilateral ECT works equally as well in depression as does right unilateral ECT, left unilateral ECT is an option that should be exercised in patients who have right-sided strokes or skull defects, or musicians, artists, and others who might desire to minimize even transitory dysfunction of their right hemisphere.

A variety of electrode positions have been used for unilateral ECT, but a consensus has developed in recent years that the most efficient one is that recommended by d'Elia and Raotma (1975). In this method, the lower electrode is placed exactly as for bilateral ECT, and the upper electrode is placed on the same side of the head adjacent to the vertex of the skull. A frontoparietal placement (Muller, 1971) has been used by clinicians because of the ease with which both electrodes can be applied with a single head-band (the d'Elia placement requires a separate, hand-held electrode for the upper position). This method raises the seizure threshold, however, because the thick frontal bones substantially impede the passage of the stimulating current, leading to more missed seizures (d'Elia and Widepalm, 1974; Erman, Welch, and Mandel, 1979; Alexopolous et al., 1984b).

Widepalm (1987) conducted an intraindividual, double-blind crossover comparison of the retrograde memory effect ''forgetting'' of fronto-frontal (modified Muller) and conventional temporoparietal placements for right unilateral ECT in connection with the second and third treatments of a course. He found no advantage for the former method.

Impedance Testing

Modern ECT instruments use minute currents, undetectable to the patient, to test the static (skin) impedance before treatment. This procedure provides information about the quality of the electrode-to-skin interface that is especially critical when administering unilateral ECT, because this method is much more likely than bilateral ECT to be vitiated by reduced stimulus levels (Sackeim et al., 1987a). The static impedance cannot be used to estimate the dynamic impedance to the treatment current, nor is it possible to provide a specific figure for the static impedance that is in the desirable range because different ECT devices use different test stimuli and are therefore not directly comparable. If the static impedance tests above the range recommended by the manufacturer, however, it should be reduced by (1) increasing the pressure on the treatment electrodes; (2) applying more electrode gel; (3) repositioning the treatment electrodes away from any hair; or (4) gently abrading the skin under the electrodes with Skin Prep tape (3M, St. Paul, MN) to remove the top layer of dead cells and sebum. The specific risk incurred in treating a patient with a high static impedance is that of skin burns; if the impedance cannot be brought into the desired range by the preceding methods, then the decision must be made whether the risk (which is actually rather modest) outweighs the potential benefits of treatment; it usually does not.

If the impedance is too low (e.g., <100 ohms) this means that a wet scalp or an electrode gel ''bridge'' has short-circuited the stimulus, usually between two unilateral ECT electrodes that have been placed too closely together. Treatment should not be given until this condition is remedied because no current will enter the brain under these circumstances.

Stimulus Selection

A detailed description of the nature of the electrical stimulus is provided in Chapter 6. Suffice it to say that the brief-pulse, square-wave stimulus is the only appropriate one for modern ECT because the older sine-wave stimulus is excessively neurotoxic, providing substantial subthreshold energy that contributes significantly to confusion and memory loss, but not to the therapeutic effect. All brief-pulse ECT devices presently manufactured in the United States deliver stimuli that have essentially identical pulse configurations and energy levels and that differ mainly in the availability of skin impedance testing, EEG monitoring capability, reliability, and ease of use (Nilsen et al., 1986; Nilsen-Stevens et al., 1990).

The seizure threshold is multidetermined. It increases with age (Kalinowsky, 1947; Shankel et al., 1960; Weiner, 1980a; Sackeim et al., 1987b,c) and with the number of ECT treatments administered in a given course (Kalinowksy and Kennnedy, 1943; Essig, 1969; Sackeim et al., 1987b,c). The threshold is higher in men than women and for bilateral than for unilateral ECT (Weaver et al., 1978; Weiner, 1980; Sackeim et al., 1987b); it is increased by long-acting benzodiazepines administered for night-time sedation (Strömgren et al., 1980); and it is decreased by pentylenetetrazol, caffeine, and theophylline (Abrams and Taylor, 1973; Shapira et al., 1985, 1987; Hinkle et al., 1987; Swartz and Lewis, 1991). For many years it was standard advice to administer ECT at a level just above the seizure threshold in order to avoid the cognitive dysfunction induced by excessive electrical stimulation (Ottosson, 1960). As described in Chapters 6 and 7, however, although just-above-threshold stimulation is effective for bilateral ECT, it fails to produce a significant therapeutic effect for unilateral ECT.

Seizure duration is highly correlated with seizure threshold and decreases with age and the number of treatments in the course (Holmberg, 1954b; Abrams et al., 1973; Sackeim et al., 1987b,c). Hyperventilation with oxygen prolongs seizure duration during ECT by about 20% to 30% compared with either no active ventilation or ventilation with 30% oxygen, without adversely affecting the cardiovascular response (Holmberg, 1953a; Bergsholm, 1984; Räsänen et al., 1988; Chater and Simpson, 1988).

According to a survey by Farah and McCall (1993), 39% of practitioners selected the initial ECT dose via stimulus titration (Sackeim et al., 1987b), 12% used a fixed dose, and 49% used a formula, mostly based on the patient's age (Abrams and Swartz, 1985c).

Stimulus Titration

Stimulus titration is one of the methods recommended in the American Psychiatric Association Task Force Report (1990) and is the most precise for a particular combination of stimulus parameters (e.g., pulse width, frequency, and stimulus train duration), allowing the operator to specify dosage in relation to the threshold if he prefers. As already noted, however, the threshold thus obtained is itself highly dependent on the methods used to assess it, with a potential variability substantially exceeding 200%. Sackeim (1994a) has suggested that this great threshold variability presents no clinical problem to the practitioner, who is advised to give his patient a 175-mC dose if a particular device or set of parameters yields a threshold of 70 mC, but a 250-mC dose in the same patient if a different device or set of parameters yields a threshold of 100 mC. In my view, however, a 250-mC dose is likely to be more effective in a particular patient receiving unilateral ECT than a 175-mC dose, regardless of the seizure threshold.

Different stimulus titration methods have been used for the two most widely used U.S. ECT devices. Coffey et al. (1995a) developed a titration schedule for the MECTA-SR1 machine (Table 8-1).

Because seizure thresholds can vary with sex and treatment electrode placement, titration is initiated at the first level for women receiving unilateral ECT; at the second level for women receiving bilat-

Table 8-1 Titration schedule for the MECTA-SR1 machine

Level	Pulse width (ms)	Frequency (Hz)	Duration (sec)	Current (A)	Charge (mC)
1	1	40	0.5	0.8	32
2	1	40	0.75	0.8	48
3	1	40	1.25	0.8	80
4	1	40	2.0	0.8	128
5	1	60	2.0	0.8	192
6	1	90	2.0	0.8	288
7	1.4	90	2.0	0.8	403
8	2.0	90	2.0	0.8	576

eral ECT or men receiving unilateral ECT; and at the third level for men receiving bilateral ECT. After the seizure threshold is established according to this schedule, the authors initiate the next treatment with a 1-level increment for bilateral ECT and a 2-level increment for unilateral ECT.

Using an empirical approach to stimulus titration with the Thymatron DGx instrument, McCall et al. (1993a), and Rasmussen, Zorumski, and Jarvis (1994) began with 25 mC in all patients—regardless of sex or treatment electrode placement—and restimulated with 25 mC increments until a seizure was obtained. Using this method, both groups of investigators obtained seizures in virtually all patients by the third stimulus (75 mC). The threshold thus obtained, the treating clinician then administers any multiple of it he wishes for the remainder of the treatment course, up to the device maximum of 504 mC.

Age-Based Dosing

Although the seizure threshold is multi-determined, a significant positive correlation with the patient's age has been one of the most consistent research findings in the field of ECT—in fact, age has been found to be a determinant of seizure threshold in every study to date. Although most studies have demonstrated moderate correlations between seizure threshold and age, fluctuating in the range 0.33 to 0.43 (Sackeim et al., 1987a, 1993; Weiner et al., 1980a; McCall et al., 1993a; Krueger et al., 1993; Beale et al., 1994; Coffey et al., 1995b; Shapira et al., 1996; Colenda and McCall, 1996), several investigators have reported substantially larger correlations, ranging from 0.52 (Watterson, 1945; Enns and Karvelas, 1995) to 0.77 (Shankel et al., 1960; Weaver et al., 1982). Coffey et al. (1995b) found that the rise in seizure threshold across a course of ECT was correlated with increasing age, but not with sex, treatment electrode placement, or initial seizure threshold. And in their statistical model predicting the seizure threshold for unilateral ECT in 106 patients, Colenda and McCall (1996) found that age contributed the most variance to the equation.

Age-based dosing (Abrams and Swartz, 1985c) uses a formula that provides a stimulus dose averaging approximately 2.5 times threshold (Weiner, 1980; Sackeim et al., 1987b; Beale et al., 1994; Enns and Karvelas, 1995): Stimulus dose (mC) = 5 × age. Thus, the initial dose for a 50-year-old patient would be 250 mC, which is approximated with one ECT device by setting the stimulus dial of the instrument to the patient's age in years.

The accuracy of this formula in producing a dose averaging approximately 2.5 times threshold was borne out in two studies comparing Abrams and Swartz's (1985c) age-based dosing method to the seizure threshold obtained via stimulus titration. Beale et al. (1994) determined by titration that the mean seizure threshold for their sample of patients receiving bilateral ECT was 134.4 mC. In the same patients, these authors calculated that the mean age-based dose would have been 337.4 mC, which is 2.5 times the threshold dose they obtained by titration. In a similarly designed study, Enns and Karvelas (1995) titrated the average seizure threshold in a sample of patients receiving bilateral or unilateral ECT to be 110.5 mC. In comparison, they calculated the mean age-based dose for the sample to be 299.8 mC, which was 2.7 times the seizure threshold value they obtained via titration.

Fixed, High-Dose Method

As described by Abrams, Swartz, and Vedak (1991), Pettinati et al. (1994), Lamy et al. (1994), and McCall et al. (1995), the fixed, high-dose method for unilateral ECT administers a dose in the 375 to 500 mC range to all patients, thus ensuring a rapid and maximal treatment response without the need for administering multiple subconvulsive stimuli.

(Of course, none of the dosing strategies described above includes consideration of the more recent attempts to optimize the treatment stimulus by employing stimulus parameters that more closely correspond to the known physiology of neuronal discharge and repolarization. For a discussion of how these factors impinge on stimulus dosing, see p. 124, this volume.)

Oxygenation

Before the introduction of succinylcholine-induced muscle relaxation for ECT, it apparently never occurred to those administering the treatment that their patients might benefit from oxygenation during the procedure, despite the fact that hemoglobin oxygen saturations routinely fell to levels of around 40 gm% (in the old terminology) and patients became profoundly cyanotic and frequently lost sphincter control before the seizure terminated. Whether this cerebral hypoxemia contributed to the occasional occurrence of late (tardive) seizures as a complication of ECT is not known; however, no more than one or two such tardive seizures have been reported since oxygenation was intro-. duced along with barbiturate anesthesia and succinylcholine for modified ECT in the 1950s. This is ironic because, in fact, succinylcholine-induced muscle paralysis attenuates much of the need for oxygenation during the seizure because muscular activity is responsible for most of the oxygen consumed during a grand mal seizure (Posner et al., 1969). Nevertheless, it is standard recommended procedure to initiate oxygenation by forced ventilation as soon as the patient is unresponsive from the barbiturate and to continue it uninterrupted throughout the treatment procedure until the return of spontaneous respirations. In patients with chronic obstructive pulmonary disease, 100% oxygen should be replaced by room air or an oxygen–carbon dioxide mixture in order not to abolish the hypoxic drive to respiration, and a pulse oximeter should be used.

Administration of Anesthetic Agents

Premedication with a parenteral anticholinergic agent prevents the slowing of the heart that results from the powerful vagal outflow that occurs during and immediately after administration of the treatment stimulus. Atropine, 0.4 to 1.2 mg intramuscularly, is recommended for this purpose, although glycopyrrolate, 0.2 to 0.4 mg intravenously, can be substituted.

The anesthetic and muscle-relaxant are administered intravenously immediately before seizure induction. The ultrashort-acting barbiturate methohexital is the anesthetic agent of choice for ECT. Although the findings of Pitts et al. (1965) showed that it induces substantially fewer cardiac arrhythmias than the older thiopental has been disputed (Selvin, 1987; Pearlman and Richmond, 1990), methohexital nonetheless has the advantages of a shorter sleep time and less postanesthesia confusion (Egbert and Wolfe, 1960; Osborne et al., 1963; Woodruff et al., 1968). The recommended initial dose of methohexital is 0.75 mg/kg of body weight (Pitts, 1982), given intravenously by rapid bolus push. The dosages for subsequent treatments should be adjusted according to the patient's response to the first injection.

Propofol is an alternative anesthetic agent to methohexital that is widely used in Europe because it is associated with a smaller hemodynamic response during ECT (Dwyer et al., 1988; Rouse, 1988; Rampton et al., 1989; Villalonga et al., 1993; Avramov, Husain, and

White, 1995). In the previous edition of this book (Abrams, 1992), I recommended against using propofol for ECT because of its systematic seizure-shortening effects (Halsall et al., 1988; Dwyer et al., 1988; Rouse, 1988; Rampton et al., 1989; Boey and Lai, 1990), a conclusion also reached by others (Swartz, 1992; Royal College of Psychiatrists, 1995). Since then, however, studies have appeared showing that the reduced seizure durations obtained with propofol are not associated with a reduced therapeutic effect in comparison with methohexital anesthesia (Mitchell et al., 1991; Malsch et al., 1994; Fear et al., 1994; Martensson et al., 1994), and this agent should be considered for ECT anesthesia in patients who have problematic preexisting hypertension or tachycardia, or who exhibit an excessive hemodynamic response during ECT. Indeed, Farah, McCall, and Amundson (1996) describe the successful use of propofol anesthesia alone to control the blood pressure surge in a patient who received ECT 4 months after undergoing repair of a posterior cerebral artery cerebral aneurysm.

Succinylcholine is the muscle-relaxant of choice for ECT and is given at a dosage of 0.6 mg/kg of body weight (Pitts, 1982), also by rapid intravenous bolus push.

The Seizure

Although the evidence for a direct therapeutic role of the electrical stimulus has been discussed above (Robin and deTissera, 1982; Abrams, 1986b; Sackeim et al., 1987a), the seizure is generally acknowledged to be the primary therapeutic agent of ECT. For this reason it is necessary to ensure that a fully developed bilateral grand mal seizure is obtained during each treatment session by employing the seizure monitoring techniques described earlier. No objective criteria have yet been established for specifying the minimum requisite seizure duration, but the consensus described above is that if a motor seizure of at least 25 seconds is not induced, the patient should be restimulated at a higher electrical dosage. Shorter seizures or those with indeterminate electrical activity are considered abortive or incompletely generalized and of reduced therapeutic benefit. The claim (Maletzky, 1978) that a specific minimum total seizure time is required for an effective treatment course is not supported by any objective data. Because most depressives require 6 to 8 treatments and the average seizure lasts about 50 seconds (Abrams et al., 1973), most patients who recover will have experienced a total of 300 to 400 seconds of seizure activity. This commonplace observation is, of course, post hoc and cannot be elevated to a general statement of principle. This point was overlooked by Calev et al. (1989) in their assertion that ECT-induced clinical improvement in depression significantly correlated with total seizure length produced by all ECTs given—the correlation is meaningless without first excluding the variance attributed to the total number of those ECTs.

Because seizure duration, once it has crossed the threshold described above, is unrelated to outcome, how else is the treating clinician to assess the quality of the induced seizure? He should look for a synchronous EEG seizure pattern with high amplitude relative to baseline, a well-developed spike-and-slow-wave midictal phase, pronounced postictal suppression, and a substantial tachycardia response (Swartz, 1996). Interhemispheric coherence (symmetry) can be estimated visually using 2-channel EEG recording. Because this important approach to seizure quality is rarely taught in residency training programs, many clinicians obtain additional training at one of the weeklong postgraduate ECT courses offered by several universities. As noted elsewhere in this volume (p. 170), computer programs have also been developed for integration in an ECT device (Abrams and Swartz, 1989, 1996; Swartz and Abrams, 1993) that automatically measure EEG amplitude, coherence, and postictal suppression, three features of the ictal EEG that have been most closely associated with seizure quality (Nobler et al., 1993; Krystal et al., 1992, 1995).

Postictal Care

With termination of the seizure, the therapeutic portion of the treatment also ends; the goal of the postictal phase is primarily that of maintaining an adequate airway until the return of spontaneous respirations and, eventually, alertness. The anesthetic specialist continues forced ventilation until the patient is breathing on his own, at which time he is transferred to a recovery area under the observation of trained staff until awakening.

Frequency and Number of Treatments

In the United States, ECT is invariably given three times per week, whereas in the United Kingdom semi-weekly treatment is the rule

(Pippard and Ellam, 1981). In the only controlled comparison to date of these two treatment schedules, McAllister et al. (1987) found that fewer treatments were required with twice-weekly (mean 6.5 ECTs) than thrice-weekly (mean 8.9 ECTs) unilateral ECT to achieve the same antidepressant effect (6.5 ECTs, incidentally, is precisely the median number of ECTs administered in the 80% of British clinics that use a twice-weekly treatment schedule). This difference probably reflects national character more than any theoretical bias: Americans are impatient for results. The more leisurely pace of treatment enjoyed by the British, however, permits more time for the full effect of each treatment to develop, resulting in a generally shorter course of treatments and less cumulative memory loss—at least where bilateral ECT is concerned. The advent of Diagnosis Related Groups to determine third-party reimbursements in the United States makes it quite unlikely that Americans shall ever adopt a more temperate rate of treatment. This is a shame, because the optimal rate of administration of ECT has yet to be objectively determined (Lerer and Shapira, 1986, 1989; Sackeim, 1989; Strömgren, 1990), and McAllister et al. (1987) found that unilateral ECT was just as effective—but produced less visual memory disturbance—when administered twice as thrice weekly.

Treatment may be given even more rapidly with right unilateral or anterior bifrontal ECT, two methods with reduced effects on memory and cognition. Abrams (1967) demonstrated that a course of 20 right unilateral ECTs given daily on weekdays did not result in significant dysmnesia, a finding later confirmed by Strömgren (1975); Abrams and Taylor (1973) reported similar results for a course of 8 anterior bifrontal ECTs admininistered daily. That daily treatment has not been universally adopted for unilateral ECT is probably testimony to the general disinclination of psychiatrists to start their day at 8:00 A.M. any more frequently than is required by custom. Support for this hypothesis derives from the increasing tendency of some psychiatrists to surrender the administration of ECT to the anesthesiologist, establishing their role in the procedure only at billing time.

It is not unusual for psychiatrists to administer two treatments per session (Swartz and Mehta, 1986), usually for conditions that constitute a serious threat to the patient's physical integrity. Delirious mania, melancholia with intense suicidal symptoms, and catatonic stupor may justify administering double bilateral ECTs in a single session, spaced 1 to 2 minutes apart to allow for the refractory period following a seizure. Double unilateral ECTs, on the other hand, are frequently given in an attempt to increase the therapeutic yield of this method.

Required Number of Treatments

The total number of treatments administered to a patient in a single treatment course is a function of the diagnosis, rapidity of response, response to any previous course of ECT, severity of illness, and the quality of the response to treatments already received. Clinicians are readily able to weigh these variables in practice and treat them accordingly as long as their patients improve with treatment. It is more difficult to specify the maximum number of treatments that should be given to a patient who is not showing the expected treatment response. Although 6 to 8 treatments achieve the desired result in the majority of melancholics receiving bilateral ECT, it is not unusual to give up to 12 to a patient who has all the clinical features generally associated with a good response but has not yet achieved one or who exhibits at least a small incremental improvement with each additional treatment. It is only a rare melancholic (perhaps fewer than 1 in 20) who requires or substantially benefits from more than 12 ECTs in a single course; when this number has been given without substantial effect and the question arises whether or not to continue, it is generally prudent to withhold further treatment for several days while observing the patient and perhaps obtaining another opinion before proceeding with additional treatments.

Manics may require more treatments than melancholics, with 8 to 12 ECTs sufficing in most cases, and only a rare patient requiring more than 16.

Catatonics typically show an initial dramatic response to the first few ECTs, only to relapse if treatment is terminated at this point. It is advisable, therefore, to continue to 6 or 8 treatments in catatonia, which is not infrequently a manifestation of melancholic stupor (Abrams and Taylor, 1976a).

The common clinical wisdom of giving two additional ECTs after maximal improvement has been achieved was not borne out by the controlled study of Barton et al. (1973). These authors found no difference in improvement at 2, 6, and 12 weeks between those patients who stopped receiving ECT at the point of full improvement and those who received two additional treatments.

Multiple Monitored Electroconvulsive
Therapy (MMECT)

In 1966, Blachly and Gowing introduced the novel procedure of administering multiple seizures in a single treatment session, while monitoring the patient's ECG and EEG. Their aim was to accelerate the treatment course and to reduce the required number of anesthesia inductions for a course of treatments. They treated 46 patients with 3 to 8 bilateral ECTs each session and claimed that the memory-loss produced by a single session was no greater than that observed after single treatments. They further claimed a specific relation between the EEG pattern of the seizure end point and the point of maximum improvement from treatment. Because these authors measured neither the memory loss nor the therapeutic effect of their method, however, their claims cannot be evaluated. Although the therapeutic and cognitive effects of MMECT have yet to be studied in a controlled, prospective design, the use of ECG and EEG monitoring that Blachly and Gowing (1966) pioneered has become standard during conventional ECT.

White, Shea, and Jonas (1968) gave an average of 3.3 sessions of MMECT-5 (the standard notation for MMECT with 5 seizures per session) to 27 patients in an open clinical trial; bilateral treatment electrode placement was used in every patient but one. These authors presented no data to support their claim that MMECT shortened the average hospital stay, reduced memory loss, or increased safety in comparison with conventional ECT. Bidder and Strain (1970) gave two sessions of bilateral MMECT-4 to 14 patients and reported an excellent clinical response in only one. Four patients who were tested before and after their treatment course exhibited only minimal impairment on a verbal paired-associates learning task, but the authors noted frequent periods of prolonged postictal confusion, drowsiness, and disorientation, and described one patient who became severely confused after each treatment session. One year later (Strain and Bidder, 1971) these authors reported the occurrence of status epilepticus of approximately 53 minutes duration during the first session of MMECT-4 in a 62-year-old woman who had received prior conventional ECT without untoward event. A left hemiparesis ensued that cleared substantially over 24 hours, but neurologic examination 3 weeks later revealed a residual mild left supranuclear weakness, and the patient continued to feel that her vision and left arm were ''not quite right'' when she was discharged 4 weeks after the episode.

Abrams and Fink (1972) treated 38 patients with an average of 2.5 sessions each of MMECT-4 or MMECT-6 in an open, uncontrolled clinical trial that employed bilateral, right unilateral, or anterior bifrontal placements. Only one patient showed a dramatic response to a single session of MMECT; the remainder showed varying responses that were mostly similar to those obtained with conventional

ECT. Postictal sleep was frequently prolonged after MMECT, and one 35-year-old woman was rousable only to deep painful stimuli for 10 hours after her first treatment. Post-ECT confusion and memory loss were often very prominent, and two patients developed prolonged organic confusional states, with high-voltage, generalized EEG delta activity, that cleared slowly but completely over 1 to 2 weeks posttreatment. Bridenbaugh, Drake, and O'Regan (1972) treated 17 schizophrenic patients in an open clinical trial with an average of 4.5 sessions of MMECT-5. They reported 16 seizures lasting more than 15 minutes each, one episode of aspiration pneumonitis, and 5 episodes of supraventricular tachycardia. A paper by Yesavage and Berens (1980) purporting to compare MMECT and conventional ECT by a retrospective chart review is rendered uninterpretable by the fact that most patients studied received both forms of treatment. Another paper from a private-practice setting (Maletzky et al., 1986) claims to demonstrate that right unilateral MMECT and conventional ECT are equally effective and that MMECT is associated with fewer adverse effects and a shorter hospital stay. However, the study—presented by an enthusiastic practitioner of MMECT (Maletzky, 1986)—is rendered methodologically unsound by nonrandom assignment to treatment methods and nonblind assessment of adverse effects. Further studies have not appeared in over a decade, and MMECT must now be considered an unwarranted risk until proven otherwise.

Record-keeping

Two permanent records should be kept of each treatment, one in the patient's chart and the other in the ECT unit. The latter should be maintained in a permanent ledger that sequentially records the essential data for each patient each treatment day, including the date, name, age, sex, hospital number and unit, ordinal treatment number, methohexital dose, succinylcholine dose, treatment electrode placement, stimulus setting(s), seizure type and duration, and pertinent comments concerning future adjustments in drug dosages or stimulus or individual peculiarities (e.g., "slow circulation time" or "develops emergence delirium"). The same information should be entered in the patient's chart, which can most conveniently be done with a rubber stamp that has information headings followed by blanks to be filled in by the attending physician or his delegate.

Maintenance Electroconvulsive Therapy

Because few illnesses are permanently relieved by a brief exposure to a therapeutic agent, most medical treatments consist of an acute phase followed by a maintenance phase. No one prescribing tricyclic antidepressants for melancholia, for example, would consider terminating therapy immediately after the patient had improved or recovered—the usual course of treatment continues for 6 months—yet this is precisely how patients are frequently treated with ECT. Relapse rates under these circumstances are quite high, ranging from 30% to 60% over 6 months. Fortunately, maintenance drug therapy with lithium or tricyclic antidepressants after a successful course of ECT reduces these rates by at least two thirds (Seager and Bird, 1962; Wilson et al., 1963; Hordern et al., 1965; Imlah et al., 1965; Kay et al., 1970; Mindham, Howland, and Shepherd, 1973; Perry and Tsuang, 1979; Coppen et al., 1981). Examples of effective maintenance regimens for unipolar or bipolar patients are amitriptyline, 150 to 200 mg at bedtime for 4 to 6 months post-ECT, or lithium in doses that provide blood levels in the neighborhood of 1.0 mEq/L for the same period of time (or longer if the prior illness course warrants conventional lithium prophylaxis). Of course, failure with either compound is cause for a trial with the other.

Maintenance ECT is an outpatient procedure for patients who have already exhibited satisfactory improvement with a conventional course of ECT and who have previously failed or do not tolerate maintenance drug therapy. The goal of continued treatment is to maintain the patient in remission by administering additional ECT at a frequency sufficient to prevent relapse without incurring cumulative memory loss. The ideal vehicle for this purpose is right unilateral ECT, which should be given an initial trial in the maintenance phase regardless of which method originally induced remission. The advantage of right unilateral ECT is that it can be given virtually as often as desired—even daily—without producing clinically significant dysmnesia (Abrams, 1967; Strömgren, 1975).

That the widespread prescription and general efficacy of lithium prophylaxis for both bipolar and unipolar illness substantially reduced the use of maintenance ECT is suggested by the virtual 25-year hiatus in articles on the topic after a number appeared stressing its value (Moore, 1943; Geoghegan and Stevenson, 1949; Stevenson and Geoghegan, 1951; Bourne, 1954, 1956; Wolff, 1957; Hastings, 1961; Holt, 1965). Recently, however, a flurry of uncontrolled reports testifies to the efficacy of maintenance ECT for the 10% to 15% of patients with affective disorder who relapse during the 6 months post-ECT despite adequate maintenance drug therapy (Kramer, 1987, 1990; Loo et al., 1988, 1991; Dubin et al., 1989; Thornton et al., 1990; Grunhaus, Pande, and Haskett, 1990; Jaffe et al., 1990a; Thienhaus, Margletta, and Bennett, 1990). Although favorable results are almost invariably presented in these case reports and retrospective chart and literature reviews, all agree that prospective trials are sorely needed and that concurrent pharmacotherapy confounds the ability to draw firm conclusions on the efficacy of the procedure.

A disturbing note is heard, however, in the mention (Kramer, 1987) of one practitioner who gave approximately 2,400 maintenance ECTs to a single patient who was allegedly "still receiving them without problems," a highly doubtful assertion. The potential for abuse of maintenance ECT thus highlighted remains an unresolved problem; maintenance ECT, like psychoanalysis, should not be interminably prolonged. Such a practice is unwarranted and if performed with bilateral placements may produce severe, continuous, cognitive deficits (Regestein et al., 1975). In my view, a second opinion should be sought before continuing maintenance ECT for more than 1 year or 12 treatments, whichever comes first.

A typical schedule for maintenance ECT provides a treatment 1 week after the initial course is successfully completed, a second in 2 weeks, a third in 3 weeks, and the fourth and subsequent treatments at monthly intervals for up to 6 months. Some patients may not remain well on monthly-interval maintenance ECT and will require treatments at 3-week intervals or, rarely, biweekly. This latter spacing should only be given with unilateral ECT, for 2 to 3 consecutive treatments, before again attempting to decrease the seizure frequency.

Maintenance ECT patients are included in the treatment schedule together with inpatients. They should receive written instructions not to have breakfast, and although they may come to the hospital alone, they should leave with a responsible person. Many patients on maintenance ECT find that they are able to go to work later that morning, especially if they have received right unilateral ECT or monthly interval bilateral ECT. Regardless of who accompanies them from the hospital, each patient should be cleared for release that morning by a physician or nurse. The usual records are maintained in the ECT unit and in the patient's outpatient chart. Laboratory tests other than those already obtained for the original treatment course are unnecessary.

Ambulatory Therapy

This phrase refers to outpatient administration of the entire course of ECT: The patient is never hospitalized. Although it is frequently performed in the United Kingdom, ambulatory ECT is remarkably underutilized in the United States. This balance should change as free-standing outpatient treatment facilities (e.g., Surgicenters) flourish in response to universal cost-containment pressures on medical practice. ECT is ideally suited to the outpatient setting. It is brief, safe, and well tolerated—far more so than the variety of endoscopic, plastic, and dental surgical procedures now routinely performed on outpatients (e.g., extraction of 4 wisdom teeth, venous stripping). Ambulatory ECT is only unsuitable for patients whose illness severity and consequent risk mandate inpatient observation and care (e.g., suicidal, agitated, or delusional melancholics; catatonics; acute manics).

Treatment Complications and Their Management

Neurological Phenomena

Transient neurologic abnormalities, including aphasias, apraxias, and agnosias, which were considered normal accompaniments of ECT rather than complications, were noted by early clinicians to occur during the immediate postictal phase following bilateral ECT (Hemphill, 1940; Kalinowsky, 1945; Gallinek, 1952b; Kane, 1963), but were never systematically investigated. Jargon aphasia has been reported after left-unilateral ECT (Gottlieb and Wilson, 1965), as have other dysphasias (Pratt et al., 1971; Annet et al., 1974; Clyma, 1975), all generally resolving within 30 minutes after treatment. The only systematic study was done by Kriss et al. (1978), who performed neurologic examinations on 29 dextral patients before and immediately after each of 62 left- or right-unilateral ECTs. Asymmetrical motor responses observed during the induced seizure usually consisted of more intense clonic movements of the musculature contralateral to the stimulated hemisphere, despite the induction of a generalized, bilateral seizure. Following the seizure, and before recovery of consciousness, upper limb reflexes ipsilateral to the treated hemisphere generally returned first. Limb strength tested after the return of consciousness revealed upper limb weakness in 80% of the observations, with a gradual return to normal over the ensuing 15 minutes. Motor and visual inattention contralateral to the treated side also occurred, as well as corresponding tactile inattention. All patients receiving left-sided ECT showed signs of dysphasia (dysnomia) immediately afterward. Overall, patients took longer to respond and to open their eyes after left- compared with right-unilateral ECT, supporting claims for the major role played by the dominant hemisphere in the maintenance and manifestation of consciousness. Anosognosia (unawareness or denial of impairment) was profound and striking after right-unilateral ECT, even after patients had become fully alert and cooperative.

Electroconvulsive Therapy–Emergent Dyskinesias

Dyskinetic movements appearing during ECT take several forms, the most ubiquitous of which are the typical postictal chewing and lip-smacking automatisms that physicians who administer ECT have long observed during the postictal phase and which Liberzon et al. (1991) characterized as "mild bilateral orobuccolingual dyskinetic movements lasting 1 to 3 min." The other oral and limb dyskinesias these authors observed during the immediate postictal period in three patients generally resolved within minutes, but lasted 24 hours in one instance. Their report is difficult to interpret because 2 of their patients were already neurologically damaged; one exhibited preexisting facial grimacing and carried a diagnosis of choreoathetotic cerebral palsy, and the other was a Wilson's disease carrier whom childhood meningoencephalitis had left with hemispheric cerebral atrophy.

Of longer duration were the 3 instances described by Flaherty et al. (1984), in which ECT-emergent involuntary facial-bucco-lingual movements took weeks or months to resolve. Although each patient had a history of neuroleptic drug administration, it was too far in the past for neuroleptic withdrawal to have caused the dyskinesias. The most likely explanation for these cases is an interaction between neuroleptic-sensitized dopamine receptors and a dopamine-receptor stimulating effect of ECT.

Different still are the ECT-emergent dyskinesias reported by Douyon et al. (1989) and M. Fink (personal communication) that materialized in patients with Parkinson's disease who continued to receive levodopa during ECT; the dyskinesias disappeared with a reduction in the dose of levodopa.

The clinical data reviewed elsewhere in this volume suggests that Liberzon et al. (1991) are correct in their attribution of the ECT-emergent dyskinesias to ECT-induced increases in postsynaptic dopamine receptor sensitivity.

Elevated Seizure Threshold—Short Seizures

Seizures may be increasingly difficult or impossible to obtain even at maximum electrical dosage in older men during the latter part of their treatment course, especially if they are receiving long half-life benzodiazepines. In a retrospective investigation of seizure duration in patients receiving unilateral ECT, Strömgren et al. (1980) found that administration of long half-life benzodiazepines (e.g., diazepam, nitrazepam) was associated with shorter seizures and the apparent need for more of them. More recently, Pettinati et al. (1990) found less improvement in depression in patients taking benzodiazepines during high-dose, brief-pulse unilateral ECT compared with those who were not, although the mean total number of ECTs prescribed did not differ. Seizure duration is unaffected, however, by short half-life benzodiazepines such as oxazepam (Olesen, Lolk, and Christensen, 1989).

There is evidence that methohexital itself shortens seizure duration compared with unmodified ECT (Witztum et al., 1970). Jones and Callender (1981) have suggested that this may lead to inadequate treatment. Although Lunn et al. (1981) obtained longer seizures with ketamine in an ECT patient than he had previously exhibited with methohexital, the former compound's hallucinogenic properties seriously limit its use for ECT. Droperidol is also problematic because coma ensued when this drug was administered immediately following ECT (Koo and Chien, 1986).

Parenteral caffeine, 125 to 2,000 mg, provides a way to lengthen short seizures (Shapira et al., 1985, 1987; Hinkle et al., 1987; Coffey et al., 1987a, 1990b; Kellner and Batterson, 1989; Lurie and Coffey, 1990; McCall et al., 1993b; Rosenquist et al., 1994) and has been recommended for this purpose by the APA Task Force on ECT (American Psychiatric Association, 1990).

The method is not without risk, however. Acevedo and Smith (1988) reported tachycardia and hypertension in a patient who had received caffeine pretreatment for ECT; Jaffe et al. (1990b) described 3 elderly patients who demonstrated multifocal VPCs and bigeminy, atrial ectopy and a junctional rhythm, and fusion beats and ventricular tachycardia; Beale et al. (1994) reported an instance of supraventricular tachycardia during an ECT with caffeine pretreatment (subsequent treatments given without caffeine were unremarkable); Kellner and

Bachman (1992) reported an instance of olfactory hallucinations; and Liebowitz and El-Mallakh (1993) reported an instance of a 15-second cardiac arrest.

Increasing the stimulus dose for brief-pulse unilateral ECT by about 30% whenever seizure duration falls between 20 and 30 seconds also effectively maintains seizure duration in the accepted therapeutic range (Coffey et al., 1990b), a strategy I believe to be preferable to administering caffeine. Coffey et al. (1990b) observed that caffeine pretreatment allowed a reduction in stimulus charge in almost half their patients, a doubtful advantage in view of the dosage sensitivity of unilateral ECT described elsewhere in this volume (p. 124).

However, an increase in stimulus dosage without giving additional stimuli is only feasible in patients who are not yet receiving the device maximum, as most patients will be who are being considered for caffeine pretreatment. As discussed in Chapter 6, administering the maximum stimulus dose via a longer stimulus train (e.g., over 6 to 8 seconds) may be an alternate effective strategy for inducing longer seizures.

The use of caffeine to lengthen seizures in ECT was pioneered at a time (Shapira et al., 1985) when it was still believed that seizure duration bore a direct relation to the therapeutic impact of ECT. Now that it is clear that no such relation exists—except perhaps at the seizure versus no seizure level—I believe it is time to reconsider the argument for using caffeine to lengthen seizure duration.

Caffeine might have a useful role in ECT if the propositions were true both that dosage in excess of seizure threshold determined the clinical potency of ECT (Sackeim et al., 1987a, 1993) and that caffeine lowered the seizure threshold. But the former proposition has yet to be proved, and Shapira et al. (1987) did not find evidence to support the latter. In the only study specifically designed to examine the effect of caffeine on the seizure threshold, McCall et al. (1993b) studied 12 depressed inpatients serving as their own controls who received right unilateral ECT with, or without, caffeine pretreatment in a balanced, randomized design, with seizure threshold titration. Although caffeine indeed lengthened seizures, it did not lower the seizure threshold.

Rosenquist et al. (1994) took the interesting tack of examining the effects of caffeine pretreatment in 12 depressed patients on some proposed measures of seizure quality and impact: EEG voltage suppression, seizure regularity, and heart rate response. None of these measures differed significantly between patients randomly assigned to receive intravenous retreatment with either caffeine or saline placebo.

Regardless of whether caffeine affects the seizure threshold, one might ask the empirical question whether it affects treatment outcome (although the legitimacy of this question is unclear because there is no a priori reason to believe that caffeine might augment the efficacy of ECT independent of any effects on seizure duration or threshold).

Interestingly, although a literature search back to 1987 reveals several controlled trials demonstrating the efficacy of caffeine in lengthening seizures, I found none specifically investigating whether the therapeutic outcome is thereby augmented. One controlled assessment of caffeine pretreatment for unilateral ECT (Coffey et al., 1990b) failed to find a significantly faster or better antidepressant response with, than without, caffeine, albeit using a treatment method that lowered the stimulus dose in the caffeine-treated group, thereby potentially reducing the therapeutic outcome. In an uncontrolled, naturalistic survey of practice on a University Hospital service, Calev et al. (1993) reported that 8 patients receiving bilateral ECT with caffeine pretreatment required fewer ECTs and exhibited greater improvement of depression scale ratings than others who did not receive caffeine, a report that requires a planned experiment to confirm.

In short, there is a dearth of hard data supporting the use of caffeine augmentation of ECT-induced seizures to enhance the therapeutic effect of ECT, and in view of the occasional untoward cardiovascular effects of such therapy, there appears to be little justification for its continued use. Instead, as described above, clinicians administering ECT should look to other measures of seizure adequacy than seizure duration (e.g., EEG postictal suppression, amplitude, coherence) and seek out methods that specifically enhance these features (e.g., stimulus train lengthening, shortening of pulse width and frequency).

The same is true for the related compound theophylline, which also lengthens seizures (Swartz and Lewis, 1991). Additionally, status epilepticus was reported in two asthmatic patients who received ECT while taking a long-acting preparation of this drug (Peters et al., 1984; Devanand et al., 1988a), and I am aware of three additional, unpublished, instances: One of a patient who eventually died from complications of status epilepticus that developed during ECT received while taking concomitant long-acting theophylline, and two others of patients who sustained permanent brain damage. Despite the fact that Rasmussen and Zorumski (1993) administered ECT without any adverse reaction in 7 patients taking theophylline for medical conditions, it remains my view that ECT should not be administered to a patient with significant theophylline blood levels without unequivocal evidence for a high seizure threshold. In any event, if threshold-lowering medications are planned, it is prudent to have a syringe ready containing 15 mg of diazepam for intravenous administration in the event of a prolonged seizure. The administration of diphenylhydantoin under such circumstances is ineffective, wastes precious time, and creates a false sense of having taken definitive action.

Prolonged Seizures

Although sporadic instances are reported of status epilepticus or other paroxysmal EEG abnormalities developing during or immediately after ECT (Roith, 1959; Strain and Bidder, 1971; Bridenbaugh et al., 1972; Ray, 1975; Small et al., 1980; Weiner et al., 1980a,b; Weiner, 1981; Prakash and Leavell, 1984; Peters et al., 1984; Kaufman et al., 1986; Finlayson et al., 1989), almost all can be attributed to some unusual aspect of the patient or the treatment: Mental deficiency secondary to brain damage at birth (Roith, 1959); a preexisting paroxysmal EEG abnormality (Weiner et al., 1980a; Kaufman et al., 1986); old stroke (Strain and Bidder, 1971); the administration of MMECT (Strain and Bidder, 1971; Bridenbaugh et al., 1972; Maletzky, 1978, 1981); the coadministration of lithium (Ray, 1975; Small et al., 1980; Weiner et al., 1980b); theophylline (Peters et al., 1984); trazodone (Kaufman et al., 1986); or hyponatremia due to self-induced water intoxication (Finlayson et al., 1989). The only instance of ECT inducing status epilepticus in a patient known to have epilepsy occurred after the administration of MMECT (Maletzky, 1981).

The clinical significance of the report of numerous prolonged seizures with brief-pulse unilateral ECT (Greenberg, 1985) is difficult to interpret as EEG seizure monitoring only became routine at about the time this latter treatment technique was introduced into general use. Nonetheless, no prolonged seizures were observed during EEG monitoring of hundreds of consecutive unilateral and bilateral ECTs administered with both brief-pulse and sine-wave stimuli (Abrams et al., 1973, 1983, 1992; Weiner, 1980a; Swartz and Abrams, 1984, 1986).

In recent years, the diagnosis of nonconvulsive generalized status epilepticus has been applied to certain events occurring during the days following the induced seizure (Weiner et al., 1980a; Varma and Lee, 1992; Rao et al., 1993; Weiner and Krystal, 1993; Grogan et al., 1995). The typical presentation is of a patient who leaves the ECT suite in a state of apparent recovery from the effects of the seizure and anesthesia, returns to the unit, and is later found mute or partially communicative, with fluctuating levels of alertness and responsivity. An EEG is taken and shows generalized delta activity, sometimes with spike-and-wave complexes. The clouded state and EEG abnormalities last for many hours or days and may be completely or partially abolished with intravenous diazepam. The diagnosis is not easy to make, however, partly because specific inclusion and exclusion criteria are lacking. Grogan et al. (1995), for example, applied the diagnosis despite the fact that their patient had a hypothalamic brain tumor and exhibited no EEG spike activity. The patient in the case reported by Weiner et al. (1980a) was also receiving lithium, a compound capable of causing severe EEG abnormalities on its own. The cases of Varma and Lee (1992) and Rao et al. (1993) were published only as letters; both patients were receiving neuroleptics, a class of drugs with known epileptogenic properties, and both first exhibited the abnormal EEG patterns in question late in the course of ECT (e.g., after 9 or 10 treatments), at a time when interictal EEGs typically show bursts and runs of generalized delta activity with superimposed spike and sharp-wave activity.

According to Weiner and Krystal (1993), nonconvulsive status epilepticus must be distinguished from the typical ECT-induced delirium, and the EEG is not always diagnostic in this regard. Weiner (personal communication) believes the definitive finding to delineate convulsive status from ECT-induced delirium is the disappearance of both the paroxysmal EEG activity and the cognitive dysfunction upon administering an anticonvulsant agent. However, the patient of Varma and Lee (1992) clearly does not meet this criterion, as a fluctuating mental status continued for some time despite therapeutic phenytoin levels and an improved EEG. And the patient of Rao et al. (1993) never showed cognitive dysfunction, but remained in a deep coma for several hours after ECT, despite the fact that the abnormal EEG discharges were terminated by intravenous diazepam; no mention is made of cognitive status after resolution of the coma.

Although no specific guidelines exist for determining when a given seizure has become excessively long, one study (O'Connell et al., 1988) showed that neuronal lesions could be produced in rats after as little as 10 minutes of continuous seizure activity induced by mercaptopropionic acid, a neurotoxic chemical. The relevance of this to ECT is unclear. However, since most ECT-induced seizures last less than 90 seconds by EEG criteria, and no relation has been established betweeen seizure duration and therapeutic impact once a 30-second threshold has been passed, it seems prudent to terminate seizures exceeding 120 seconds (Abrams, 1990). Intravenous diazepam, 10 to 15

mg, has long been the drug of choice for terminating prolonged seizures, although administration of additional barbiturate anesthetic (e.g.,
methohexital, 25 to 50 mg) or midazolam, 1 to 3 mg intravenously, is
similarly effective.

Prolonged Apnea

There is no antidote for succinylcholine and no specific treatment to
reverse prolonged apnea. Assisted respiration is simply continued for
as long as it takes the patient's own limited pseudocholinesterase activity to metabolize the succinylcholine (usually 30 to 60 minutes).
Intubation is not required as long as good pulmonary exchange documented by oximetry is achieved by face mask. If it seems that apnea
may be prolonged for more than an hour, consideration should be given
to the administration of a unit of typed and cross-matched fresh whole
blood or plasma to supply an exogenous source of pseudocholinesterase (Matthew and Constan, 1964). Although it is possible to continue
to use succinylcholine for subsequent treatments, albeit at a much
lower dose (Impastato 1966; Hickey et al., 1987), a more rational approach is to switch to atracurium for further treatments, because it is
not dependent on serum pseudocholinesterase for its metabolism (Stack
et al., 1988; Kramer and Afrasiabi, 1991).

Emergence Delirium

About 10% of patients develop a self-limited delirium or acute confusional state during the immediate postictal phase, characterized by
all of the following clinical features occurring in concert:

1. Restless agitation
2. Disorientation
3. Clouded consciousness
4. Repetitive stereotyped movements
5. Impaired comprehension
6. Failure to respond to commands
7. Subsequent amnesia for the episode

The anesthesia, electrical stimulation, and seizure each presumably
contribute their part to causing the syndrome, in which the dazed,
restless patients mutter incoherently while fumbling with the bed-
clothes, rubbing and pulling at their skin, moaning loudly, flopping

about, and even trying to climb off the stretcher. The physical restraint required to prevent this behavior only seems to make things worse, and Kellner et al. (1991) were able to divert the patient's attention with a water-filled rubber glove. The delirium generally lasts from 10 to 45 minutes untreated and resembles nothing so much as a psychomotor seizure. It is readily terminated by intravenous benzodiazepines or barbiturates if a vein can be found and the patient held still long enough to inject it—both unlikely propositions. Since patients who develop emergence delirium manifest it during more than a third of their treatments (Devanand et al., 1989b), many therapists prefer routinely to prevent recurrent episodes by administering diazepam, 5 to 15 mg intravenously, as soon as the induced seizure terminates. Midazolam, 1 to 3 mg intravenously, was recently shown by Liston and Sones (1990) to be an effective alternative treatment with the potential advantages of less venous irritation and a shorter duration of action. However, since fewer than 10% of patients manifest the syndrome after each treatment, it is equally prudent, albeit more time-consuming, to retain the patient in the treatment room for several minutes longer than usual—intravenous access line carefully kept patent and benzodiazepine-filled syringe at the ready—and to administer the syringe contents only at the first clinical manifestations of delirium.

Devanand et al. (1989b) were unable to identify predictors of emergence delirium from among the variables of age, pre-ECT agitation or excitement, number of ECTs administered, barbiturate anesthetic or succinylcholine dosage, or mean seizure duration (unaccountably missing from this list—considering the authors' major research interest—is the variable of stimulus charge). Among 5 patients switched from unilateral to bilateral ECT for lack of a treatment response, 3 developed emergence delirium only after bilateral ECT. It is clear, however, that the syndrome occurs with equal frequency after bilateral, right unilateral, and left unilateral ECT (Leechuy, Abrams, and Kohlhaas, 1988; Liston and Sones, 1990).

Based on the hypothesis that emergence delirium is a form of lactate-induced panic secondary to seizure-induced skeletal muscle metabolism, Swartz (1990) effectively prevented the syndrome in 5 patients by increasing the succinylcholine dose by about 45%, an intriguing strategy that awaits confirmation in a controlled comparison with placebo.

In the rare patient who fails to respond to benzodiazepine inhibition or prophylaxis, the intravenous line can be left in place following the treatment and a 2% solution of methohexital infused at a rate sufficient to prevent the delirium from emerging. This procedure should be directly supervised by a physician or registered nurse.

Mania or Organic Euphoria

Years ago, Kalinowsky (1945) described the emergence of organic psychotic states during the course of bilateral ECT—additional ECTs would typically attenuate the syndrome, which might then transiently reappear during the post-ECT convalescence. As noted elsewhere in this volume, Fink and Kahn (1961) described a euphoric-hypomanic response to ECT that they considered highly favorable. Devanand et al. (1988) described 3 patients who developed maniform states while undergoing right unilateral or bilateral ECT, 2 of whom exhibited no concurrent cognitive impairment and were therefore diagnosed as having true hypomanic or manic syndromes; the third exhibited significant disorientation and impaired cognitive examination scores and was designated to be suffering from an organic-euphoric state. Andrade et al. (1988c) reported that 4 out of 32 endogenous depressives developed transient, nonorganic, self-limited manic syndromes during the course of bilateral ECT, followed by recovery from their depressions. A fifth patient (Andrade et al., 1990) fared similarly at first, but then relapsed and required two additional courses of ECT, with concurrent pharmacotherapy, to achieve a sustained remission.

In my experience, the occurrence of a maniform syndrome during ECT—regardless of the associated cognitive status—is favorable, and an indication to withhold further treatment while closely observing the patient. The majority go on to enjoy full remission of all symptoms, including cognitive impairment; the few who slip back into depression or remain in a maniform state can then be treated either with additional ECT or pharmacotherapy—the rationale for combining the two, however, is obscure.

Aspiration Pneumonitis

Since the introduction of muscle relaxants, no cases of aspiration pneumonitis were reported until Zibrak, Jensen, and Bloomingdale (1988) described two patients with gastroparesis—one of whom had not eaten for 12 hours—who suffered aspiration of gastric contents during ECT, followed by adult respiratory distress syndrome. (I had a similar case in my practice of a depressed woman in her 70s who had not eaten for over 12 hours prior to ECT, but nevertheless vomited copious amounts of gastric contents immediately following termination of her first seizure and developed aspiration pneumonitis that took almost 2 weeks to resolve.) The authors recommend that ECT candidates with concurrent disorders judged to put them at high risk for gastroparesis (e.g., diabetes mellitus, hypothyroidism, amyloidosis, scleroderma) should have a careful gastrointestinal history taken, followed by a GI series or radionucleotide gastric emptying study, if indicated. The only sure way to prevent vomiting—and aspiration of gastric contents—in patients with documented gastroparesis is to remove the stomach contents by nasogastric tube before induction of anesthesia.

Ruptured Bladder

Irving and Drayson (1984) reported rupture of the urinary bladder during the 10th ECT in a 74-year-old man with a history of prostatism. The only other case in the literature is that of O'Brien and Morgan (1991), who described a 55-year-old man on amitriptyline, 150 mg/day, who had failed to void before treatment and who sustained a 3-cm tear in the bladder fundus during the extremely vigorous muscular contractions of an apparently unmodified seizure. These cases amply support the standard recommendation for patients to void their bladder before coming to ECT.

Nausea or Vomiting

These are infrequent after ECT and can be prevented by dimenhydrinate, 50 mg intramuscularly, given at the end of the seizure.

Headache

Headache occurs in about one third of all patients after ECT and usually responds to aspirin or, if severe, ibuprofen. Acting on the theory that electrically induced temporalis muscle spasm contributes to the development of post-ECT headache, Swartz (personal communication) has successfully prescribed heat and massage for this symptom.

Precautions and Contraindications; Drug Interactions

Reserpine is contraindicated in patients receiving ECT because several deaths and near-deaths due to cardiovascular collapse or respiratory depression have been reported with the combination (Foster and Gayle, 1955; Kalinowsky, 1956a; Bracha and Hess, 1956; Bross, 1957). Although the combination of chlorpromazine and ECT is believed to be safer (Berg, Gabriel and Impastato, 1959), a number of deaths and life-threatening incidents have also occurred with such coadministration (Weiss, 1955; Kalinowsky, 1956a,b; Gaitz, Pokorny, and Mills, 1956; Grinspoon and Greenblatt, 1963), which must therefore be considered contraindicated and, in any case, has no justification from controlled trials. If a neuroleptic must be combined with ECT (as in a manic patient who is early in the treatment course and has not yet responded adequately), neither fluphenazine nor haloperidol has been associated with ECT-related hypotensive reactions, although the latter compound seems inordinately represented among neuroleptics precipitating neuroleptic malignant syndrome (NMS).

As noted earlier, lithium prolongs the neuromuscular blockade of succinylcholine (Hill, Wong, and Hodges, 1976) and has also been implicated in the causation of acute, reversible, delirious states after ECT, variously characterized by confusion, disorientation, lethargy, EEG slowing, and seizures (Jephcott and Kerry, 1974; Hoenig and Chaulk, 1977; Mandel et al., 1980; Small et al., 1980; el-Mallakh, 1988; Penney et al., 1990). The case of Ray (1975), often cited as an early example of this phenomenon, is not relevant because the patient first developed neurotoxic symptoms only several days after receiving combined therapy. In my own experience, I treated one man in his 30s on lithium therapy who developed a pronounced organic confusional state lasting for several days after receiving only 2 or 3 ECTs. The fact that some patients have safely received this combination (Martin and Kramer, 1982; DeQuardo and Tandon, 1988; Penney et al., 1990) or that no demonstrable pharmacokinetic or drug-interaction factors are known to preclude prescribing it (Rudorfer et al., 1987), proves only that the combination does not constitute an absolute contradiction. The central consideration, however, is that the absence of experimental data demonstrating an advantage of combined therapy over either agent given separately renders the substantial morbid risk of the combination unjustifiable.

Tricyclic antidepressants may be safer than lithium or neuroleptic drugs in combination with ECT, although Freeman and Kendell (1980) noted that the only 2 deaths in a sample of 243 patients who received ECT occurred in patients with preexisting cardiac disease who were taking tricyclic antidepressants. Inasmuch as there is no controlled study demonstrating a synergistic effect of such combined therapy and there is some evidence that it may actually antagonize the effects of ECT given alone (Price et al., 1978), there seems little reason to prescribe it. Despite concerns frequently expressed over the safety of administering ECT to patients receiving MAOIs, the literature provides no specific evidence for an increased risk of such combined therapy (el-Ganzouri et al., 1985; Freese, 1985). As is true for tricyclics, however, no therapeutic advantage has been demonstrated for combining ECT and MAOIs.

9

Technique of Electroconvulsive Therapy: Praxis

The following is a specific treatment sequence that I find useful for administering ECT. It assumes that the patient has been properly prepared for treatment as outlined earlier and is lying on a stretcher in the treatment room, that vital signs have been recorded, and that all necessary staff personnel are in attendance.

At the beginning of the treatment day, each patient's individual doses of intravenous medications and saline should be drawn up into separate syringes, labeled with the patient's name, date, type and dose of medication, and placed together in a small container marked with the patient's name. One can identify each syringe with stick-on, color-coded dots: For example, green for anticholinergic, yellow for anesthetic, red for muscle-relaxant, and white for saline flush. To further facilitate identification, use a particular size syringe for each medication: 3 cc for anticholinergic, 10 cc for anesthetic, 5 cc for muscle-relaxant, and 30 cc for saline flush.

1. Apply blood pressure cuff and record baseline blood pressure. The same cuff will later be reinflated just before administration of succinylcholine to block this drug from the muscles distal to the cuff and permit safe observation of the unmodified seizure. For this reason, if unilateral ECT is contemplated, the cuff should be applied initially to the arm ipsilateral to the placement of the unilateral treatment electrodes in order to document that a generalized, rather than a focal contralateral, seizure has occurred (Welch, 1982). Avoid the cuffed-limb method in the presence of severe osteoporosis to obviate the possibility of unmodified muscle contraction causing fracture (Levy, 1988).

2. Apply ECG electrodes. Self-stick ECG recording electrodes are applied precordially—above and below the heart—with a third applied to the shoulder as a ground. It saves time to apply them while the patient is waiting for treatment. The appropriate ECG leads are then connected and a baseline rhythm strip obtained.

3. Apply EEG electrodes. Disposable, pregelled, stick-on electrodes are now available in a small size especially for EEG monitoring. They save time because they do not have to be smeared with electrode jelly first or cleaned up afterward; they will not pull loose during the seizure; and their adhesive surface allows them to be placed anywhere on the skin rather than just under the perforated rubber headstrap, unlike the older type that only permits recording from bifrontal forehead leads. This is an important advantage because bifrontal leads cannot differentiate focal contralateral seizures from generalized ones. Frontal-to-mastoid electrodes on the same side of the head are often preferred for EEG monitoring during ECT because they produce a high-voltage, easily read record (despite occasional ECG artifact) and can be placed contralateral to the treatment electrodes during unilateral ECT to verify that a generalized seizure has occurred. The same ground electrode applied for ECG monitoring can be used for the EEG.

Patients should shampoo their hair the night before and wash their faces with soap and water on treatment mornings. Careful rubbing of the skin over the recording sites with an alcohol-soaked swab followed by drying with a gauze pad is the only other preparation necessary to remove the oily residues and provide artifact-free recordings. The EEG leads are then connected; ECT instruments with integral EEG automatically initiate monitoring when the stimulus is administered at the time of treatment.

4. Start intravenous line. An intravenous line is most conveniently started with a 21-gauge, thin-walled ''butterfly'' needle assembly attached to a saline-filled, 20-mL syringe. When blood flows into the syringe receptacle of the butterfly assembly, connect the saline-containing syringe, flush the intravenous line with a few milliliters of saline, and apply a plastic clamp to the tubing while keeping pressure on the syringe plunger. Be sure not to start the intravenous line in the arm with the blood pressure cuff, because it will infiltrate when the cuff is inflated.

5. Apply treatment electrodes. For bilateral ECT, the electrode sites are on the bare skin over both temples. A perforated elastic strap is usually used to hold flat steel disk electrodes in place, although

two nonconductive electrode handles can be used as well. Before applying the electrodes, wipe the skin and scalp sites with alcohol and dry. Lay the headstrap over the forehead and determine the perforations into which you will insert the electrodes. Insert the electrodes, apply conductive gel to the prepared skin sites and the electrode surfaces, position the electrodes over the temples, and wrap the strap around the head, fixing it firmly in place by inserting each electrode post through a second perforation.

For unilateral ECT the d'Elia placement is standard: The lower site is over the right temple and the upper—or paravertex —site is on the scalp just to the right of the vertex. A concave para-vertex electrode is manually applied with an electrically insulated handle, and the lower electrode is held in place with an elastic strap or another handle. When treating a patient with a skull defect, be sure to place the treatment electrodes far from the defect to avoid the possibility of excessively high current density at the brain surface.

For anterior bilateral ECT, Letemendia et al. (1993) positioned the stimulus electrodes 5 cm above the lateral angle of each orbit, about 14 cm apart. However, Manly and Swartz (1994) prefer an asymmetrical placement, with the right-sided electrode situated in the conventional frontotemporal site for bilateral ECT and the left-sided electrode placed 5 to 7 cm anterior to the conventional frontotemporal site—above the left eye—with the lateral electrode edge bordering the intersection ridge between the forehead and the temple.

The electrode sites should be carefully rubbed with alcohol and dried and then rubbed again with a small amount of conductive electrode gel. The electrode treatment surfaces are then covered with a generous layer of conductive gel and applied firmly to the skin or scalp. To maximize contact, extra care must be taken to part the hair and expose the scalp when applying the upper unilateral ECT electrode. Clipping the hair to expose a circle of scalp is ideal for this purpose (Weiner et al., 1980a) but is unlikely to be well received by patients at non–Veterans Affairs facilities.

For self-adhesive, solid gel disposable stimulus electrodes, simply rub the skin sites with a saline-moistened pad—do not clean with alcohol or other organic solvents—and apply directly to the skin without additional electrode gel. When applying disposable stimulus electrodes to hair-covered scalp areas—as for unilateral ECT—thoroughly moisten the site first with saline

solution and press the electrode firmly in place with an electri-
cally-insulated handle.

6. Test impedance. Checking the static impedance tests the quality
   of the skin-to-electrode contact. An impedance of zero ohms suggests a short circuit between the two electrodes, formed by wet
   hair, electrode gel, or saline solution. This is corrected by washing
   and drying the skin and scalp and using less gel or solution on
   the electrodes. A high impedance—3000 ohms or more, for
   example—should be reduced by the following steps.
   a. The connection between each banana plug and its receptacle
      on the back of the electrode should be checked for rust, for-
      eign material, or corrosion and cleaned as needed.
   b. A loose connection can result from flattening of the metal
      spring leaves of the banana plug; these can be restored to
      shape with the point of a knife.
   c. If there is long hair on the scalp beneath the electrodes, the
      electrodes should be repositioned.
   d. The rubber headstrap can be tightened or the pressure on the
      electrodes otherwise increased.
   e. If necessary, gently abrade the skin at the electrode site with
      Skin Prep tape (3M, St. Paul, MN) or abrasive gel such as
      Omniprep (Weaver Co., Aurora CO).
   f. If applying disposable solid gel electrodes, massage the skin
      again with a saline-soaked pad and leave it moist.
   If the impedance remains high after all these procedures, treatment should only be given if the patient is so ill that the (small)
   risk of skin burn is of less importance than that of the untreated
   disorder.

7. Administer atropine, 0.4 to 1.2 mg intravenously, by rapid bolus
   push. Patients with myocardial ischemia may benefit from a few
   minutes of oxygenation before anesthesia induction with the mask
   held slightly away from the nose and mouth to avoid a claustro-
   phobic response. Pulse oximetry is now routinely recommended
   by many anesthetic specialists to monitor oxygen delivery to patients with pulmonary diseases, sickle cell trait, or myocardial ischemia or failure; increasingly, it is used in all patients.

8. Administer methohexital. While the patient counts aloud from 1
   to 100, and after determining that the needle is still patent and in
   the vein by gently aspirating the saline syringe and observing
   backflow of blood, replace the saline syringe with one containing
   an initial dose of 0.75 mg/kg methohexital (about 40 to 70 mg),

which is then given by rapid bolus push. The methohexital dose may require adjustment for subsequent treatments depending on the patient's response to the initial injection (e.g., substance abusers require larger doses; patients with prolonged circulation times may take longer to fall asleep). As soon as the patient has stopped counting and is unresponsive to questions, the empty methohexital syringe is replaced by one containing an initial dose of 0.6 mg/kg succinylcholine.

9. Inflate blood pressure cuff to 10 mm Hg above the systolic pressure to occlude the succinylcholine to be administered next from reaching the distal muscles (Fink and Johnson, 1982).

10. Administer succinylcholine by rapid bolus push. The empty syringe is then replaced with the saline syringe, and the tubing is flushed and clamped again for later availability in the event that additional intravenous therapy is required. The dose of succinylcholine may also require subsequent adjustment.

11. Insert mouthguard and administer oxygen. As soon as the succinylcholine has been given, the rubber mouthguard is inserted between the teeth and 100% oxygen is administered by positive pressure and continued throughout the treatment (including the seizure) until spontaneous respirations have returned.

12. Observe muscular fasciculations of the first (depolarization) phase of succinylcholine. These will appear first in the muscles of the head, neck, and upper chest and spread to those of the trunk and limbs before reaching the small muscles of the feet and hands. When the fasciculations have died down in the small muscles of the feet (generally about 1 minute after the succinylcholine injection), the patient is ready to be treated. If the adequacy of muscle relaxation is in doubt, abolition of the patellar reflex can provide complementary information. A more precise method for testing muscle relaxation entails the use of a nerve-muscle stimulator set to provide intermittent pulses to a peripheral nerve (e.g., radial) at a rate of one or two per second. When the resultant muscle contraction response is abolished, muscle relaxation is adequate.

13. Administer the treatment stimulus. When adequate muscle relaxation has been achieved and the stimulus settings are adjusted (accounting for patient age and sex, number of previous treatments in the course, stimulus type, treatment electrode placement, type and dose of nighttime sedative, and barbiturate anesthetic dose), oxygenation is temporarily interrupted, the patient's head and neck are hyperextended with the jaw held tightly shut (a properly

inserted mouthguard will automatically prevent the tongue from protruding between the teeth), and the stimulus is administered.

The tonic and clonic muscle contractions observed in the cuffed limb or EMG indirectly substantiate the occurrence of a cerebral seizure. If a clearly discernible tonic-clonic progression is not apparent—and this is judged not to be the result of an excessive dose of succinylcholine—restimulation should be performed in about 20 seconds (H. Sackeim, personal communication), generally at the device maximum. Although such a clear tonic-clonic progression will usually last at least 15 to 25 seconds, it is not possible to specify with any degree of certainty what the minimum duration should be, other than to note that seizures below about 20 seconds tend to exceed 2 standard deviations from the mean (Sackeim et al., 1993). If a missed, or abortive (e.g., <5 sec.), seizure occurs, restimulation at maximum dosage should be immediately accomplished without a waiting period.

The EEG should exhibit qualitative evidence of good seizure intensity and generalization (a synchronous or coherent pattern with high amplitude relative to baseline, well-developed midictal spike-and-slow-wave morphology, and pronounced postictal suppression); the tachycardia response should be prominent. If one or more of these are deemed clearly insufficient, restimulation as described above is also indicated.

Perhaps the most important reason to monitor the EEG during ECT is to assure that the seizure ends completely, since paroxysmal brain electrical activity commonly continues after motor activity has ended. The approaching end of the seizure is heralded by progressive slowing of the spike-and-wave bursts of clonus; a classical seizure end point occurs when these are abruptly replaced by electrical silence or when the paroxysmal clonic activity is suddenly replaced by lower amplitude mixed frequencies. The auditory EEG signal becomes increasingly irregular, and the staccato tones that accompany each muscular contraction change abruptly to a nearly steady tone at seizure termination. About 10% to 15% of ECTs do not have a clear-cut end point on the EEG. The paroxysmal activity gradually wanes, blending indistinguishably into low-amplitude postictal activity. When this occurs, both the end of the motor seizure and the sudden decline in the ECT-induced heart-rate elevation can aid in estimating seizure duration. It is prudent to be sure that all seizure activity has ended before stopping EEG monitoring.

14. Initiate routine postictal care. In medically unstable patients or those who have experienced emergence agitation, the intravenous line should be left in place until the patient awakens, in case medications need to be given rapidly. A full-length arm-board can preserve the intravenous line; just before the patient is taken to the recovery area, the tubing is flushed with saline and clamped, and the clamp and saline syringe are taped to the armboard. In the recovery area, the staff should keep an eye on the intravenous line. After spontaneous respirations have returned and full ventilatory exchange has been established, the patient is wheeled on a stretcher to a recovery area to be observed by trained staff until alert, oriented, and able to walk without assistance. The patient should be turned on his side and carefully observed for any respiratory obstruction or distress. Stertorous breathing can be alleviated by hyperextending the neck with the jaw held tightly shut; excessive secretions may require suctioning, and the appropriate device should be maintained in readiness at all times in the recovery area. A manual assisted-respiration bag and mask (e.g., Ambu) should also be available.

Patients should be examined for cognitive impairment between ECT sessions with a simple bedside test of orientation, recall, and retention of newly learned material (e.g., Swartz and Abrams, 1991b). A reduction in treatment frequency from three to two times per week or a change to unilateral from bilateral ECT should be considered if the patient develops cognitive impairment that requires extra nursing attention.

10

Memory and Cognitive Functioning After Electroconvulsive Therapy

Several aspects of cerebral functioning can be affected for varying intervals by ECT, depending on the number, frequency, and duration of the induced seizures, the anatomical placement of the stimulating electrodes, and the stimulus type and charge. Depending on which particular combination of these variables they receive, patients during the immediate postictal period may experience confusion and neurological dysfunction that occasionally progresses to delirium. After the postictal confusion has cleared, two specific types of memory impairment can be demonstrated: A retrograde amnesia for events preceding the seizure and an anterograde amnesia for events following it. Nonmemory cognitive impairments may also be detectable in the interictal period using various modern neuropsychological procedures. Finally, patients may experience subjective memory dysfunction that may or may not be objectively confirmed. Studies of the various aspects of ECT-induced disruption of functioning naturally divide themselves into those conducted during the immediate postictal period and those conducted after full alertness and orientation have been reestablished.

Our general understanding of the relative roles of the electrical charge and the induced seizure in causing the memory disturbance of ECT is derived largely from the work of Ottosson (1960), who compared the amnesic effects of a very high stimulus dose, a moderately suprathreshold dose, and the latter dose in which the seizure was shortened by pretreatment with intravenous lidocaine (Figure 10-1). His as yet unconfirmed conclusion that electrical dose, rather than seizure duration, determines the amnesic effects of ECT applies only to the method studied: partial sine wave bilateral ECT.

Thus, Weiner et al. (1986b) found that stimulus dose correlated significantly with autobiographical amnesia after sine-wave, but not

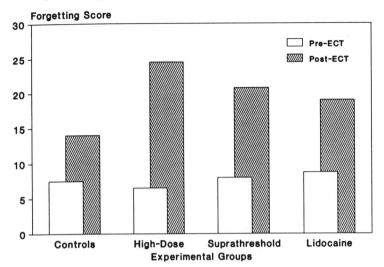

**Figure 10-1   ECT-induced forgetting: seizure versus stimulus.
(Adapted from Ottosson, 1960.)**

brief-pulse, ECT; Sackeim et al. (1986b) found no relation between
electrical dosage and memory loss for low-dose right unilateral or bilateral ECT; and Coffey et al. (1990b) found no relation between electrical dosage and either time to reorientation or Wechsler Memory
Scale scores for brief-pulse, right unilateral ECT administered at systematically higher or lower stimulus dosing over a treatment course
(mean charge at the final ECT of 199 vs 124 mC). Conversely, Miller
et al. (1985) found a significant correlation between seizure duration
and the amnesic effects of right unilateral ECT; Sackeim et al. (1986b)
found the duration of postictal disorientation directly related to seizure
duration with low-dose right unilateral, but not with bilateral, ECT;
and Calev et al. (1991b) reported a significant correlation between
seizure duration and the duration of postictal disorientation after low-
dose bilateral ECT. In a later study, Sackeim et al. (1993) found that
high-dose unilateral ECT delayed reorientation more than low-dose
unilateral ECT.

An exclusive role for the electrical stimulus in causing the amnesia of ECT is also inconsistent with the substantial memory impairment reported for nonelectrical methods of induction—pentylenetetrazol and flurothyl (Fink, 1979)—and by the extensive literature

demonstrating that the amnesic effects of bilateral ECT can be sharply reduced simply by repositioning the treatment electrodes anteriorly, or over the right hemisphere, an effect that is independent of stimulus dose (Weiner et al., 1986b; Squire and Zouzounis, 1986; Lawson et al., 1990).

These data suggest to me that when markedly suprathreshold electric currents traverse the temporal lobes and diencephalon—as with bilateral ECT (Weaver et al., 1976)—the electrical stimulus is then anatomically well-positioned to impair memory functions, which it does in relation to its intensity and to a much greater extent than the seizure that it induces. With reduced dosage, or diversion of the electrical stimulus from the structures subserving memory, however—as in low-dose bilateral ECT, unilateral ECT, or anterior bilateral ECT—the cognitive impact of the stimulus relative to the seizure is markedly reduced, and the seizure then assumes preeminence. (This argument is analogous to that previously presented concerning the relative therapeutic effects of stimulus and seizure.)

Just as no monolithic entity "ECT" was valid for the discussion of therapeutic efficacy, so arguments on the nature of ECT-induced disorientation, dysmnesia, and impaired cognition are contingent on knowledge of stimulus type, dosage, and application site.

Confusion

Although the imprecise term confusion as generally applied to ECT subsumes mainly disorientation, a patient recovering consciousness after ECT might understandably exhibit multiform abnormalities of all aspects of thinking, feeling, and behaving, including disturbed memory, impaired comprehension, automatic movements, a dazed facial expression, and motor restlessness. The term disorientation is also misleading because its "time, place, and person" components are actually memories, some recent (e.g., age and date) and some remote (e.g., name). True orientation, that is, the ability properly to locate one's self in space and time solely by environmental cues, has not been studied with regard to ECT.

Lunn and Trolle (1949) studied 21 patients during a 2-hour, post-ECT period at intervals of 10, 30, 60, and 120 minutes. Personal orientation items of name and marital state were most resistant to the effects of ECT. At the 10-minute assessment interval, 90% of the patients could give their name, whereas only 10% could give their age. This finding nicely demonstrates a temporal gradient of retrograde amnesia because a lifetime elapses between the learning of these two variables. Improvement in all functional areas was rapid but only reached 100% accuracy by the end of the 2-hour interval for items testing agnosia, visual perception, and apraxia. At the same test interval, five items of time orientation were responded to with less than 60% accuracy. The observation by Daniel and Crovitz (1986) of a close correspondence between the curves for postictal recovery of these orientation items and the temporal resolution of retrograde amnesia reported by Cronholm and Lagergren (1959) are consistent with the view that conventional tests of orientation simply measure memory.

Wilcox (1955) administered various tests of intellectual functioning at 15, 30, and 45 minutes post-ECT in 51 patients and confirmed Lunn and Trolle's (1949) results, reporting that memory for name was present in 97% of the observations made immediately on awakening, but that memory for time was often still impaired when tested 45 minutes later. Mowbray (1959) studied the recovery of consciousness after ECT in 30 patients by a method of continuous systematic interrogation from the period of postictal stupor to the re-establishment of full consciousness. Again, memory for name was present almost immediately, followed in short order by address, marital status, and birthplace, whereas memory for age, year, and date was not restored until an average elapsed time of slightly more than 45 minutes. Similar results were obtained by later investigators (Lancaster et al., 1958; Daniel and Crovitz, 1986; Daniel et al., 1987; Calev et al., 1991b).

Moreover, Daniel et al. (1987) observed that during the postictal period following ECT, patients gave responses to age and current year that were displaced backward in time, supporting the notion that such disorientation represents retrograde amnesia. With postictal clearing, however, the backward displacement became compressed, similar to the shrinking of the retrograde amnesia observed following head injury and consistent with the widely reported temporal gradient of retrograde amnesia.

The temporal gradient for memories affected during the postictal recovery period was demonstrated in a different way by Rochford and Williams (1962), who asked patients emerging from ECT to name a series of simple common objects, the names of which are acquired at different ages in childhood. Whereas *comb* (a word usually learned by 4 years of age) could be named by about 90% of patients shortly after being able to give their own names, the *teeth* of the comb (not learned until about 11 years of age) could not be named until 12 minutes later.

Relation to Treatment Electrode Placement

Early workers were unanimous in describing less postictal confusion after unilateral than after bilateral ECT (Goldman, 1949; Bayles et al., 1950; Blaurock et al., 1950; Impastato and Pacella, 1952; Liberson, 1953; Liberson et al., 1956; Thenon, 1956; Lancaster et al., 1958; Cannicott, 1962; Impastato and Karliner, 1966), although their reports can be faulted for lack of a systematic methodology and for confounding the effects of electrode placement with stimulus type (usually brief-pulse). Numerous subsequent investigators have used the time required for the postictal return of full orientation to measure more precisely the confusion induced by different treatment techniques (Gottlieb and Wilson, 1965; Valentine et al., 1968; Halliday et al., 1968; Sutherland et al., 1969; d'Elia, 1970; Fraser and Glass, 1980; Daniel and Crovitz, 1986). With the exception of the study of Gottlieb and Wilson (1965), the results confirm the earlier observations that reorientation occurs more rapidly after right unilateral ECT than after bilateral ECT. Moreover, investigators who included a left unilateral ECT group for comparison reported that this method, along with bilateral ECT, was associated with slower reorientation or more postictal confusion than right unilateral ECT (Halliday et al., 1968; Sutherland et al., 1969; Cronin et al., 1970; d'Elia, 1970). A similar advantage for right unilateral ECT is obtained when patients emerging from ECT are required to recall words or sentences learned shortly before the seizure (Lancaster et al., 1958; Cannicott and Waggoner, 1967; Valentine et al., 1968).

More recently, Sackeim et al. (1986b) studied time to reorientation in a sample of depressives receiving brief-pulse, right unilateral or bilateral ECT with stimulus charge titrated to just-above-threshold levels. With this low-dosage technique, recovery of full orientation was rapid in both treatment groups, but significantly more so after right unilateral (mean, 8.6 minutes) than after bilateral ECT (mean, 26.7 minutes). Spontaneous respirations also returned significantly earlier after unilateral than after bilateral ECT. In a subsequent comparison of low- and high-dose unilateral or bilateral ECT, Sackeim et al. (1993) found that recovery of orientation took longest with bilateral ECT regardless of dose, but that when unilateral ECT was considered separately, recovery of orientation took longer for the high-dose than the low-dose group.

Relation to Stimulus and Seizure

In addition to assigning patients randomly to unilateral or bilateral electrode placements, two groups of investigators also split assignment by stimulus type: sine-wave or brief-pulse (Valentine et al., 1968; Daniel and Crovitz, 1986). The method of statistical analysis employed by Valentine et al. (1968) does not permit a precise separation of the effects on postictal reorientation of the two treatment variables. Reorientation, however, always occurred earlier after brief-pulse than after sine-wave stimulation. Daniel and Crovitz (1986) used analysis of variance to separate treatment effects and found that full orientation was regained significantly earlier after brief-pulse than after sine-wave stimulation, an effect distinct from the equally significant advantage described earlier for unilateral compared with bilateral electrode placement. In neither of these studies is it possible to determine whether stimulus type (sine-wave versus brief-pulse) or charge is the critical determinant of postictal confusion.

Calev et al. (1991b) separately examined the effects of the stimulus charge and the duration of the induced seizure on postictal and interictal disorientation in 37 major depressives who received titrated, low-dose bilateral ECT. None of the correlations between stimulus charge and disorientation reached significance, whereas longer seizures were associated with longer disorientation times, a relationship that was independent of stimulus charge.

Delirium

Although postictal (emergence) delirium regularly occurs in patients receiving ECT (Fink, 1979; Abrams and Essman, 1982), it has received scant attention in the literature. Sackeim et al. (1983b) described two patients who manifested transient postictal delirium after bilateral and right unilateral ECT (but not after left unilateral ECT), exhibiting agitation, restlessness, clouded sensorium, disorientation, and failure to respond to commands. Based on these cases and on a proposed similarity to acute confusional states occurring after right middle cerebral artery infarction, these authors hypothesized that postictal delirium reflected a primary disruption of right-sided cerebral systems with resultant increased neurometabolic activity. Daniel (1985) reported the contradictory case of a patient who developed postictal delirium after bilateral but not after right unilateral ECT and claimed that the syndrome was nonspecific. An initial report of postictal delirium occurring in a fully-dextral man who received left unilateral ECT (Leechuy and Abrams, 1987) suggested that it was indeed premature to attribute this syndrome exclusively to right hemisphere mechanisms. This caveat was subsequently confirmed in two reports that ECT-induced postictal delirium was a random effect that occurred with equal frequency after bilateral, right unilateral, or left unilateral ECT (Leechuy, Abrams, and Kohlhaas, 1988; Liston and Sones, 1990).

Effects on Memory

The side effect of ECT principally responsible for its continued lack of full acceptance among laity and professionals alike is the disturbance in memory functioning caused primarily by sine-wave, bilateral ECT. This is no mean point, because as will be discovered later in this chapter, a fully therapeutic course of brief-pulse, right unilateral ECT typically does not induce any measurable degree of amnesia. Thus, the history of ECT research has largely been characterized by attempts to reduce the undesirable and unnecessary effects of sine-wave, bilateral ECT on memory, while retaining its beneficial action on depression and other psychiatric syndromes.

This research spans two broad eras of about 25 years each. The first era, extending roughly from the introduction of sine-wave, bilateral ECT in 1938 to the spreading acceptance of right unilateral ECT in the early 1960s, attempted to characterize the amnesic effects of sine-wave, bilateral ECT, often (but by no means always) using tasks and methodologies that were conceptually simple by today's standards. The second, extending to the present, has concentrated mainly on demonstrating the differential effects on memory of bilateral, right unilateral, and left unilateral ECT, employing more rigorous methodology (e.g., random assignment, blind assessment, and untreated control groups) and increasingly sophisticated and precise neuropsychological measures often developed for the study of lateralized hemispheric processes.

The results of the the first era of investigation have been summarized or reviewed by several authors (Campbell, 1960; Williams,

1966; Cronholm, 1969; Dornbush, 1972; Dornbush and Williams, 1974; Fink, 1979) and will generally be referred to here only in abbreviated form or for historical clarification. The second era of investigation, which provides the most important clinical and theoretical data, is covered in more detail.

In assessing the literature on ECT-induced memory loss, a distinction must be made between learning and retention (Cronholm and Ottosson, 1961a; Harper and Wiens, 1975). This is because the depressive syndrome (specifically, melancholia), either through attentional-motivational deficits or some more integral biological dysfunction, generally impairs the ability to acquire new information, and the relief of this syndrome by ECT tends to reverse this impairment. For example, the ability to learn nonsense syllables increases remarkably throughout a course of ECT (Thorpe, 1959), as does the ability to reproduce a complex visual figure (Rossi et al., 1990). Thus, a standard "memory" test, such as the Wechsler Memory Scale (Wechsler, 1945) is variously estimated to contain only 13% to 22% of memory-specific variance (Cannicott and Waggoner, 1967; Zung et al., 1968; Harper and Wiens, 1975) and measures predominantly new learning, or acquisition.

Investigators studying the effects of ECT using the Wechsler Memory Scale (and other similar instruments such as the Babcock or Gresham inventories) may incorrectly conclude simply that ECT improves memory. The same holds true for paired-associate learning tasks, also widely used to study ECT-induced amnesia. The real memory variable of interest in the context of ECT is, of course, retention: The ability to recognize, relearn, or recall (in order of increasing difficulty) previously learned material (Ottosson, 1968; Dornbush and Williams, 1974). Impaired retention for material learned before a disruptive event (in this case, ECT) constitutes retrograde amnesia; impaired retention of material learned after a disruptive event constitutes anterograde amnesia. Anterograde amnesia is tested under conditions in which patients are required to learn new material (immediate memory) and then to recognize or recall it after a timed interval has elapsed (delayed memory). The difference between immediate and delayed memory constitutes the hypothetical variable forgetting (Cronholm and Ottosson, 1961a), and it is precisely differences in forgetting induced by ECT that should be of primary interest to investigators. Naturally, forgetting (or memory decay) is inherent to all memories, and it is therefore necessary to design studies that control for normal forgetting, or baseline decay, when investigating the effects of ECT on retention.

Unfortunately, only a few investigators (e.g., Zinkin and Birtchnell, 1968; d'Elia, 1970) have done so.

Retrograde Amnesia

Cronholm and Lagergren (1959) tested the ability of endogenous depressives (among others) to recall a number learned 5, 15, and 60 seconds before a single bilateral ECT; recall was better the greater the interval between learning and ECT, clearly demonstrating a temporal gradient of retrograde amnesia and supporting the consolidation hypothesis of memory formation. In a more complex design, Cronholm and Molander (1961) used three sets of verbal and nonverbal paired associate tasks to test learning and then retention 6 hours later, on the day before the first ECT. This procedure was repeated with parallel test forms of equal difficulty on the next day, but with ECT administered 1 hour after learning. On all three tests (word pairs, figure pairs, and letter-symbol pairs), performance 6 hours after learning was much worse following the interposition of ECT, consistent with a significant adverse effect of sine-wave bilateral ECT on retention of recently learned material. Miller (1970) found a similar retrograde disruption of verbal paired-associates learned 30 minutes before bilateral ECT. Daniel and Crovitz (1983a,b) analyzed the raw data from nine published studies of ECT-induced retrograde amnesia and found that material presented 20 to 60 minutes before ECT was recalled better than that presented up to 10 minutes before ECT, and that recall of material learned before ECT was more difficult in the immediate postictal period (up to 22 minutes post-ECT) than 23 minutes or more afterwards.

Interestingly, Daniel et al. (1985) reported that the presence of postictal EEG suppression was associated with amnesia for a story told to patients 50 minutes before receiving ECT. In their study, however, it is difficult to determine whether seizure generalization or treatment electrode placement was the critical intervening variable, because bilateral ECT was strongly associated with both postictal EEG suppression and amnesia.

Although such studies of very recently learned material are of theoretical importance in defining precisely the nature of ECT-induced retrograde amnesia, they do not evaluate retention of memories acquired some time before ECT, and it is disturbed memory for such past events that is of major concern to patients, their families, and their physicians. Studies of the effects of ECT on autobiographical and other remote memories are therefore of primary clinical relevance. The first

such study was reported by Janis (1950), who obtained extensive an-
amneses concerning early schooling, travel, employment, and other life
experiences, from 19 patients scheduled to have ECT as well as from
control subjects. Four weeks after a mean course of 17 bilateral ECTs,
every patient exhibited deficits for some of the previously reported
memories, whereas such deficits rarely occurred in controls. Five of
the ECT patients were followed over a subsequent 10- to 14-week
period and continued to show such deficits in autobiographical memory. For reasons that are unclear, this excellent study was mostly discounted or ignored, perhaps because its results were inconsistent with
the prevalent clinical view of the time that ECT simply did not cause
long-term or persistent memory loss (Kalinowsky and Hoch, 1952)—
except, perhaps, in patients with preexisting marked histrionic personalities (Stengel, 1951)—or because Janis himself felt that the observed
memory deficits were related more to the patient's emotional state than
to any lasting cerebral effects of ECT.

In any case, almost 20 years elapsed before any formal attempt
was made to study this problem again (Strain et al., 1968). These
authors studied the effects of sine-wave unilateral and bilateral ECT
on several tasks, including scores derived from a Personal Data Sheet
that included 25 questions pertaining to personal experiences from the
remote past and 25 questions about recent events leading up to and
including the index hospitalization. Both treatment groups exhibited
significant retrograde amnesia (that was worse for bilateral than for
unilateral ECT) for personal memory data 36 hours after the last ECT
received. Ten days after the last treatment, both groups still showed
significant impairment, although between-treatment differences had
disappeared by this time. A 1-year follow-up study unfortunately did
not include assessment of the personal memory items (Bidder et al.,
1970), although Brunschwig et al. (1971) alluded to persistent deficits
in personal memory scores after 1 year in an abstract devoted to methodological issues in the assessment of post-ECT memory changes. In
any event, no untreated group had been included to control for "normal" forgetting.

In a comprehensive follow-up study of memory and nonmemory
cognitive impairment 1 week, and 4 and 7 months after sine-wave,
right unilateral or bilateral ECT, Weeks et al. (1980) included a 28-
item personal remote memories schedule modeled after the one used
by Strain et al. (1968). One week after a course of ECT, personal
memory recall was no different from that before starting treatment;
moreover, there were no differences between ECT patients and a

matched no-ECT control group for the number of personal memory items recalled at either of the longer follow-up intervals.

Squire et al. (1981) asked 10 depressed patients who were scheduled to receive bilateral ECT (stimulus unstated), and 7 drug-treated depressed controls, a series of personal history questions covering events in their lives occurring from 1 week to 20 years previously and ranging from naming the teachers in their first six grades to reporting everything they could remember about the day of hospitalization for their present admission. Shortly after they had ECT, there was a marked reduction in the number of autobiographical facts that the patients could recall, although about 7 months later there was no difference between ECT and control subjects for the total number of items correctly recalled. On closer examination, however, it became clear that ECT patients performed substantially worse than controls on the more recent memory items, especially those pertaining to the day of admission. Moreover, the ECT patients were less likely than controls to recognize omitted information when reminded of it by the examiners, and although this unrecognized information was mainly from recent time periods, half of the ECT patients denied recognizing some material about remote events that they had spontaneously recalled during the initial interview. In contrast, the 7 control subjects never failed to recognize such information.

Perhaps the most specific demonstration of persistent retrograde amnesia for autobiographical information after ECT appears in the conference proceedings of a 1985 meeting at the New York Academy of Sciences (Weiner et al., 1986b). These authors employed a personal memory questionnaire that was constructed from an individualized inventory of a number of items relevant to the patient's own life experiences, concentrating on the several years before the time of testing and including such items as last birthday, last New Year's Eve, favorite television program, last overnight trip out of town, and last movie seen. The questionnaire was administered before ECT, 2 to 3 days after a course of ECT, and 6 months later, to a sample of depressed patients who had been randomly assigned to receive unilateral or bilateral ECT with either brief-pulse or sine-wave stimulation (Figure 10-2).

Shortly after ECT, all patients except those receiving brief-pulse unilateral ECT were significantly impaired in the recall of these personal memory items. More importantly, only patients who had received bilateral ECT (regardless of stimulus type) continued to exhibit significant deficits on this questionnaire 6 months later.

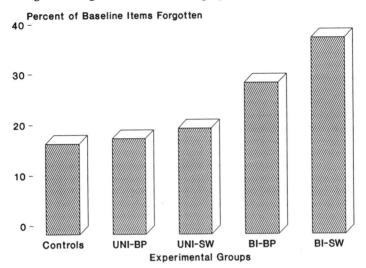

Figure 10-2   Effects of ECT treatment parameters on autobiographical amnesia. (Adapted from Weiner et al., 1986b.)

Bilateral ECT also impairs retention of nonautobiographical memories. In order to avoid the sampling bias introduced by the fact that questions about the remote past tend to sample a greater time interval and to be more general than questions about the recent past, Squire et al. (1975) developed a test in which subjects were asked to recognize the names of television programs that had been broadcast nationally between 6 and 11 P.M. for a single season between 1957 and 1972. After 5 sine-wave, bilateral ECTs, amnesia occurred for the names of programs broadcast 1 to 3 years before treatment but not for programs broadcast 4 to 17 years before treatment (Figure 10-3), demonstrating a temporal gradient of retrograde amnesia in very long term memory, once again confirming the nineteenth-century proposition that the susceptibility of a memory to disruption is proportional to its age (Ribot, 1882).

The amnesia for recently broadcast television programs, as well as that for public events of an overlapping time period, gradually subsided during the weeks after treatment and was not detectable after 7 months (Squire et al., 1981). Pre-ECT performance for the entire 15-year period was not significantly poorer in patients than in controls, demonstrating little or no effect of depressive illness on the retention

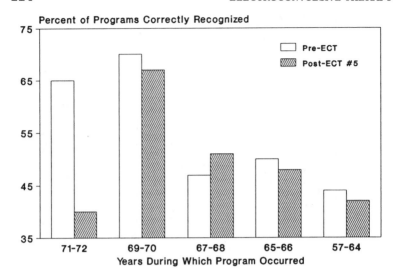

Figure 10-3   ECT and memory for TV programs broadcast during the years 1957–1972. (Adapted from Squire et al., 1975.)

of memories (in contrast to the previously described adverse effect of depression on new learning). Moreover, the fact that amnesia could occur for material learned 3 years, but not 4 years, previously suggests that the process of consolidation of memories continues for years. (In the same study, a group of 8 depressed patients who had received a course of sine-wave, right unilateral ECT showed no impairment in memory for past television programs, even as early as 1 hour after the fifth treatment.)

The study of Weeks et al. (1980) included a Famous Personalities test that required subjects to identify 50 names of famous or obscure personalities from the 1930s to the 1970s. Although no significant change in scores on this task was observed 1 week after ECT, the ECT group scored significantly lower than the no-ECT controls at the 4-month follow-up testing. By 7 months, this difference had disappeared.

EFFECTS OF ELECTRODE PLACEMENT

Retrograde amnesia for test items learned before treatment is less pronounced after right unilateral than after bilateral ECT. Lancaster et al. (1958) found that a test sentence given immediately before the first ECT was more readily recalled 15 minutes after the fourth right unilateral ECT than after the fourth bilateral ECT, and Cannicott and Waggonner (1967) reported that four words learned immediately before ECT were more readily recalled 30 minutes after right unilateral than after bilateral ECT. Valentine et al. (1968) found that free recall of verbal paired-associates learned 10 minutes before treatment was much more impaired after bilateral than after right unilateral ECT when sinusoidal current was used. Zinkin and Birtchnell (1968) also found a right unilateral ECT advantage 2 to 3 hours after treatment for recognition of pictures of common objects learned 2 to 3 minutes before ECT. d'Elia (1970) reported a similar right unilateral versus bilateral ECT advantage in the recall 5 hours after ECT of paired-associates and biographical facts learned 1 hour before treatment.

The reduced retrograde amnesic effects of right unilateral ECT compared with bilateral ECT occur regardless of whether identification of the test items learned before ECT (in this case, verbal paired-associates) is accomplished by recognition, relearning, or recall (Costello et al., 1970). A substantial and similar advantage for right unilateral compared with bilateral ECT, although not statistically significant, was also reported by Valentine et al. (1968), Sutherland et al. (1969), and Fleminger et al. (1970b). Wilson and Gottlieb (1967) provide the only contrary data in the literature, reporting less retrograde amnesia after bilateral than after right unilateral ECT for the recall, immediately on regaining consciousness, of four digits and a proverb learned 30 minutes before each of six treatments.

In their investigation of the effects of titrated low-dose brief-pulse, right unilateral and bilateral ECT, Sackeim et al. (1986b) tested patients 5 minutes after full post-ECT reorientation for the recall or recognition of words, geometric and nonsense shapes, and faces learned 15 minutes before the administration of ECT. The recall and recognition of words and the recognition of geometric and nonsense shapes were all significantly better after right unilateral than after bilateral ECT; no between-group differences occurred on the facial recognition task. The effects of ECT on these memory variables were also examined over the course of treatment, revealing that neither method was associated with cumulative impairment of retrograde memory. In fact, bilateral ECT, but not unilateral ECT, was associated with a significant cumulative improvement of nonsense shape recognition that was entirely attributable to the patients who showed marked improvement over the treatment course. Thus, low-dose brief-pulse ECT seems to have little if any effect on memory functions, regardless of treatment electrode placement.

In a subsequent study comparing bilateral with right unilateral ECT at two dosage levels, Sackeim et al. (1993) reported that bilateral ECT and high dosage both caused more impairment of performance on the memory tests for facial expression and geometric shapes, and that within the unilateral ECT group, the amnesia was greatest under the high-dose condition. Although the greater amnesic effects of bilateral ECT were still observed 1 week post-treatment, no dosage effects could be detected at that time, and no intergroup differences were found 2 months later.

EFFECTS OF THE STIMULUS

Daniel et al. (1983) studied retrograde amnesia in a sample of depressives who had been randomly assigned to right unilateral or bilateral ECT administered with either brief-pulse or sine-wave stimuli. Twenty-four hours after the fifth ECT, retrograde amnesia for events occurring 30 minutes before treatment was significantly greater with sine-wave than with brief-pulse ECT, regardless of the electrical energy (sine-wave ECT generated significantly more energy than brief-pulse ECT). This provocative finding suggests that the reduced amnesic effects of brief-pulse, square-wave therapy are inherent in differences in the stimulus configuration (e.g., its faster rise-time) rather than in the smaller charge it generally introduces into the brain compared with sine-wave stimuli. This study also confirmed prior reports of lesser retrograde amnesia after right unilateral than after bilateral ECT.

EFFECTS OF SEIZURE DURATION

In the same study, Daniel et al. (1983) found no correlation between seizure duration and retrograde amnesia. Miller et al. (1985), however, studied recall of verbal paired-associates and block designs that had been learned 20 minutes before each treatment, 20 minutes and 4 hours after each of six right unilateral ECTs, and found that seizure duration correlated modestly but significantly with retrograde amnesia for block designs, but not for verbal paired-associates, at both retesting intervals ($r = 0.4$ and 0.5, respectively).

Anterograde Amnesia

A series of deceptively simple studies on memory function in endogenous depressives before and after ECT were conducted by Cronholm and his associates at Stockholm's Karolinska Institute during the late

1950s (Figure 10-4) (Cronholm and Molander, 1957, 1961; Cronholm and Blomquist, 1959; Cronholm and Ottosson, 1960, 1961a).

These investigators introduced a procedure requiring patients to recall verbal and nonverbal materials immediately after presentation and then again after a delay of 3 hours. The immediate memory score was taken as a measure of learning ability, the delayed memory score as a measure of retention, and the difference between them as a measure of forgetting. Testing intervals and conditions varied among the substudies, but their overall conclusion was that endogenous depression was associated with an impairment of learning ability (but not retention) and that this learning impairment was reversed by the clinical improvement caused by ECT, which itself impaired retention but not learning ability. This retention deficit, however, was no longer detectable 1 month later (Cronholm and Molander, 1964). Thus, ECT converted a disorder (melancholia) characterized by poor learning and normal retention into one characterized by normal learning and poor retention (Ottosson, 1968).

In a notably sophisticated study, Korin, Fink, and Kwalwasser (1956) examined the ability of patients over a course of 12 sinewave, bilateral ECTs to learn and then recall word lists after either an

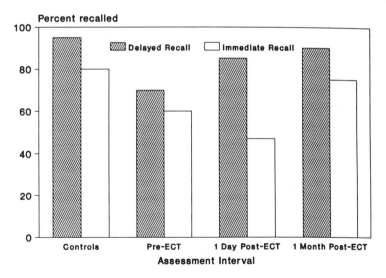

Figure 10-4   Learning versus retention in the Karolinska Institute studies. (Adapted from Cronholm et al., 1957–1961.)

interpolated nonsense-syllable learning task or a 10-minute rest period filled by reading a popular magazine. Compared with untreated controls, patients showed sharp and significant retention decrements throughout the treatment course under both delayed-recall conditions, but more markedly so after the interpolated learning task. Scores under both conditions returned to baseline 1 week post-ECT and surpassed it 2 weeks later. In this study, no relation was found between anterograde amnesia and clinical improvement.

The severity of the anterograde amnesia induced by sine-wave, bilateral ECT depends, in part, on how long ECT precedes the new learning. Squire et al. (1976) tested the ability of patients to recognize material learned up to 1 hour after ECT or 3 hours after ECT and found retention significantly better under the latter condition. Conversely, Squire and Miller (1974) demonstrated that ECT had less of an effect on the ability to retain memory contents over short retention intervals (e.g., 30 minutes) than over long ones (e.g., 24 hours), probably because consolidation of memories is a dynamic, evolving process. However, when learning occurs 6 to 10 hours after treatment, immediate retention can be normal, but delayed retention as tested 24 hours later can be markedly impaired (Squire and Chace, 1975). This means that patients who have recovered the ability to retain some newly learned material for more than 30 minutes or so, and therefore appear normal on casual observation, may actually be markedly amnesic at the time as demonstrated by their inability to reproduce that material the next day (Squire, 1982).

EFFECTS OF ELECTRODE PLACEMENT

Often included in reviews of ECT-induced anterograde amnesia (e.g., Price, 1982a; Daniel and Crovitz, 1983b), but actually more appropriately considered studies of learning, are the many investigations of the effects of left or right unilateral and bilateral ECT that employ the Wechsler Memory Scale (or similar memory inventories) or paired-associate learning tasks without a delayed-recall condition (Martin et al., 1965; Zamora and Kaelbling, 1965; Cohen et al., 1968; Levy, 1968; Sutherland et al., 1969; Cronin et al., 1970; Fleminger et al., 1970a,b; Fromholt et al., 1973). Without exception, these studies show greater impairment in verbal learning after bilateral or left unilateral ECT than after right unilateral ECT. Moreover, several studies using these and other verbal tasks actually find an improvement in verbal learning after right unilateral ECT (Martin et al., 1965; Zamora and

Kaelbling, 1965; Sutherland et al., 1969; Costello et al., 1970; Strömgren et al., 1976).

The following investigators specifically studied anterograde amnesia. Halliday et al. (1968) used verbal and nonverbal learning tasks with a 30-minute delayed-recall condition to assess anterograde amnesia after sine-wave, left and right unilateral and bilateral ECT. No differences in delayed recall were found between right unilateral and bilateral ECT; left unilateral ECT was associated with the greatest recall decrement among the three methods. Zinkin and Birtchnell (1968) assessed delayed recall after 5, 20, and 60 minutes in their picture-recognition task and found anterograde amnesia to be significantly worse after sine-wave bilateral than after right unilateral ECT. d'Elia (1970) used the Cronholm and Molander (1957) memory battery to study anterograde amnesia after right unilateral and bilateral ECT. When he calculated before- and after-ECT change scores for the variables of forgetting and delayed recall, he was unable to demonstrate increased verbal forgetting with either method, although delayed recall scores were significantly lower after bilateral ECT. The importance of this study lies in the fact that changes in forgetting before and after ECT are arguably the most appropriate measure of anterograde amnesia induced by this treatment. This is also the only comparison of the verbal anterograde amnesic effects of right unilateral and bilateral ECT to account for baseline decay when assessing retention differences.

Dornbush, Abrams, and Fink (1971) examined the short-term (18 seconds) and long-term (3 hours) retention of verbal and visual memory in endogenous depressives with delayed recall tasks presented before and 24 hours after four to five sine-wave, right unilateral or bilateral ECTs. Short-term auditory verbal memory was tested by asking the patients to recall nonsense consonant trigrams (e.g., DLG) presented by tape at intervals of 0, 6, 12, and 18 seconds after learning, with retention intervals filled with an interposed rote task (number reading) to prevent rehearsal.

Neither method impaired trigram learning (the 0-second interval), and unilateral ECT did not affect retention at any of the other test intervals. Bilateral ECT, however, significantly impaired retention at the 6-second interval and thereafter, presumably by disrupting the holding period required for transfer of information from short-term to long-term memory store (Figure 10-5).

The paired-associate learning task of the Wechsler Memory Scale was also administered, with a delayed-recall requirement introduced 3

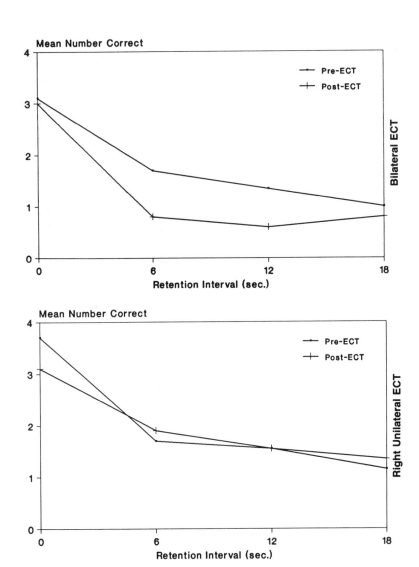

Figure 10-5   Auditory short-term memory for bilateral and uni-lateral ECT. (Adapted from Dornbush, Abrams, and Fink, 1971.)

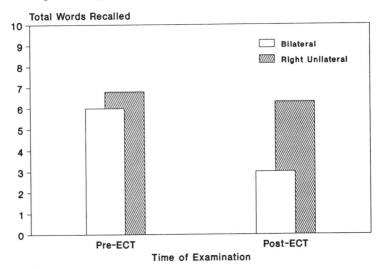

Figure 10-6   Paired-associate recall with bilateral and unilateral ECT. (Adapted from Dornbush, Abrams, a..d Fink, 1971.)

hours post-testing. As expected, bilateral, but not right unilateral ECT significantly impaired delayed recall of the second half of the word-pairs learned 3 hours earlier (Figure 10-6).

We also devised a visuospatial short-term memory task with low verbal encodability for this study that required patients to reproduce the location of a circle on a straight line after the same filled retention intervals described earlier (Figure 10-7). Neither unilateral nor bilateral ECT impaired retention at any of the filled intervals, but immediate retention at 0 seconds was significantly better with unilateral than bilateral ECT (performance improved with the former and worsened with the latter).

This result suggests that this task may require the time-dependent, sequential processing skills of the left hemisphere (Horan, Ashton, and Minto, 1980). Longer-term verbal retention was also studied using the paired-associates subtest of the Wechsler Memory Scale presented in the usual three learning trials and then 3 hours later to measure delayed recall, a variable that was significantly impaired by bilateral but not right unilateral ECT.

Fromholt et al. (1973) included a delayed-recall task (the Logical Memory subtests of the Wechsler Memory Scale) in their comparison

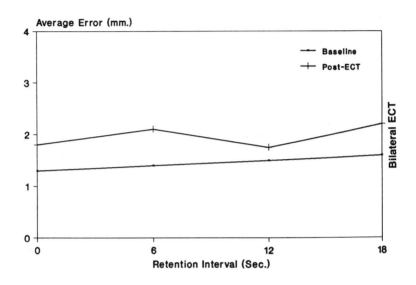

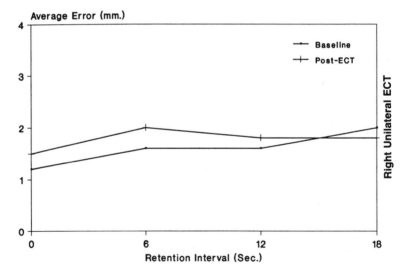

Figure 10-7 Visual memory effects of bilateral and unilateral ECT. (Adapted from Dornbush, Abrams, and Fink, 1971.)

of the relative effects of sine-wave, right unilateral and bilateral ECT on the Wechsler Memory Scale, and found that six right unilateral ECTs were followed by better retention of the memory passages 20 minutes after learning, as well as by the higher Wechsler Memory Scale scores previously noted.

Squire and Slater (1978) also compared the effects of sine-wave, right unilateral and bilateral ECT using the short-term retention tasks of Dornbush, Abrams, and Fink (1971), adding an additional long-term (16 to 19 hours) verbal task of paragraph recall and a visual one requiring recall of the complex Rey-Osterreith geometric figure. These authors confirmed the reported impairment in short-term verbal memory retention after bilateral, but not after right unilateral, ECT, as well as the advantage of right unilateral compared with bilateral ECT in retention of visuospatial material. In addition, they reported that bilateral ECT (but not right unilateral ECT) markedly reduced the number of paragraph segments retained after 16 to 19 hours and that both methods impaired the ability to reproduce the Rey-Osterreith figure at the same interval, bilateral ECT significantly more so than right unilateral ECT.

Using visually presented stimuli of systematically varying verbal encodability (low- and high-imagery nouns, pictures of common objects, geometric designs, and nonsense figures), and including no-ECT patient controls, normal controls, and a delayed-recognition condition, Robertson and Inglis (1978) found that bilateral ECT induced similar retention deficits across all tasks, whereas the deficits after right unilateral ECT rose with increasing nonverbal task mediation, reaching significance only for nonsense figures. Bilateral ECT induced significantly greater retention deficits compared with right unilateral ECT for low- and high-imagery nouns and pictures of common objects, but not for geometric designs or nonsense figures. The results of this model study were interpreted by its authors to support Paivio's (1969, 1971) dual-encoding model of verbal learning that specifies those stimulus and task attributes that vary the extent to which memory and learning depend upon symbolic (verbal) and imagery (nonverbal) encoding. Symbolic encoding is evoked by verbal and abstract stimuli and by demands for the sequential processing of information. The imagery system is evoked by concrete stimuli and by demands for parallel processing.

This portrayal of the mechanisms or processes involved in information acquisition and retention clearly overlaps with the material-specific view (verbal versus nonverbal) of human cerebral asymmetry:

The symbolic and imagery systems relate strongly to the left and right hemispheres. It finds support in the later study of Horan, Ashton, and Minto (1980), who demonstrated in two separate samples that right unilateral ECT, but not bilateral ECT, significantly improved performance on a relatively pure sequential processing task, the Knox Cube Imitation test. These authors suggest that right unilateral ECT suppression of right hemisphere interference allowed the left hemisphere's sequential processing mode to operate more efficiently. Such reasoning can explain a variety of otherwise puzzling reports that right unilateral ECT improves verbal memory performance (Martin et al., 1965; Zamora and Kaelbling, 1965; Sutherland et al., 1969; Costello et al., 1970; Strömgren et al., 1976). The findings of Zinkin and Birtchnell (1968) and Halliday et al. (1968) that bilateral and left unilateral ECT caused greater difficulty than right unilateral ECT on visual recognition tasks of relatively high verbal encodability likewise fit the model, as does Williams' (1973) demonstration that patients receiving right unilateral, but not bilateral, ECT more frequently recognized nominal compared with pictorial representations of pictures of common objects learned before treatment, and Ashton and Hess' (1976) report that right unilateral and bilateral ECT induced equivalent retrograde amnesia for complex geometric forms of low verbal encodability. In the same vein, Weeks et al. (1980) included a delayed recall task that required patients to remember nine pictorially presented common objects after a 10-minute interval that was filled with another memory task. One week after a course of treatment, patients receiving bilateral ECT recalled significantly fewer items than those receiving right unilateral ECT, a difference that was no longer apparent 4 and 7 months post-ECT.

Sackeim et al. (1986b) included measures of delayed recall to test anterograde effects of low-dose ECT (separate analyses for unilateral and bilateral groups were unfortunately not presented in this report), and included a normal control group for comparison. Before the first ECT, after the seventh ECT, and 4 days after the last ECT of their course, patients were tested for their performance on verbal and nonverbal (faces) paired-associate learning tasks; 4 hours later recognition memory for these pairs was tested again, providing a measure of delayed recall. At the pretreatment session, patients performed significantly worse than controls on immediate recognition memory (learning), but did not exhibit a greater rate of forgetting over the 4-hour delay, confirming the work of earlier investigators (e.g., Cronholm and Ottosson, 1961a). Although there was a significant reduction in immediate recognition memory scores after the seventh ECT compared with baseline, 4 days after the last ECT no such deficit could be demonstrated. In contrast, delayed memory scores were reduced following both the seventh and final treatments, also supporting the claim of earlier workers that ECT had different effects on the acquisition and retention of information (Cronholm and Ottosson, 1961a).

Calev et al. (1989) showed that the anterograde amnesia induced by titrated, low-dose, bilateral ECT for verbal paired-associates was not significantly different from that with imipramine: ECT increased forgetting by 77%, compared with 60% for imipramine. Neither treatment method significantly impaired nonverbal recall of a complex figure.

EFFECTS OF SEIZURE DURATION

The study of Miller et al. (1985) of right unilateral ECT described earlier in the retrograde amnesia section also included a delayed recall condition in which patients learned verbal and nonverbal material 4 hours post-ECT and were tested for recall 20 hours later. As was true for retrograde amnesia, anterograde amnesia for block designs, but not for verbal paired-associates, significantly correlated with seizure duration: The longer the seizure, the greater the forgetting.

COGNITIVE EFFECTS OF SUBCONVULSIVE STIMULATION

Ottosson's (1960) original elegant experiment demonstrating that bilateral ECT-induced memory loss is primarily a function of the electrical dosage administered has been confirmed by Sackeim et al. (1993), and also extended to unilateral ECT. Because subconvulsive stimulation also involves passing an electric current through the brain, it is reasonable to predict adverse memory consequences from this form of stimulation as well. Fortunately, Cronholm and Ottosson (1961b) also examined this possibility in a study of the effects on retrograde amnesia of three different forms of electrical stimulation for bilateral ECT: (1) conventional suprathreshold seizure induction; (2) conventional suprathreshold seizure induction followed by 1 minute of weak subconvulsive stimulation; and (3) conventional suprathreshold seizure induction followed by 1 minute of strong subconvulsive stimulation. The experimental variable ''forgetting'' (immediate recall minus delayed recall) was evaluated before and 1 hour after ECT using memory tests of verbal paired associates, figural reproduction, and autobiographical data. Compared with simple seizure induction, the addition of weak subconvulsive stimulation increased the combined forgetting score for the three tests by 24%, and the addition of strong subconvulsive stimulation increased the combined forgetting score by 71% (only the latter increase was statistically significant), thus nicely demonstrating a graded effect of prolonged subconvulsive stimulation in aggravating the retrograde amnesia consequent to a single induced seizure.

In view of the American Psychiatric Association Task Force (1990) recommendation concerning stimulus titration via multiple sub-convulsive stimulations, and the report (Farah and McCall, 1993) that about 40% of U.S. practitioners routinely employ this method, it is important to know how this procedure affects memory and orientation. The expectation I expressed in the previous edition of this book was that multiple subconvulsive stimuli administered in the same treatment session via bilateral electrode placement would inevitably have a dysmnesic effect.

It is therefore disappointing that the only modern article to study the cognitive effects of subconvulsive stimulation did not examine the stimulus titration procedure per se but, because of problems relating to the uniqueness of the first seizure of a treatment course, limited its investigations to single subconvulsive stimuli that chanced to occur later on in treatment (Prudic et al., 1994). In this study, which com-pared treatment sessions in which generalized seizures were preceded by a single subconvulsive stimulation with those in which only single, convulsive stimulations were administered, no adverse cognitive con-sequences of single unilateral or bilateral subconvulsive stimulations were found, despite the fact that the total charge administered in convulsive-only sessions was less than half that administered in ses-sions containing a subconvulsive stimulus.

Although questions remain concerning the cognitive conse-quences of the full stimulus titration procedure, which often entails the administration of multiple subconvulsive stimuli with requisite dosage increments at each step, the study of Prudic et al. (1994) makes it unlikely that such consequences will be substantial.

PERSISTENCE OF ANTEROGRADE AMNESIA

Anterograde amnesia for recently learned material diminishes fairly rapidly after ECT. Squire, Shimamura, and Graf (1985) presented word lists to patients 45 minutes, 60 minutes, 85 minutes, and 9 hours after four or five ECTs, testing retention by recognition of the words 15 minutes after each presentation. After bilateral ECT, retention was in-itially no better than chance but increased to about 80% correct rec-ognition by the 9-hour test interval (a control group of depressed patients not receiving ECT obtained a mean of 95% correct answers). Patients receiving unilateral ECT were not significantly impaired on this test, obtaining 80% to 90% correct answers at all test intervals.

Comparison with Antidepressant Drugs

In an open clinical trial, Calev et al. (1989) compared the anterograde and retrograde amnesic effects of 3 weeks of imipramine, 200 mg/day, with those of a course of 7 titrated, low-dose, brief-pulse, bilateral ECTs. Both treatment methods produced similar and significant deficits in performance on a verbal anterograde memory task (paired-associates retention), but only ECT impaired retrograde memory for autobiographical and public events. Neither treatment induced deficits in either immediate memory span (digit recall) or visual retention (complex figure reproduction).

Nonmemory Cognitive Effects

Neuropsychological issues of lateralized hemispheric specialization of function that were raised by the introduction of unilateral ECT stimulated most of the studies of ECT-induced nonmemory cognitive impairment reviewed in this section. Earlier studies have been reviewed elsewhere (e.g., Campbell, 1960; Fink, 1979; Price, 1982b) and are difficult to assess because they were not blind, often contained mixed diagnostic groups, and frequently tested patients after much longer courses of ECT (e.g., 20 or more) than would be given today. In general, however, impairments in various perceptual and psychomotor performance tasks were observed immediately after sine-wave, bilateral ECT, recovering to pretreatment levels or better by about 2 weeks after the last seizure.

McAndrew, Berkey, and Matthews (1967) were the first to use lateralized neuropsychological tests to study the effects of sine-wave left or right unilateral ECT and bilateral ECT in a small sample of depressives (8 per group). Cognitive functions generally improved after ECT, and these authors found no differences among or within the three treatment groups for performance on Halstead categories, finger tapping, sandpaper roughness discrimination, maze coordination, the grooved pegboard, finger agnosia, and the WAIS similarities, vocabulary, digit span, block design, and picture arrangements subtests. It is doubtful, however, that their sample was large enough to permit them to detect an existing real difference among the methods. They observed a tendency for improvement in performance on hemisphere-related tasks to occur following unilateral stimulation of that hemisphere.

Using a similar battery of tasks to study patients randomly assigned to receive either left or right sine-wave, unilateral ECT, Small et al. (1972) found that five right unilateral ECTs improved performance on a number of right-hemisphere Halstead subtests, but the reverse was not true following left unilateral ECT. In an extension of this study that included a bilateral ECT group, Small et al. (1973) found that all three electrode placements were associated with improved performance on nonverbal cognitive tasks.

Annett et al. (1974) employed naming and visual discrimination tasks administered before and 30 minutes after sine-wave, left or right unilateral ECT and found that although left unilateral ECT impaired naming ability, right unilateral ECT did not impair visual discrimination. Berent et al. (1975) found significant impairment on a verbal task 5 hours after a single left unilateral ECT, and significant impairment on a nonverbal task after right unilateral ECT under the same conditions. Interestingly, this latter degree of nonverbal impairment was similar to that observed after 5 ECTs in an earlier study from the same laboratory (Cohen et al., 1968), whereas the verbal impairment consequent to five left unilateral ECTs in that study had been much greater than that observed by Berent et al. (1975) after a single treatment. This observation led these authors to suggest that the left hemisphere was more susceptible than the right to the cumulative effects of a series of ECT.

Kronfol et al. (1978) studied the effects of sine-wave, left and right unilateral ECT on verbal and nonverbal tests after both a single ECT and a course of eight treatments. The neuropsychological measures were chosen to be relatively hemisphere-specific on the basis of prior studies in patients with lateralized brain damage and had all been developed in the neuropsychology laboratory at the University of Iowa. They included left hemisphere tasks of Digit Sequence Learning, Controlled Word Association, Sentence Repetition, and the Token Test, and right hemisphere tasks of Form Sequence Learning, Judgment of Line Orientation, Three-Dimensional Constructional Praxis, and Facial Recognition. Despite considerable variability in right and left hemisphere task performance observed after single ECTs given with either treatment method, the statistically significant and clinically relevant findings of this study are limited to the observations that eight left unilateral ECT impaired performance on one left hemisphere task, and eight right unilateral ECTs improved performance on one right hemisphere task. The most striking aspect of this study is the absence of systematic lateralized hemispheric effects of either left- or right-sided unilateral ECT even when carefully studied by a highly trained research neuro-psychologist using sophisticated and well-validated measures. The relatively meager results obtained are consonant with results of several other studies demonstrating a decline in left hemisphere task performance after left unilateral ECT (Cronin et al., 1970; d'Elia and Raotma, 1975; Berent et al., 1975) and an improvement in right hemisphere task performance after right unilateral ECT (McAndrew et al., 1967; Small et al., 1972; Dornbush, Abrams, and Fink, 1971; Horan, Ashton, and Minto, 1980). However, they are likewise dissonant with studies showing that right unilateral ECT improves performance on some left hemisphere tasks (Zamora and Kaelbling, 1965; Martin et al., 1965; Cannicott and Waggoner, 1967; Halliday et al., 1968; Costello et al., 1970; Fromholt et al., 1973; Strömgren et al., 1976) and impairs performance on right hemisphere tasks (Cohen et al., 1968; Robertson and Inglis, 1978) and that left unilateral ECT improves performance on right hemisphere tasks (Small et al., 1973).

In fact, the findings by Kronfol et al. (1978) that right unilateral ECT improved performance on three ''right hemisphere'' tasks (Form Sequence Learning, Three-Dimensional Constructional Praxis, and Judgment of Line Orientation, with only the last reaching statistical significance) suggests that these tasks may demand substantial sequential processing by the left hemisphere (Robertson and Inglis, 1978). This is clearly the case for the Form Sequence Learning task, and anyoné taking the Judgment of Line Orientation test can readily testify that it requires an iterative, and therefore sequential, mental matching of the pair of test lines with each pair in the array of choices. The Three-Dimensional Constructional Praxis task does not at first blush seem to require sequential processing, but it is notably the only one of the tasks to show impairment after left hemisphere lesions. Weeks et al. (1980) also included a variety of nonmemory cognitive tasks in their study and found significant improvement in choice reaction time and visual perceptual analysis 1 week after a course of ECT.

Taylor and Abrams (1985) studied primarily nonmemory neuro-psychological functioning in a sample of 37 melancholic patients who were randomly assigned to receive either right unilateral or bilateral sine-wave ECT. Patients were examined before ECT and again 48 to 72 hours after their sixth ECT on an extensive test battery that included evaluation of neurological soft signs, aphasia testing, the Mini-Mental

State Examination (Folstein et al., 1975), tachistoscopically presented verbal and nonverbal materials, and a variety of tasks selected from the Halstead-Reitan (Reitan, 1955) and Luria-Nebraska (Golden et al., 1978) test batteries. Test protocols were scored blindly and assigned global, hemispheric, and regional cortical impairment scores.

In this sample, 6 ECTs with either electrode placement did not significantly increase global cognitive impairment scores, nor were increases in regional hemispheric cortical impairment scores observed after right unilateral ECT (Figure 10-8). Bilateral ECT worsened only the right temporal lobe score; this finding, coupled with a nonsignificant improvement in the same score induced by right unilateral ECT, led to the only real cognitive difference between electrode placements observed in the study.

Jones, Henderson and Welch (1988) used a battery of 10 neuropsychological tests (20 variables) known to be sensitive to frontal-lobe lesions (e.g., Wisconsin card-sorting test, controlled word-association test) to examine unipolar depressives before and after courses of ECT administered with the four possible combinations of stimulus waveform and treatment electrode placement, all of which were unfortunately combined in the data analysis. The immediate effect of ECT on

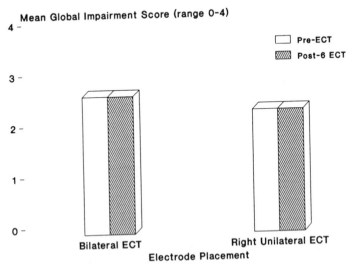

Figure 10-8   Immediate nonmemory cognitive effects of ECT. (Adapted from Taylor and Abrams, 1985.)

the 20 variables tested was significant only for performance on the Thurstone word fluency test, which was worse 48 hours after treatment.

Williams et al. (1990) studied dichotic perception and a mixed battery of 3 immediate and 2 long-term memory tasks before and after a course of 8 to 12 right unilateral sine-wave ECTs in a sample of 11 acutely depressed patients. In contrast to the authors' study hypothesis, dichotic listening errors fell in both ears after ECT—significantly so only in the right ear—and performance on the 3 immediate memory tasks improved slightly, all confirming the previously reported ECT-induced normalization or improvement of hemispheric functioning presumably related to improvement in the depressed state.

Intelligence Quotient

Intelligence quotient (IQ) tests are mixed neuropsychological test batteries that contain only modest numbers of memory-related items. The Wechsler Memory Scale, although not specifically an IQ test, correlates very highly with the Wechsler-Bellevue and Wechsler Adult Intelligence Scales (WAIS), so it should come as no surprise that the older literature shows that bilateral ECT does not impair (and may improve) performance on these and similar instruments (Huston and Strother, 1948; Fisher, 1949; Stieper, Williams, and Duncan, 1951; Foulds, 1952; Summerskill, Seeman, and Meals, 1952). More recently, Squire et al. (1975) demonstrated that the verbal IQ and arithmetic subtests (the latter considered to be particulary sensitive to cerebral dysfunction) of the WAIS tested 1 hour after 6 sine-wave, bilateral ECTs were the same as before ECT (Figure 10-9).

Follow-up Studies

Squire and Chace (1975) examined memory functions in a retrospective follow-up study of patients who had received courses of right unilateral or bilateral ECT 6 to 9 months earlier and in control patients who had never received ECT. To maximize test sensitivity, 1-day and 2-week intervals were interposed between learning and retention, and assessments of memory functions were made with six different tests of new learning and remote memory capacity. No objective evidence for persisting memory impairment (e.g., the ability to learn and retain) could be found on any of the tests (Figure 10-10).

The Squire et al. (1981) study reviewed earlier was part of a larger, prospective, follow-up study of retrograde amnesia induced by

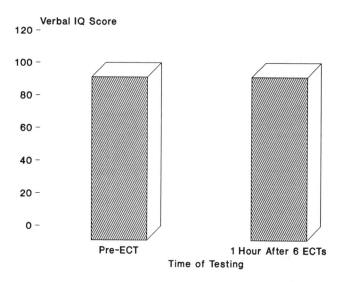

Figure 10-9 Effects of ECT on verbal IQ. (Adapted from Squire et al., 1975.)

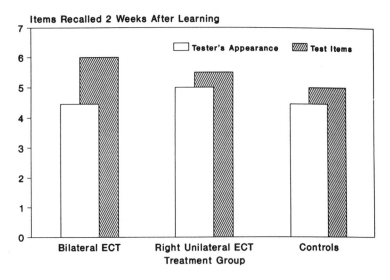

Figure 10-10 Memory function 6 to 9 months after ECT. (Adapted from Squire and Chace, 1975.)

bilateral ECT. In addition to the autobiographical memory items already discussed, the authors included tests of recognition and recall of public events and recall of previously broadcast television programs, all administered before ECT, 1 week after completion of treatment, and about 7 months later (Figure 10-11). At this latter test interval, no persistent deficits could be demonstrated in the recognition or recall of the public events or television program items. As already noted, strong evidence for persistent memory loss was limited to personal events that had occurred a few days or weeks before treatment.

The study by Weeks et al. (1980) was also the first controlled, prospective study of enduring nonmemory cognitive deficits in depressed patients after right unilateral and bilateral ECT. One week after a course of ECT, patients did not exhibit any cognitive worsening compared with their pretreatment performance; indeed, they improved significantly on certain tasks. Compared with the performance of non-ECT treated depressives and with matched normal controls, on a comprehensive test battery, patients who had ECT showed no impairment at 4 or 7 months post-treatment (Figure 10-12). There was a significant cognitive advantage for right unilateral ECT compared with bilateral ECT at 1 week post-treatment (right unilateral ECT patients were

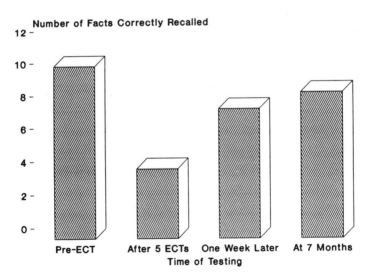

Figure 10-11   Memory for public events at various post-ECT intervals. (Adapted from Squire et al., 1981.)

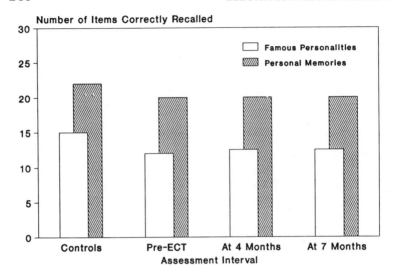

Figure 10-12   Effect of ECT on memory for personal and public events. (Adapted from Weeks et al., 1980.)

actually quite similar to controls on many tasks) that was no longer present at 4 and 7 weeks.

A subsequent long-term follow-up study of nonmemory cognitive functions after ECT confirmed these results. Abrams and Taylor (1985) examined 13 patients before ECT, 1 day after 6 right unilateral or bilateral ECTs, and 30 days, 6 months, 1 year, and 2 years after completion of a treatment course, comparing their scores on a global impairment index (calculated from a comprehensive cognitive test battery) with those of a sample of age-equated normal controls. Because no significant cognitive differences were found between right unilateral and bilateral ECT in this sample, the two groups were combined for analysis.

Patients exhibited significantly more global cognitive impairment than controls at baseline and 1 day after 6 ECTs, but were not significantly different from controls at the 30-day, 6-month, and 1- to 2-year follow-up intervals. Within patients, global impairment scores were reduced (but not significantly) from baseline levels 1 day after 6 ECTs, with further reductions observed during the follow-up period, so that 1 to 2 years later impairment scores were very substantially reduced below pre-ECT levels (Figure 10-13).

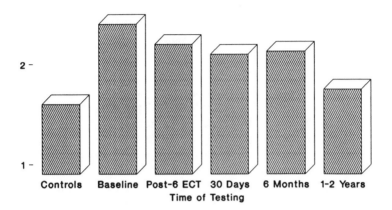

Figure 10-13   One to two-year follow-up of cognitive functions after ECT in 13 patients. (Adapted from Abrams and Taylor, 1985.)

Williams et al. (1990) found that although autobiographical and logical memory were impaired during 2 weeks after sine-wave, right unilateral ECT, no evidence for persistent cognitive dysfunction on verbal or visuospatial memory or dichotic listening performance was found in a sample of 15 patients tested at least 6 months after their last ECT.

In the only follow-up study of patients who have received unusually large numbers of ECTs, Devanand et al. (1991) compared 8 patients who had each received more than 100 lifetime treatments with sine-wave, bilateral ECT (mean of 12 courses and 160 ECTs) with a closely matched control group who had never received ECT. The two groups did not differ on any measure of objective or subjective cognitive functioning, including an abbreviated version of the subjective memory rating of Squire et al. (1979).

Notable in a personal, but unusually forceful, context is the experience of Janet Frame, who received over 200 applications of unmodified bilateral ECT during 8 years of hospitalization for "chronic schizophrenia" (in fact, she was never mentally ill) and who then narrowly escaped leucotomy to become New Zealand's most acclaimed writer and winner of two coveted literary awards (Frame, 1984).

Prediction of Post-ECT Cognitive Impairment

Scant attention has been paid in the literature to predictors of ECT-induced cognitive impairment other than age, treatment electrode placement, seizure duration, and stimulus dose. In the first study of whether preexisting cognitive impairment constitutes a risk factor, Sobin et al. (1995) examined a sample of 71 depressed patients randomly assigned to high- or low-dose right unilateral or bilateral ECT, and found that pretreatment global cognitive status assessed via Mini-Mental State Examination (Folstein et al., 1975), and postictal orientation recovery time, were both significantly associated with retrograde amnesia for autobiographical memories 1 week and 2 months after their treatment course, regardless of treatment group assignment. These findings suggest that the Mini-Mental State Examination might be used as a screening test to guide the selection of ECT treatment parameters demonstrated to affect cognition—treatment electrode placement, stimulus characteristics, and frequency of administration—and that postictal disorientation should be routinely assessed for the same purpose.

Subjective Memory Dysfunction

In one of the Cronholm and Ottosson (1963a) studies of immediate and delayed recall and retention after ECT, patients were asked 1 week after a course of treatment whether they felt their memory was worse, unchanged, or better. The experience of relief from depression was associated with a subjective sense of improved memory and correlated with improved performance on the immediate recall (learning) tasks, but not on retention, and with verbal, but not visuospatial, performance. The finding of subjective improvement in depression-sensitive memory complaints after ECT has been confirmed by Pettinati and Rosenberg (1984) and Mattes et al. (1990).

Although, as noted earlier, Squire and Chace (1975) could not detect objective evidence of impaired learning, retention, or remote memory 6 to 9 months after right unilateral or bilateral ECT, 63% of the bilaterally treated sample complained of impaired memory since their treatment, compared with 30% of the right unilateral group (and

17% of the no-ECT controls). The authors interpreted the patients' subjective experiences in terms of their expectation that they might suffer long-term memory difficulties.

Subsequently, Squire et al. (1979) developed a new self-rating instrument for assessing subjective memory functioning after ECT, requiring subjects to rate themselves on a continuum from "worse than ever before" to "better than ever before" on 18 items reflecting recognition, recall, retention, comprehension, concentration, and alertness. These authors found persistent complaints of memory impairment in some patients as long as 6 months after an average course of 11 bilateral ECTs. These complaints closely resembled those occurring 1 week after treatment had ended but were sharply different qualitatively from those observed before ECT, suggesting to the authors that the patient's experience of altered memory 6 months after the course of bilateral ECT could not be attributed solely to illness variables (e.g., depressed mood, low self-esteem). Freeman, Weeks, and Kendell (1980) examined a nonsystematically obtained sample of patients who complained of persistent cognitive dysfunction a mean of 10 years after having had a course of ECT, most with bilateral electrode placement. These patients generally performed as well as no-ECT controls on most subtests of a battery of 19 memory and nonmemory cognitive tasks but were significantly impaired on several tasks, a few even scoring in the organic impairment range. The authors concluded that a small subgroup of patients receiving ECT might suffer permanent memory impairment.

In a 3-year follow-up study of the sample of Squire et al. (1979), Squire and Slater (1983) found that patients who had received bilateral ECT generally felt that they had difficulty remembering events from about 6 months before ECT to 2 months afterward. In fact, 50% of the patients who had received bilateral ECT felt that their memory had never returned to normal. Again, the pattern of memory complaints resembled much more closely the one reported 1 week after ECT, when patients were amnesic, than the pattern before treatment, when they were depressed. The significance of the patients' subjective estimate that ECT induced 6 months' retrograde amnesia is doubtful because they reported nearly the same phenomenon (5 months' retrograde amnesia) when examined before ECT 3 years earlier. Right unilateral ECT was generally not associated with the subjective experience of memory impairment.

These reports contrast with patients' subjective self-ratings of memory function immediately following ECT. Sackeim et al. (1993)

observed that despite demonstrated objective cognitive deficits, their patients reported marked (mean = 43%) subjective improvement in their memory, a phenomenon that was related to improvement in depressive symptoms. Even more striking, because of the much higher stimulus doses used (fixed high dose = 403 mC) is the observation of McCall et al. (1995) that their patients reported significantly fewer problems in subjective global memory after, than before, ECT.

Management of Memory Impairment

No specific treatment is available to reduce the memory impairment of ECT, which occurs in its most pronounced form after bilateral ECT, especially when administered at a high dosage or frequency (e.g., with a sine-wave stimulus or as multiple seizures in a single-treatment session). The hope generated by early case reports (Weingartner et al., 1981; Partap et al., 1983) that vasopressin might attenuate ECT-induced memory impairment proved ephemeral: A recent random-assignment, double-blind, placebo-controlled trial of intranasal vasopressin provides no evidence that this hormone attenuates bilateral ECT-induced anterograde or retrograde amnesia or the related subjective memory complaints (Mattes et al., 1990).

The physician is thus left with several practical measures to take in the event that emergent confusion and memory loss become problematic during a course of ECT. If sine-wave or conventional bilateral ECT are being used, the obvious step is to switch to a brief-pulse stimulus and unilateral or anterior bilateral ECT. If a thrice-weekly treatment schedule is in force, reducing the frequency to twice a week will help. The physiological principles discussed in Chapter 6 governing neuronal discharge and recovery can also be applied here, because increasing the efficiency of the stimulus parameter package should reduce cognitive side effects as well as augment the therapeutic impact. Lowering the pulse width to the 0.25 msec to 0.5 msec range, and the frequency to the 40 to 70 Hz range, without altering the dosage, should reduce memory loss and confusion by reducing the charge rate. If bilateral ECT is being used, the dosage can be reduced to the lowest level that is compatible with inducing a well-developed EEG seizure pattern. However, I recommend against lowering the dosage with unilateral ECT for reasons already specified in Chapters 6 and 7. Fortunately, cognitive dosage effects of unilateral ECT are reported to be undetectable 1 week after the treatment course (Sackeim et al., 1993).

Summary

A remarkable amount of knowledge has accumulated on the effects of ECT on memory, and the day is now past when the physician administering sine-wave, bilateral ECT can blithely assure his patient that "the memory-loss will only be temporary." True, many who receive such therapy will not complain of persistent dysmnesia, either because none exists or because they are characteristically the ones with the highly favorable therapeutic responses, who are likewise known for their denial-prone personality structure and the development of anosognosia after treatment (Fink et al., 1959b; Kahn and Fink, 1959).

Although more studies are needed to confirm and extend those of essentially two investigators and their associates (see Squire, 1986), the data now at hand are adequate to provide patients a reasonably accurate indication of what to expect with bilateral ECT: At best, transient memory disturbances for events immediately before and after the course of treatment, clearing within a few weeks; at worst, significant memory deficits for a period extending from 6 months or more before ECT to 2 months afterward, which may persist objectively for as long as 6 months or more and subjectively for as long as several years afterwards. Moreover, all patients receiving bilateral ECT will experience permanent memory gaps (anterograde amnesia) for some events occurring during the course of treatment, especially on treatment days. Patients can be assured, however, that no permanent effects on memory functioning will occur (that is, the ability to learn and retain new information) and that nonmemory cognitive functions, including intelligence and its components of reasoning, judgment, comprehension, and abstract thinking—as well as visual-motor and perceptual skills—will also be unaffected and will likely improve in comparison to their pretreatment status.

The situation with right unilateral ECT is far more favorable. Patients can be assured that little or no retrograde or anterograde memory disturbance will occur during or immediately following the treatment course and that whatever dysmnesia does occur will be transient and undetectable, objectively or subjectively, 6 months later. The most striking finding in this context in recent years has been the even more benign effects on memory that result when right unilateral ECT is administered with brief-pulse stimulation (Weiner et al., 1986b). Among all stimulus and electrode combinations, one finds that only patients receiving brief-pulse, right unilateral ECT were found to be no different from untreated controls on every measure of amnesia studied, either 2 or 3 days after a treatment course or 6 months later. This was most apparent in the very sensitive Personal Memory Recall questionnaire that included, among other items, recent outstanding experiences as well as events of the current hospitalization: All groups except controls and patients receiving brief-pulse, right unilateral ECT patients exhibited significant levels of impairment when tested 2 to 3 days after ECT. Of equal importance, of course, is the fact that, in this study, patients receiving brief-pulse, right unilateral ECT had just as good a clinical response as those assigned to other treatment combinations. As increasingly higher doses become routine for unilateral ECT in order to maximize therapeutic impact, objective memory deficits may become manifest. However, my expectation, based on all the data surveyed to date in which high-dose right unilateral ECT has been employed, is that these memory effects will be short-lived, of minimal intensity, and essentially limited to nonverbal, right hemisphere functions. As the dosage limits of modern brief-pulse devices are reached, and a switch to bilateral ECT becomes imperative to maintain or achieve the desired therapeutic effect, strategies directed toward improving the concordance between the stimulus parameters and the known physiology of the cerebral neuron, together with changes in treatment frequency and the site of treatment electrode application, should help limit the intensity and duration of amnestic side effects.

11

Neurochemical Correlates

In this chapter, the word ''neurochemical'' subsumes all of the following terms unless more particularly specified: neurochemical, neurohumoral, neurotransmitter; neuroendocrine, neurohormonal, neuropeptide. The correct individual designations are, of course, used in the sections describing the particular substance, although it seems to make little difference whether, for example, corticotropin-releasing factor is called a hormone, a neuropeptide, a neurotransmitter, or a neuropeptide neurotransmitter.

The literature on neurochemical correlates of induced seizures contains a dearth of human ECT studies compared with ECS trials in animals, yet normal animal data have not helped to explain how ECT works in mentally ill patients. Moreover, although animal brains are unarguably better suited than their human counterparts to prodding, chopping, grinding, and liquefying, one searches in vain for a single supporting structure of our present, painfully limited, neurochemical understanding of how ECT works that requires the underpinning of animal data. Discrepant results abound, and the few consistently replicable observations in animals simply do not generalize to man. Thus, electrically induced seizures have opposite effects in man and in rodents on beta-adrenergic receptors (Mann et al., 1990), serotonin-2 receptors (Newman and Lerer, 1988), and plasma insulin (Thiagarjan et al., 1988); naloxone lowers baseline and postictal prolactin levels in rats but not in humans (Swartz, 1991a); and if seizure termination is mediated by opioid systems in rats, it almost certainly is not in man (Sperling et al., 1989).

The first edition of this book included a concise review of the animal data on ECS for completeness' sake and to avoid accusations of philistinism, cynicism, and anthropocentrism, but such reasoning no longer seems justified. A literature search reveals paper after paper reporting the effects of ECS on total or regional rodent brain concentrations of a dizzying variety of substances for no better reason than that the techniques now exist for measuring them. Moreover, when the multiple statistical tests invariably employed chance to reveal a significant change in one or another of these substances, the authors hasten to suggest the relevance of their "finding" to the mode of action of ECT in psychiatric patients:

> . . . which of the many established pharmacological actions of ECS are important to the behavioral changes [in depression]? This is a difficult question to address in patients, so for the most part, one has to make inferences from animal studies of nondepressed rodents. (Nutt et al., 1989)

The list of animal preparations thus recently employed is extensive, and includes—but is far from limited to—serotonin inhibition of forskolin-stimulated adenyl cyclase in rat hippocampal membranes; postsynaptic serotonin-2 receptor binding in rabbit prefrontal cortex; cyclohexyladenosine, ethylcarboxyamidoadenosine, forskolin, and nitrobenzylthioinosine binding in rat cerebral cortex, cerebellum hippocampus, and striatum; desmethylimipramine binding in pooled rat cerebral cortex membrane preparations; blood glucose levels in C57BL/6J ob/ob obese mice; clonidine-induced hypoactivity in female rats; dihydroalprenolol binding in cerebral cortex of dihydroxytryptamine-lesioned rats; immunoreactivity of a metenkephalin fragment in rat cerebrospinal fluid; regional distribution of substance P, neurokinin, neurotensin, neuropeptide Y, vasoactive intestinal peptide, and galanin in rat frontal cortex, striatum, occipital cortex, hippocampus, hypothalamus, and pituitary; changes in messenger RNA coding for corticotropin-releasing factor and arginine vasopressin in selected neuroendocrine neurone populations; changes in mouse rectal temperatures; the firing rates of and density of 8-hydroxy-2-(di-n-propylamino) tetralin binding in rat hippocampal and dorsal raphe neurons; regional distribution of gamma-aminobutyric acid in rat brain; and so forth.

The problem presented by such studies is not only their apparently abstruse or occasionally risible subject matter—which on closer inspection often turns out to be quite relevant—but that the extreme variability in results within and between studies renders them so difficult to interpret. Tortella et al. (1989) explain why this might be so:

> Disparities in these [receptor] data most likely reflect the neurobiological complexities of ECS-induced receptor alterations coupled

with interpretive difficulties stemming from the methodological variables involved in the detection of these changes. . . . Thus, experimental outcomes may to some degree be dictated by the extent of membrane purification, perhaps by influencing the composition of receptor sites available for assay. In addition, the relative receptor selectivities of the different radioligands, and their susceptibilities to the influence of the binding assay ionic composition are important factors determining experimental outcome.

A few examples illustrate these points: One research group finds that transauricular ECS increases gamma-aminobutyric acid levels in rat brain in all areas except the hippocampus and nucleus accumbens, whereas transcorneal ECS increased it in hippocampus, frontal cortex, hypothalamus, and olfactory bulb, but reduces it in the nucleus accumbens (Ferraro et al., 1990). The authors conclude that selective activation of neuronal pathways may be achieved by altering the placement of ECS stimulating electrodes.

One study finds that ECS increases cyclohexyladenosine binding sites in rat cerebral cortex for 14 days and reduces forskolin binding in hippocampus and striatum for 2 days (Gleiter et al., 1989). After substantial discussion on how differences in rat strain or assay method might account for their failure to reproduce other investigators' results, the authors conclude that different seizure-inducing agents and antidepressant treatments seem to have different effects on the mouse adenosine neuromodulatory system.

Another study finds that ECS does not significantly change rat brain regional concentrations of substance P, neurotensin, or vasoactive intestinal polypeptide in the hypothalamus, pituitary, or left or right frontal or occipital cortices, but does significantly elevate neuropetide Y in hippocampus and occipital cortex. Multiple additional trends, tendencies, and marginal changes are offered, all fluctuating about $p = 0.05$ (Stenfors et al., 1989). The authors conclude that regional increments in neuropeptide Y might constitute, in part, the therapeutic mode of action of ECT.

To make matters worse, it now appears that the extensive literature on rodent brain neurotransmitters so widely cited when the first edition of this book appeared must now be discounted because the studies relied on, of all things, data from dead animals!

There is considerable conflicting earlier literature on the changes in neurotransmitter turnover produced by ECS [the entire animal neurotransmitter literature through 1989 is cited]. These studies relied on postmortem neurochemical studies of neurotransmitter concentrations and turnover to infer the effect of ECS on transmitter release. (Nutt et al., 1989)

It is therefore puzzling that half of a recent NIMH-sponsored special issue of *Psychopharmacology Bulletin* (Public Health Service, 1994), entitled "New Directions for ECT Research," is devoted to a review of the animal ECS literature (Fochtmann, 1994a) that includes 30 pages of references and a 62-page appendix tabulating all published articles of each and every effector, receptor, and parameter ever studied. It is discouraging that NIMH so clearly intended this topic to be the main thrust of the publication—and by implication, the future of ECT research—because not a single one of the 850 studies tabulated bears any known relevance to ECT in man.

The situation is, in fact, even more dismal because despite a subsequent apologia by Fochtmann (1994b), other than the 60-year-old observation in a Rome slaughterhouse confirming that an electric current passed through the head is not fatal, there is not a single piece of the admittedly meager accumulation of hard data that we have concerning ECT in man that was derived from animal research. This being said, Fochtmann's (1994a) article is a tour de force, absolutely required reading for anyone doing research in ECS, or who wishes to use animal data to attempt to explain how ECT works in man.

Human data are plentiful enough for our purposes, if only they can survive the close scrutiny prescribed by Kety (1967) before incorporating them into our understanding of the ECT process:

> . . . the difficulty lies not in demonstrating such changes, but in differentiating between those which are more fundamental and those which are clearly secondary, and also in attempting to discern which of the changes may be related to the important antidepressive . . . effects and which are quite irrelevant to those. (Kety, 1967)

Unfortunately, the disorders for which ECT is prescribed are quite possibly the result of pathological states that derive from, or cause, changes in the particular neurochemical studied—either before, during, or after ECT—thus increasing the chance that a given "finding" will be spurious.

> An important assumption, which is very hard to test, is that the observed alterations in pharmacological processes precede rather than are a consequence of the behavioral changes. (Nutt et al., 1989)

The problem is compounded by the frequently small sample sizes studied and the multiple statistical—especially correlational—tests employed (usually without appropriate correction for multiple testing), and by the inclusion of "trends," "tendencies," and "near-significant" results that, within a year or two of publication, are widely cited as fact by other investigators desirous of establishing the probity of their own trends, tendencies, and near-significant results. Tenuous theoretical constructs from other studies with equally inadequate methods are elevated to the level of "supporting data," thus creating the general illusion of a rather substantial and compelling body of knowledge. To insist that studies meet standard methodological and statistical (including power analysis) requirements and include an untreated or sham-treated control group to be accepted as valid would eliminate virtually every reference on the subject. This melancholy excercise has, in fact, been twice performed for the literature on ECT compared with antidepressant drugs (Abrams, 1982b; Rifkin, 1988), each time with devastating results.

Measurement of various brain monoamines and their myriad derivatives in blood and urine is at once the easiest and least productive approach to elucidating neurotransmitter mechanisms of action of ECT because of the confounding effects of diagnostic heterogeneity, previous and concomitant drug adminstration, effects of peripheral neurotransmitter production and metabolism, and uncontrolled motor activity level. Even spinal fluid studies are bedeviled by active transport of metabolites into the cerebrospinal fluid and the effect of motor activity—especially including body position at the time of the tap—on cephalad-caudad concentration gradients. Still further removed from cerebral events are the studies of lymphocyte or platelet neurotransmitter receptors. No compelling data on possible mechanisms of action of ECT have been forthcoming from any of these lines of investigation (e.g., Linnoila et al., 1984; Lerer, 1987; Buckholtz et al., 1988; Rausch et al., 1988; Cooper et al., 1988; Devanand et al., 1989a; Lykouras et al., 1990), which have mostly been abandoned in favor of indirect neuroendocrine release and challenge studies of monoaminergic function.

For example, ECT-induced pituitary hormone release—alone and in response to drugs that have known effects on central monoaminergic systems—can reflect ECT-induced changes in receptor functioning. In such studies, care must be taken to choose hormones that are not altered in depressive illness because changes in hormonal responses that are due to relief from depression may be interpreted incorrectly as reflecting changes in receptor sensitivity (Swartz, 1991a). Growth hormone, thyrotropin, oxytocin, vasopressin, corticotropin, luteinizing hormone, follicle-stimulating hormone, endorphins, and prolactin responses to ECT have all been studied, with remarkably—and often disappointingly—variable results.

Prolactin

By far the most consistent neurochemical result of ECT-induced seizures is the 10- to 50-fold increase in immediate postictal serum prolactin levels, which peak at 10 to 20 minutes post-stimulus and return to baseline within 2 hours (Ryan et al., 1970; Ohman et al., 1976; Klimes et al., 1978; O'Dea et al., 1978; Meco et al., 1978; Arato et al., 1980; Skrabanek et al., 1981; Balldin, 1982; Whalley et al., 1982, 1987; Linnoila et al., 1984; Swartz and Abrams, 1984; Haskett et al., 1985; Swartz, 1985; Papakostas et al., 1985, 1990; Scott et al., 1986; Taubøll et al., 1987; Johansson and von Knorring, 1987; Turner et al., 1987; Weizman et al., 1987; Markianos et al., 1987; Cooper et al., 1989; Sperling et al., 1989; Devanand et al., 1989a; Zis et al., 1991, 1993; McCall et al., 1996; Lisanby et al., 1997). Markianos et al. (1987) have also reported that the amounts of prolactin released by ECT and thyrotropin-releasing hormone are similar and significantly correlated. Although many of the 25 studies cited included patients under the influence of neuroleptic drugs—which Swartz (1991b) has correctly identified as a potentially confounding variable—their findings are essentially identical to those from studies conducted in drug-free subjects; in fact, no contradictory data exist.

ECT-induced prolactin release is not blocked by naloxone (Haskett et al., 1985; Papakostas et al., 1985; Turner et al., 1987; Weizman et al., 1987; Sperling et al., 1989), so it is not dependent on opioid receptor mechanisms; it is not enhanced by phentolamine (Klimes et al., 1978), so it is not an alpha-adrenergic phenomenon; and it is not blocked by ketanserin or ritanserin (Zis et al., 1989a; Papakostas et al., 1990), so it is not mediated by serotonin-2 receptors. The fact that methysergide, a nonselective serotonin receptor blocker that also exhibits dopaminergic properties, attenuates ECT-induced prolactin release (Papakostos et al., 1988; Zis et al., 1989b), suggested to these authors that such release is either serotonin-1–mediated or secondary to acute antidopaminergic mechanisms, as proposed by Deakin et al. (1983). The latter hypothesis received support from Cooper et al.

(1989), who asserted that their finding of a sharp increase in ECT-induced prolactin and luteinizing hormone levels without concomitant release of follicle-stimulating hormone favored "a powerful acute antidopaminergic action for ECT" (although they found significant increases in cerebrospinal fluid homovanillic acid levels induced by the first ECT). The primacy of serotonergic mechanisms in ECT-induced prolactin release finds support in the study of Shapira et al. (1992), who reported that ECT enhanced fenfluramine-induced prolactin release, suggesting an increase in central serotonergic responsivity (that was not, unfortunately, correlated with the treatment response to ECT). Whalley et al. (1987), likewise conclude that ECT-induced increases in plasma prolactin and adrenocorticotropic hormone, with little or no effect on luteinizing hormone or thyrotropin, probably reflect the activation of serotonergic neurones.

Because pituitary prolactin release is under tonic dopaminergic inhibitory control, the many studies showing a fall in ECT-induced prolactin release across a course of treatment (Meco et al., 1978; Whalley et al., 1982, 1987, 1989; Balldin, 1982; Deakin et al., 1983; Abrams and Swartz, 1985a; Aperia et al., 1985; Haskett et al., 1985; Scott et al., 1989b) suggest that repeated ECTs produce a sustained increase in postsynaptic pituitary dopamine receptor sensitivity, an effect that—if it also occurs in the brain—neatly explains the phenomenon of ECT-emergent dyskinesias, the need for the reduction of levodopa dose in some patients with Parkinson's disease who receive ECT (Balldin et al., 1980b; Douyon et al., 1989), and the almost universally favorable effects of this treatment on the motor manifestations of Parkinson's disease (Rasmussen and Abrams, 1991, 1992). The report of Balldin et al. (1982) is consistent with this view. They found that ECT systematically, but not significantly, increased apomorphine suppression of serum prolactin in depressed subjects. Other reports are, however, inconsistent or equivocal: Coppen et al. (1980a), found that ECT increased—rather than decreased—the prolactin response to thyrotropin-releasing hormone in depressed patients; Christie et al. (1982) failed to demonstrate an ECT-induced increase in apomorphine suppression of prolactin release; and Lerer and Belmaker (1982) and Linnoila et al. (1983) failed to demonstrate enhanced dopaminergic function after a course of ECT.

ECT-induced prolactin release is a function of seizure duration in some studies (Skrabanek et al., 1981; Balldin, 1982; Johansson and von Knorring, 1987; Mitchell et al., 1990) but not in others (Aperia et al., 1985; Swartz and Abrams, 1984; Swartz, 1985; Papakostas et al.,

1986a,b, 1990; McCall et al., 1996; Lisanby et al., 1997). However, although Balldin (1982) proposed that ECT-induced prolactin release was a biochemical marker of seizure activity because it correlated significantly with motor seizure but not ECT stimulus duration, we have reported evidence for a prolactin-releasing effect of the electrical stimulus that is separate from the induced seizure (Abrams and Swartz, 1985b).

The finding of Linnoila et al. (1984) that ECT-induced prolactin elevations did not correlate with changes in plasma levels of the dopamine metabolite, homovanillic acid, suggests either that the phenomenon is independent of pituitary dopamine metabolism, or—more likely—that the contribution of tuberoinfundibular dopamine metabolism to plasma homovanillic acid concentration is trivial. Papakostas et al. (1986a) found a close correlation between the prolactin responses to ECT and to thyrotropin-releasing hormone, suggesting a possible common underlying prolactin-releasing mechanism.

Most investigators have failed to find a significant correlation between ECT-induced prolactin release and clinical improvement (Deakin et al., 1983; Scott and Whalley, 1986; Whalley et al., 1987). Abrams and Swartz (1985a), however, reported such a correlation in 12 melancholic patients, between mean prolactin elevations induced by four consecutive ECTs and both a blind global improvement rating after 6 ECTs and the total number of ECTs prescribed by the attending psychiatrist. Further inspection of the data revealed that 4 patients with a slow ECT response had a sharp initial prolactin reponse that attenuated substantially across the 4 ECTs measured, whereas the 12 patients with a rapid treatment response exhibited small initial prolactin elevations that changed little with successive ECTs. No correlation was found between motor seizure duration and ECT-induced prolactin release.

The most recent (and largest, N = 79) study, however—despite finding greater prolactin release with bilateral than unilateral ECT, and with high-dose compared with low-dose stimulation—nevertheless failed to detect any direct evidence that the ECT-induced prolactin surge was associated with clinical improvement in depression (Lisanby et al., 1997). The authors therefore concluded that their data provided no support for the diencephalic theory of the mechanism of action of ECT proposed by Abrams and Taylor (1976b) and Abrams (1992).

However, immediately after the treatment course, patients classified as responders, and those who showed the greatest improvement in depression scale scores, exhibited a significant reduction in their prolactin surge across the treatment course. Nonresponders exhibited no such change, suggesting to me, at any rate, an association between blunting of the hypothalamic inhibition of pituitary prolactin release and clinical response—that is, a diencephalic effect of ECT.

Prolactin is also released by thyrotropin-releasing hormone, and Coppen et al. (1980b) reported that a course of ECT significantly increased the peak prolactin response to intravenous thyrotropin-releasing hormone in a sample of severely depressed patients, all of whom recovered. In unpublished data collected by Dr. Conrad Swartz and me however, there was no change in mean prolactin response to thyrotropin-releasing hormone across a course of 6 bilateral or unilateral ECTs in a sample of 32 melancholic men, most of whom recovered with treatment.

Swartz (1991b) argues that because ECT-induced prolactin release probably primarily reflects pituitary chemistry, its study is unlikely to reveal much about neurochemical mechanisms of ECT. However, because more prolactin is released by bilateral than unilateral ECT (Swartz and Abrams, 1984; Abrams and Swartz, 1985a; Papakostas et al., 1984, 1986a,b; Swartz, 1985; Zis et al., 1991, 1996; McCall et al., 1996; Lisanby et al., 1997), and by higher than lower dosage electrical stimuli (Robin et al. 1985; Abrams and Swartz, 1985b; Zis et al., 1993; Lisanby et al., 1997), the amount of prolactin released may reflect the physiological impact of the ECT technique used. The results of the study of Zis et al. (1992) support this view. These authors examined the effects of ECT on prolactin release with and without prior administration of metoclopramide to block dopamine receptors. Following metoclopramide (which induced a substantial prolactin surge), no further increase in prolactin levels was seen with ECT, and the authors concluded, in contrast to Swartz's (1991a) view, that ECT-induced prolactin release was not merely an extracerebral phenomenon but resulted from decreased hypothalamic dopaminergic inhibition of the pituitary lactotroph.

Moreover, there is evidence from depth electrode studies in patients with partial epilepsy for a specific relation between intracerebral stimulation or seizures and prolactin release. In one study (Sperling and Wilson, 1986), electrical stimulations were administered to amygdala, hippocampus, and frontal cortex: Only stimulations producing a high-frequency regional limbic afterdischarge resulted in serum prolactin elevation. In a second study (Sperling et al., 1986), serum prolactin levels always rose after complex partial seizures—all of which involved limbic discharges—and only rose after simple partial seizures if they induced limbic discharges. The authors concluded that prolactin release during partial seizures resulted from spread of discharges from mesial temporal structures to ventromedial hypothalamus. Just as occurs after ECT, postictal serum prolactin levels after complex partial seizures peaked at 15 minutes and returned to baseline in about 1 hour, without significant correlation with seizure duration.

Thyrotropin, Thyrotropin-releasing Hormone

Acute release of thyrotropin (thyroid-stimulating hormone) from the posterior pituitary during ECT is reported by some investigators (Aperia et al., 1985; Taubøll et al., 1987; Dykes et al., 1987; Scott et al., 1989b; Papakostas et al., 1990) but not others (Thorell and Adielsson, 1973: O'Dea et al., 1979; Whalley et al., 1987; Cooper et al., 1989). Cooper et al. (1989) nevertheless reported a significant correlation between the average changes in thyrotropin and prolactin across 4 ECTs.

The amount of thyrotropin released falls across a course of ECT (Aperia et al., 1985; Scott et al., 1989), although the thyrotropin response to thyrotropin-releasing hormone is variously reported diminishing (Decina et al., 1987), increasing (Kirkegaard et al., 1977; Nerozzi et al., 1987), or remaining unchanged (Coppen et al., 1980b) over the treatment course. Cooper et al. (1989) found less thyrotropin released after the last than after the first ECT of a series, but the reduction was not significant. As occurs for prolactin, the attenuation in thyrotropin release across a treatment course has been attributed to an ECT-induced increase in postsynaptic dopamine receptor function (Aperia et al., 1985). Although Scott et al. (1989b) found no relation between ECT-induced thyrotropin release and antidepressant efficacy as measured by the change in Hamilton depression scale score, they did obtain a perfect correlation between summed total EEG spike activity and change in thyrotropin release across a course of treatment. This confirmed an earlier finding (Dykes et al., 1987) that significant thyrotropin release does not occur during seizures lasting less than about 30 seconds, and provides a potential biological rationale for the arbitrary clinical dictum to repeat ECT-induced seizures that fail to last this long. However, because thyrotropin release was correlated with seizure duration rather than with clinical efficacy, Scott et al. (1989b) concluded that ECT-induced thyrotropin release is probably an epiphenomenon of seizure activity and unlikely to provide insights into the antidepressant mode of action of ECT.

The effect of a course of ECT on the thyrotropin response to exogenous thyrotropin-releasing hormone has also been studied, with the usual conflicting results. Kirkegaard and Carroll (1980) reported an increase in the thyrotropin response to thyrotropin-releasing hormone following ECT, the extent of which was inversely correlated with the risk of relapse. However, not only were Decina et al. (1987) unable to find a single patient who met Kirkegaard and Carroll's (1980) criterion for predicting relapse among 23 patients studied, but they observed the same change in thyrotropin response in responders as in nonresponders: No patient with a pretreatment blunted thyrotropin response showed normalization after ECT, and—most striking of all—the mean thyrotropin response became significantly more blunted after ECT, despite a generally favorable response to treatment. Thyrotropin-releasing hormone is not reported to be released by ECT (Whalley et al., 1982).

The most recent studies on the subject have been entirely negative. In a sample of 42 unipolar depressives, Lykouras et al. (1993) found no difference between responders and nonresponders for the thyrotropin response to TSH, and Hofmann et al. (1994) reported similarly disappointing results in a sample of 20 patients. Based on currently available data, therefore, further investigation of this topic appears to be unwarranted.

Corticotropin-releasing Factor, Corticotropin, and Cortisol

It was already known by the late 1960s that elevated plasma cortisol levels accompanied the stress of depressive illness; that ECT temporarily induced acute postictal increases in plasma levels of corticotropin and cortisol; that the elevated baseline cortisol levels fell with improvement in the depressed state; and that the cortisol response to ECT was unrelated to this improvement (Gibbons and McHugh, 1962; Hodges et al., 1964; Berson and Yalow, 1968). Our understanding of this subject has not increased since then.

Although ECT does not release corticotropin-releasing factor into the blood (Widerlöv et al., 1989), it nevertheless acutely elevates plasma levels of corticotropin (Berson and Yalow, 1968; Whalley et al., 1987; Widerlöv et al., 1989) and cortisol (Gibbons and McHugh, 1962; Hodges et al., 1964; Elithorn et al., 1968; Arato et al., 1980; Deakin et al., 1983; Haskett et al., 1985; Whalley et al., 1987;

Weizman et al., 1987; Mathe et al., 1987; Widerlöv et al., 1989; Mitchell et al., 1990) and increases the cortisol response to intravenous infusions of the alpha-2 receptor agonist, methylamphetamine (Slade and Checkley, 1980). Turner et al. (1987) provide the only contradictory data.

Basal and ECT-induced cortisol levels fall across a course of ECT (Whalley et al., 1982; Christie et al., 1982; Linkowski et al., 1987; Widerlöv et al., 1989), as do the cortisol (but not the corticotropin) response to exogenous corticotropin-releasing factor (Dored et al., 1990) and the cerebrospinal fluid levels of corticotropin-releasing factor itself (Nemeroff et al., 1991).

Numerous investigators have studied the effects of ECT on the response of the elevated plasma cortisol levels in depressed patients to exogenously administered dexamethasone, examining the phenomenon as either continuous (postdexamethasone plasma cortisol levels) or dichotomous (suppressor compared with nonsuppressor status). Four studies (Albala et al., 1981; Papakostas et al., 1981; Varma et al., 1988; Palmer et al., 1990) found that a course of ECT significantly reduced postdexamethasone plasma cortisol levels; one found that it did not (Devanand et al., 1987). Similar variability has been reported for the effects of ECT on suppressor status (Coryell and Zimmerman, 1983; Lipman et al., 1986a,b; Fink et al., 1987; Devanand et al., 1987; Katona et al., 1987). Swartz and Saheba (1990) found that doubling the standard dexamethasone dose to 2 mg sharply reduced interpatient variability in postdexamethasone plasma cortisol levels after but not before a course of ECT; in fact, all of their patients tested with the 2-mg dose showed post-ECT suppression.

Presumably because melancholia is associated with a state-dependent, stress-related, hypercortisolemia that attenuates with clinical improvement regardless of treatment method, changes in basal and postdexamethasone levels of cortisol—as well as in its antecedents—have been uniformly uninformative with regard to mechanisms of action of ECT. Thus, the reliable observation that a course of ECT reduces elevated baseline plasma cortisol levels in depressed patients is most likely due to a nonspecific reduction in stress-induced corticotropin release associated with relief of depression.

Growth Hormone

Growth hormone levels are generally reported unchanged or reduced immediately after ECT (Yalow et al., 1969; Ryan et al., 1970; O'Dea et al., 1979; Arato et al., 1980; Whalley et al., 1982, 1987, 1989; Deakin et al., 1983; Linnoila et al., 1984; Robin et al., 1985; Haskett et al., 1985; Scott et al., 1986; Linkowski et al., 1987; Turner et al., 1987; Weizman et al., 1987), although contradictory data exist (Skrabanek et al., 1981; Aperia et al., 1986).

Oxytocin, Vasopressin, Neurophysins

Because oxytocin and its associated neurophysin are cosynthesized and released stochiometrically, plasma oxytocin-associated neurophysin concentrations accurately reflect oxytocin release. Whalley et al. (1982) initially found that plasma levels of oxytocin–associated neurophysins were increased immediately post-ECT; they later reported that this effect diminished across a course of treatments (Whalley et al., 1987). Scott et al. (1986) and Whalley et al. (1987) reported that the release of ECT-induced neurophysin correlated significantly with improvement in depression. They subsequently extended their original findings using an alternative neurophysin assay from an independent laboratory, while at the same time demonstrating that the neurophysin response to ECT did not correlate significantly with seizure duration (Scott et al., 1989b). In a preliminary communication, Smith et al. (1990) reported a 10-fold increase in both plasma oxytocin and vasopressin levels 5 minutes after ECT in a sample of 11 elderly patients.

Plasma levels of arginine vasopressin rise abruptly and significantly after ECT, peak at about 5 to 10 minutes postictally, and return to baseline within 30 minutes (Raskind et al., 1979; Sorensen et al., 1982; Widerlöv et al., 1989). The observation that ECT-induced corticotropin and cortisol release followed increases in arginine vasopressin but not in corticotropin-releasing factor led Widerlöv et al. (1989) to conclude that arginine vasopressin was responsible for ECT-induced pituitary corticotropin release (although hypothalamic releasing factors are unlikely to be detectable in the peripheral circulation using existing methods).

Endorphins

ECT reliably increases baseline (Alexopoulos et al., 1983; Misiaszek et al., 1984; Weizman et al., 1987) and immediate postictal plasma endorphin levels (Emrich et al., 1979; Alexopoulos et al., 1983;

Misiaszek et al., 1984; Inturrisi et al., 1986; Weizman et al., 1987; Ghadirian et al., 1988; Griffiths et al., 1989; Dored et al., 1990), eight observations in search of a clinical correlation.

The possibility that endogenous opioid mechanisms mediate the termination of ECT-induced seizures and therefore the reduction in seizure threshold and duration across a treatment course (Tortella et al., 1989; Nakajima et al., 1989) is rendered unlikely by the inability of very high doses of naloxone to alter the length of ECT-induced seizures (Sperling et al., 1989).

Other Hormones

Mathe et al. (1987) reported that plasma prostaglandin E2 metabolite did not change with anesthesia without ECT, but was significantly elevated at all post-ECT sampling times. The maximum increase, about 50%, was attained at 15 and 30 minutes and did not change across a course of treaments. Positive correlations with ACTH and cortisol were obtained. The increased release of prostaglandin E2 may, in part, account for the elevated plasma ACTH and cortisol.

Neuroendocrine Challenge Tests

Drugs that release hormones from the anterior pituitary via stimulation of specific monoamine systems have been used as challenge tests in patients receiving ECT. Hormonal responses to the dopamine agonist apomorphine have been used indirectly to probe dopamine receptor changes induced by ECT, with inconsistent results. Modigh et al. (1984) found that, although all of 17 patients treated improved with ECT, some exhibited increases and some, decreases in apomorphine-induced growth hormone suppression. Costain et al. (1982) found a significant increase in apomorphine-induced growth hormone release after a course of ECT, which the authors noted was consistent with an ECT-induced increase in dopamine receptor sensitivity. Although Christie et al. (1982) claimed failure to confirm such an effect, their published figure is virtually identical to that of Costain et al. (1982b) and shows that, after a course of ECT, growth hormone levels were substantially increased at baseline and at each of 6 post-apomorphine sampling intervals, although with statistical significance found only 15 minutes post-apomorphine. Balldin et al. (1982) found that ECT enhanced apomorphine-induced suppression of prolactin levels in parkinsonian patients, although this effect did not correlate with improvement in motor symptoms.

Slade and Checkley (1980) failed to find any change in the growth hormone response to intravenous infusions of the alpha-2 receptor agonist clonidine in depressed patients before and after a course of ECT or to infusions of the alpha-2 receptor agonist, methylamphetamine; however, they did observe a significant increase in the cortisol response to this drug. However, Balldin et al. (1992) found that clonidine-stimulated growth hormone secretion was significantly blunted by ECT, suggesting down-regulation of hypothalamic alpha-2 receptors. Unaccountably, although the authors had collected depression rating scale data, they did not examine the relationship between changes in growth hormone secretion and clinical outcome.

Mechanisms of Action

Among others, Scott (1989) holds the view that neurochemical changes that do not correlate with improvement in depression cannot be central to the antidepressant effects of ECT:

> In summary, the neuroendocrine effects of ECT may be a correlate of stress, seizure activity or the antidepressant effects of ECT. The release of anterior pituitary hormones after ECT has not consistently correlated with the antidepressant effects of ECT, and is unlikely to be useful in the prediction of clinical outcome.

Scott's (1989) argument omits consideration of an earlier point made in his paper that, although the induction of a seizure is universally recognized as prerequisite to the antidepressant potency of ECT, no correlation has ever been found between the duration of the induced seizure and its therapeutic impact:

> Generalised tonic and clonic seizures are an essential component of ECT and thus it is important to ensure that such a seizure occurs at each ECT treatment. . . . There is no correlation between individual seizure length and clinical outcome and thus seizure length cannot be used to predict recovery.

Similarly, although high-frequency limbic discharges are a prerequisite for prolactin release during partial seizures (Sperling et al., 1986), the duration of such discharges is unrelated to the extent of prolactin release. Thus, it is entirely plausible (King and Liston, 1990) for neurochemical release to be central to the antidepressant action of ECT without any correlation existing between the amount of neurochemical released and the degree of clinical improvement.

The hypothetical construct of seizure generalization may be useful in integrating diverse findings reported in the complex relationships among the technical aspects of ECT administration, observed physiologic responses, and therapeutic impact (Abrams, 1991a). As noted previously, the hypothetical variable of seizure generalization is proposed to be related to the extent of postictal suppression, the duration of the induced seizure, the amount of prolactin released, and the correlation among different estimates of seizure duration (Swartz and Larson, 1986). The concept of seizure generalization may be useful in integrating diverse findings reported in the complex relationships among the technical aspects of ECT administration, observed physiologic responses, and therapeutic impact (Abrams, 1991a). As noted previously, seizure generalization is proposed to be related to EEG seizure amplitude, intensity, and coherence; the degree of postictal suppression; the duration of the induced seizure; the amount of prolactin released; the tachycardia response; and the correlation among different estimates of seizure duration (Swartz and Larson, 1986).

The view that ECT-induced EEG seizure activity is driven by a central pacemaker is supported by the increased ictal EEG coherence that is observed during, compared with following, the seizure (Krystal et al., 1995). The intercorrelation among the durations of ECT-induced motor activity, EEG spike activity, tachycardia response, and the amount of prolactin released—reflecting activity in anatomically diverse brain areas—should increase as increased efficiency of pacemaker driving produces greater seizure generalization. The obvious hypothesis is that the therapeutic—and specifically, the antidepressant—impact of ECT will increase directly with the strength of the multiple correlation among these physiological variables.

The initial reports of an increase in seizure threshold over a treatment course were partly responsible for an anticonvulsant theory of the mechanism of action of ECT (Sackeim, 1994a). Indirect support for this attractive theory was provided by the initial finding of Sackeim et al. (1987c) that patients whose seizure thresholds did not increase substantially across a course of treatment did not have a good clinical outcome. Further support has not been forthcoming, however. Coffey et al. (1995b) employed a flexible stimulus titration schedule to estimate seizure threshold change across a course of 6 unilateral or bilateral ECTs, and found that with moderately suprathreshold ECT almost half of their depressed patients showed no threshold increase. Moreover, in the patients that exhibited such an increase, there was no association between the rise in threshold and either therapeutic response status or speed of response. Likewise, Shapira et al. (1996) used a stimulus titration schedule to determine seizure threshold change across a course of ECTs and found no relation between threshold increase and improvement in treatment-resistant depressives in response to moderately suprathreshold bilateral ECT.

Modern theories of the mode of action of ECT have not advanced much beyond the general understanding of the problem that was already widely proposed by the early 1960s:

> ... many workers consider that one type of depressive illness, called variously endogeneous or physiological depression, reflects a failure of hypothalamic centres concerned with instinctive drives and adrenal stress mechanisms, and it has been frequently suggested that E.C.T. acts by stimulating these mid-brain centres. (Hodges et al., 1964)

This notion that convulsive therapies worked to reverse the vegetative changes in depression by providing ''massage of diencephalic centers'' was already clearly expressed by 1939 (King and Liston, 1990), the year of the first English-language publication on ECT. Observations, such as the one offered by Weizman et al. (1987), that

> It seems that ECT affects various neurotransmitters and neuromodulators and that the interactions among these systems result in the neuroendocrine changes observed following an ECT course.

are no more helpful in explaining the mechanisms involved than the statement that ''climate results from a complex interaction of cosmological, meteorological, and geological forces'' is in explaining the weather. It is further notable that a recent comprehensive review of the data supporting a neurobiologic mechanism for the therapeutic effects of ECT in man (Kapur and Mann, 1993) failed to uncover a single candidate for the magic bullet, concluding that ''Despite considerable investigation, the mechanism of antidepressant (sic) effect of ECT is still a mystery.''

It should be clear from this brief review that no coherent general neurochemical theory of the action of ECT yet exists. King and Liston (1990) have, in my view, correctly summarized the situation:

Taken together, however, the myriad biochemical sequelae of electroconvulsive stimulation, the gaps in our knowledge of their functional correlates, and the difficulties in extrapolating from animal to
man or from normal to pathophysiological states makes it tenuous
to entrust the therapeutic efficacy of ECT to the observable change
in specific transmitter, receptor, or system.

The broadly drawn hypotheses that ECT exerts its beneficial effects in depression through hypothalamic mechanisms (Carney and
Sheffield, 1973; Abrams and Taylor, 1973, 1974, 1976b; Fink and Ottosson, 1980) or by neurotransmitter release, otherwise unspecified
(King and Liston, 1990), are not specific enough to be heuristic—or,
in the latter case—even testable; and the more specific hypotheses
(Abrams, 1986b, 1990; Staton et al., 1988; Fink and Nemeroff, 1989;
Fink, 1990; Sackeim, 1994b) are either too narrow, premature, unconfirmed, or just plain wrong. Modern ECT researchers, regardless of
their species of predilection, do not have any more of a clue to the
relationship between brain biological events and treatment response in
ECT than they did at the time of the first edition of this book—which
is to say, none at all. Moreover, modern theories of the action of
ECT—even as formulated by sophisticated investigators with impeccable credentials—have not surpassed in conceptual elegance the 18th-
century claim that things burned because they contained phlogiston;
ECT awaits its Lavoisier.

12

Patients' Attitudes, Legal-Regulatory Issues, and Informed Consent

Patients' Attitudes Toward Electroconvulsive Therapy

Doctors who give ECT have shown remarkably little interest in their patients' views of the procedure and its effects on them, and only recently has this topic received any consideration in the literature. Gomez (1975) was the first to examine the incidence and severity of subjectively experienced side effects of ECT. She tried to understand why, as she believed, "many patients and their relatives view the prospect of ECT with horror." She interviewed 96 patients, most of them depressed, 24 hours after each treatment, for a total of 500 consecutive treatments, of which 420 were given with bilateral electrode placement. The self-reported incidence of side effects was remarkably low: Muscle pain topped the list at 8.2%, with subjective memory impairment and headache occurring only about 3% of the time. Surprisingly, subjective complaints were no less frequent in patients receiving unilateral compared with bilateral ECT. The aspect of ECT most disliked by patients who were interviewed after they had received three or four ECTs related primarily to fear—most frequently, a fear of permanent impairment of memory or intellectual abilities, followed about equally by fear of entering the ECT room, fear of death or serious damage, and the apprehension experienced while simply waiting to receive treatment. A quarter of the sample expressed no special fear or dislike of ECT.

Hillard and Folger (1977) administered a questionnaire to patients receiving ECT on two different state mental hospital wards and found that attitudes toward this treatment were significantly more favorable on the ward in which ECT was more frequently given, despite the fact that neither hospital made any effort to brief patients beforehand on the safety or therapeutic aspects of ECT.

Freeman and Kendell (1980) conducted a systematic study of the experiences and attitudes toward ECT among 166 patients who had received treatment from 1 to 6 years earlier. Almost one half of the patients either had no particular feelings before receiving their first ECT or were reassured and pleased that treatment was about to begin. Specifically, a majority (77% to 90%) had no fears at all about becoming unconscious, losing bladder control, receiving electricity, having the seizure, or experiencing brain damage as a result of the treatment. More than 80% of the patients said that having ECT was no worse than a visit to the dentist and 50% actually preferred the ECT; nevertheless, only 65% reported that they would be willing to have it again. One half of the patients felt that memory impairment was the worst side effect, and 30% felt their memory had never returned to normal afterward. Only 1.2%, however, felt that the treatment had worked by making them forget their problems. Only about 20% fully understood what the treatment involved; most had no idea or only a partial understanding (presumably as a result of the combined cognitive effects of the disorder for which they were treated and the treatment itself). Many patients could not recall ever having signed consent for ECT, did not regard the process as particularly important, and were quite willing to relinquish the responsibility to others (90% of the patients said that either the consent procedures had been adequate or were satisfied to defer to the doctor's recommendation); it was the authors' strong impression that most patients would agree to almost anything a doctor suggested.

Hughes et al. (1981) used the same questionnaire to interview 72 patients who received ECT for severe mental illness: 83% said they had improved and 81% were willing to have ECT again. Slightly more than half thought a visit to the the dentist was more distressing. Almost half reported memory impairment after treatment, and 18% said it was still present when interviewed. Half said they had received no explanation of the treatment, and 28% could not remember signing the consent form; nevertheless, only about 10% thought the consent procedure should be changed, and most thought the decision about ECT should be left to the doctors.

Results similar to those obtained in the preceding two studies were reported by Kerr et al. (1982), who also found that more than

50% of their patients denied ever having had the procedure explained to them.

A prospective study of patients' attitudes regarding ECT was conducted by Baxter et al. (1986) in Berkeley, California. More than 50% of patients who were about to have ECT for the first time were concerned about experiencing memory loss, having a seizure, or sustaining brain damage, and about 25% were worried about the anesthesia, the possibility of pain, and the use of electricity. After a course of ECT, most of these patients felt that they had received adequate information to decide about having the treatment, that they were helped by it, and that their decision to have it had been a good one. In contrast, patients who had received ECT in the past (some of them presumably without modern anesthesia techniques) were more frightened about the treatment and pessimistic about its outcome, although all consented to a new course of ECT.

More recently, Pettinati et al. (1994) surveyed patient attitudes toward ECT in a sample of 56 depressed patients before and after ECT, compared with 22 depressed patients never treated with ECT. Virtually all (98%) of the ECT-treated group stated they would be willing to have ECT if they became depressed again, compared with 70% in the no-ECT group. In a striking confirmation of the earlier studies cited above, a majority (62%) of the ECT-treated group rated the experience less upsetting than having a tooth pulled, compared with 14% of the no-ECT group. The difference between the two groups in favorable attitudes toward ECT was maintained 6 months later.

In view of the fact that most of the several hundred patients interviewed in the studies described here and in a larger review by Freeman and Cheshire (1986) had rather positive views about ECT and did not find the treatment especially frightening, upsetting, painful, or unpleasant, how is it possible to account for the widespread negative public image of ECT (Frankel, 1982; Consensus Development Conference 1985) and the history of legislative restrictions on its use (Winslade et al., 1984)? I believe there are several contributory factors.

Abuse of Electroconvulsive Therapy

Fink (1983) points out that professional concerns about ECT are hardly new, citing the critical 1947 report of the Group for the Advancement of Psychiatry (which began with the introductory statement ''In view of the reported promiscuous and indiscriminate use of electroshock therapy, your Committee on Therapy decided to devote its first meeting to an evaluation of the role of this type of therapy in psychiatry"). In 1972, Dr. Milton Greenblatt, then Commissioner of Mental Health for the State of Massachusetts, organized a Task Force to Study and Recommend Standards for the Administration of Electro-Convulsive Therapy (Frankel, 1973). This Task Force was created in response to local allegations about the excessive use of ECT, particularly for outpatient maintenance therapy, by one or two zealous practitioners, as exemplified in an article by Regestein et al. (1975) entitled "A case of prolonged, reversible dementia associated with abuse of electroconvulsive therapy." These authors described in detail the appalling (but apparently ultimately reversible) cognitive consequences in a 57-year-old woman who had received a "maintenance" ECT every Saturday morning for more than 2 years. They also briefly described the devastating effects of a similar treatment schedule on an executive, concluding with the statement that "the ready insurance payments for any number of ECT further encourage errors in judgement concerning the efficacy of such treatment." Basing their clinical recommendations largely on the in-house clinical manuals of Abrams and Fink (1969) and Salzman (1970), the Task Force responded with a series of carefully worded statements that limited, among other things, the number of ECTs to be given in a single treatment course, and further constrained the use of outpatient and maintenance ECT. Indeed, concerns over the "potential for misuse and abuse of ECT and the desires to ensure the protection of patients' rights" were central to a United States government-sponsored conference to assess the place of ECT in medical practice (National Institutes of Health, 1985).

The Anti–Electroconvulsive Therapy Lobby

Among those offering their opinions at this conference, as well as at another one earlier in the year (*Electroconvulsive Therapy: Clinical and Basic Research Issues*, New York Academy of Sciences, January 16–18, 1985), were members of lay groups such as the Mental Patient Law Project, the disingenuously named Citizen's Commission on Human Rights (actually a Scientology-funded organization), the Network Against Psychiatric Assault, and the International Network for Alternatives to Psychiatry, as well as several indefatigable individual lay and medical crusaders against the use of ECT. Anyone who was present at these meetings can readily testify that the term vocal minority aptly describes this loose coalition of ex-patients, civil libertarians, religious cultists, consumer advocates, and medical opportunists, a consortium virtually unopposed by any equivalent pro-ECT patient advocacy groups. The reasons for this imbalance are obvious: The majority of patients who receive ECT (about 100,000 each year) are well satisfied with the results and are hardly motivated to influence public opinion on the subject—they are too busy getting on with their lives and would probably prefer not to be reminded of their illness or its treatment.

It is safe to say, however, that without Scientology there would hardly be an organized anti-ECT movement in this country or any-where else. An article in the *Wall Street Journal* suggests that Scientology's vitriolic attacks on psychiatry, psychopharmacology, and ECT are financially motivated (Burton, 1991):

> Scientologists' central belief is that human beings have a soul-like entity called a ''thetan'' that is perfect and travels from galaxy to galaxy. Their goal is to help their thetans get rid of something called engrams—essentially bad memories. To this end, Scientology developed a lie-detector-like device called an E-meter, which is used to treat mental problems often at hundreds of dollars per session. Psychiatrists consider these ''treatments'' quackery.

Founded in the late 1940s by science-fiction writer L. Ron Hubbard (who reportedly died in hiding in 1986 after 5 years of success-fully evading an Internal Revenue Service indictment for tax fraud), Scientology portrays itself as a religion despite an Internal Revenue Service ruling that stripped the mother ''church'' of its tax-exempt status by arguing that it was more a business than a church (Behar, 1991; Burton, 1991). A *Time* magazine cover story described the self-styled church as ''a hugely profitable global racket that survives by intimidating members and critics in a Mafia-like manner'' (Behar, 1991). In fact, Behar continues, ''in the early 1980's, eleven top Scientologists, including Hubbard's wife, were sent to prison for infiltrating, burglarizing, and wiretapping more than 100 private and government agencies in attempts to block their investigations.'' Scientology has counterattacked with an astonishingly expensive and slick advertising campaign of public disinformation, but it is too soon to tell whether it will have the desired impact of maintaining the group's credibility.

The disproportionate effectiveness of the anti-ECT lobby is amply demonstrated by the history of the introduction and passage of the highly restrictive Assembly Bill 4481 for legislating ECT use in Cal-ifornia (Moore, 1977), as well as the saga—described later in this chapter—of the Food and Drug Administration's (FDA) effort to re-classify ECT devices (Isaac, 1990; Abrams, 1991b).

A junior student at the University of Massachusetts, who was also a member of the Network Against Psychiatric Assault, wrote Assembly Bill 4481 while participating in a special study project at the University of California. A northern California Assemblyman (Vasconcellos) was then found who was willing to present the bill, which passed both houses of the legislature with only one dissenting vote and which was signed into law by then-Governor Ronald Reagan who, when later criticized for his action, typically disclaimed responsibility and stated that he "had no respect for the type of people who had supported the Vasconcellos law," but had signed the bill at the end of the legislative session when he had had more than 1000 legislative actions to consider (Bennett, 1983). AB 4481 was successfully challenged by the International Psychiatric Association for the Advancement of Electrotherapy (now the Association for Convulsive Therapy) and was replaced by the somewhat less restrictive AB 1032, which continues in force at this time.

A few years later, in November 1982, the citizens of Berkeley, California, approved by referendum a Board of Supervisors ordinance that made administering ECT in city hospitals a crime punishable by a fine of $500 or 6 months in prison, or both (Bennett, 1983). This ordinance was subsequently reversed by the Alameda County Superior Court on a technical point of law.

Interestingly, although the availability of ECT steadily declined during the 7 years after the enactment of AB 1032, there was little year-to-year variation in its use in California: Approximately 1.12 persons per 10,000 population per year received ECT during this period (Kramer, 1985), a figure that is just below the range of the national average of 1.3 to 4.6 per 10,000 when sampled in 1978 (Fink, 1979), but less than the reported 2.42 patients per 10,000 population who received ECT in Massachusetts from 1977 to 1980 (Kramer, 1985).

In response to antipsychiatry forces responsible for the 1982 Berkeley ban on ECT, the San Francisco Board of Supervisors passed a resolution in early 1991 against the use or financing of ECT (Peterson, 1991). Although the resolution had little practical effect, it provided the impetus for the same forces to sponsor California Assembly Bill 1817 (Ferguson) that would, in addition to broadening patients' rights advocacy, permit local restrictions on the use of ECT and ban it for patients under age 16. The California Alliance for the Mentally Ill opposed the bill in its 27 April 1991 position paper to members of the California Assembly Health Committee, asserting that "For involuntarily committed patients suffering from the major mental illnesses, the *world-wide standard* of treatment is psychotropic medications or ECT."

The Assembly Health Committee was also apprised of FDA support for the safety and efficacy of ECT and received a letter from the head of the Alcohol, Drug Abuse, and Mental Health Administration, stressing that the efficacy of ECT was clearly supported by the results of scientifically controlled trials. At the Committee's hearing on 30 April 1991, patients and their families testified enthusiastically for ECT, as did a representative of the California Psychiatric Association. The opposition was so effective that the bill was withdrawn from consideration until 1992, and the anti-ECT provisions deleted by author's amendment; only the patients' rights advocacy provisions remained.

Inadequate Consent Procedures

Psychiatrists have lagged behind other medical specialists in developing and promulgating the doctrine of informed consent for medical procedures. This is likely to have resulted in large measure from the nature of the patients treated; their frequent impairments of perception, judgment, and reasoning often require others, including their physicians, to make decisions for them. A number of articles written on the subject (Salzman, 1977; Culver et al., 1980; Gilbert, 1981; Frankel, 1982; Senter et al., 1984; Winslade et al., 1984), however, make it abundantly clear that the laggard must now catch up. In fact, there is no longer any choice in the matter as state after state introduces mental health legislation with the same three themes: (1) voluntary patients may not receive involuntary treatment; (2) competent patients, even if involuntary, may not receive involuntary treatment; and (3) involuntary, incompetent patients may only receive involuntary treatment under court order (or, in some states, in the presence of a documented real and immediate threat to life or limb).

Misrepresentation of Electroconvulsive Therapy in the Media

Although the depiction of ECT in the 1940s movie *The Snake Pit* was accurate for that time, the portrayal of electricity stiffening MacMurphy's body in *One Flew Over the Cuckoo's Nest* was not, because the nature of ECT had been completely transformed by modern anesthesia techniques long before the latter movie was filmed. Nevertheless, for reasons known only to themselves, both the director of the movie and the author of the book on which it was based deliberately presented a false image of the treatment to the public. One of the more egregiously misleading images of ECT presented to the public appeared in the 6 December 1995 issue of the tabloid *USA Today*. The writer, Dennis Cauchon, who was subsequently severely reprimanded for the false and misleading statements in the article, relied almost entirely on the unsupported claims of anti-ECT activists for the material he presented, despite the fact that he had interviewed at length —in person and via telephone—most of the leading ECT researchers in the country, while posing as an objective and unbiased observer. Among the more misleading false claims made were the assertions— offered without any substantiating data—that the mortality rate for ECT in geriatric patients was 1 in 200, and that the death rate with ECT was actually 50 times higher than published figures showed. Although *USA Today* published several strong rebuttals, including one from the Medical Director of the American Psychiatric Association, the damage was already done.

Whether because public opinion is less easily swayed by such misrepresentations than many have feared or because such inaccurate portrayals are effectively countered by more balanced media presentations, public surveys have generally revealed an unexpectedly overall positive attitude toward ECT (Kalayam and Steinhart, 1981; Baxter et al., 1986).

One particularly favorable view of ECT was presented by the talk-show host Dick Cavett in public television interviews and an article in *People's Weekly* (3 August 1992). It is hard to overestimate the positive effects on public opinion of the following statement, which he made concerning his personal experience of receiving ECT for a severe depressive illness:

> In my case, ECT was miraculous. My wife was dubious, but when she came into my room afterward, I sat up and said, ''Look who's back among the living.'' It was like a magic wand. (News and Notes, 1992)

Realistic Fears of Memory Loss

As described in Chapter 9, there is substantial subjective and objective support for long-term, perhaps even permanent, memory loss in some patients who receive sine-wave bilateral ECT. Considering the appropriately high social and individual value placed on intact memory function, it is readily understandable that fears of ECT-induced memory loss are paramount among a majority of candidates for and recipients of this treatment. The facile reassurance by generations of psychiatrists (including myself) that such memory loss was ''only temporary'' not only occasionally proved inaccurate but served to inculcate a deserved sense of distrust among patients whose personal experience proved otherwise.

Regulation of Electroconvulsive Therapy Devices

When the Medical Device Amendment to the Food, Drug, and Cosmetic Act gave the Food and Drug Administration (FDA) regulatory responsibility for medical devices in 1976, it placed ECT devices in the restricted category of class III, which requires manufacturers to provide data demonstrating safety and efficacy of new devices they intend to market. However, because existing ECT devices—as well as those subsequently introduced as ''substantially equivalent'' to pre-1976 devices—were exempted from such premarket approval procedures under a grandfather clause, there was no practical significance to the FDA's action.

In 1978 the FDA's Neurological Devices advisory panel recommended reclassifying ECT devices into class II, which assumes ECT to be both safe and efficacious and requires only that devices meet a performance standard for safety of construction and instructions for use (designated ''labeling''). Under intense immediate fire from Scientologists and other antipsychiatry activists led by Marylin Rice—a former government economist and the pseudonymous Natalie Parker of Berton Roueche's (1974) remarkably biased anti-ECT *New Yorker* piece—the FDA quickly requested its advisory panel to reconsider (Isaac, 1990). When the panel duly reversed its opinion, the FDA published a final rule in 1979 classifying ECT devices into class III. At the same time, however, the FDA invited the American Psychiatric Association (APA) to petition the agency to reclassify ECT devices into class II.

The APA procrastinated 3 years before filing such a petition in 1982; the FDA advisory panel then recommended again that ECT devices be reclassified into class II, but only after a performance standard had been developed. A year later, on 5 April 1983, the FDA published notice of its intent to reclassify ECT devices into class II; there the matter stood for the next 7 years while the FDA waffled to the tune of the Scientologists and other anti-ECT activists, despite the fact that various national and international performance standards (e.g., IEC 601) had already achieved worldwide acceptance.

Finally, on 6 September 1990, the FDA proposed a definitive rule (21 CFR Part 882) to finally place ECT devices in class II—still contingent on the development of a performance standard—but this time only for devices labeled by their manufacturers as intended solely for use in patients with "severe depression," which FDA defined as DSM-III major depressive disorder with melancholia. (ECT devices intended for use in other conditions—including mania, catatonia, and schizophrenia—would remain in regulatory class III, requiring manufacturers to undertake controlled trials of safety and efficacy and to seek FDA approval for each condition.)

The FDA claimed that its decision to severely limit the clinical indication for ECT was "based on its review of new, publicly available, valid scientific evidence . . ." It formed an in-house ECT Task Force of the Center for Radiological Devices and Health (CDRH), the agency with specific responsibility for ECT devices, to "examine all of the scientific literature pertaining to ECT"—particularly those papers presented since 1982 when reclassification was first proposed by the APA—and to "determine what evidence there is for or against reclassification for any or all of the following conditions: severe depression, mania, and schizophrenia." The six-member CDRH Task Force included one medical family practitioner, one D.Sc., three Ph.D.s, and one person without a stated degree, none of whom had ever published an article on ECT.

The FDA ECT Task Force identified 715 articles on ECT published since 1982, from which they selected 200 for review—including such esoterica as "To Bedlam and Back" (*Journal of Psychosocial Nursing and Mental Health Services*), and "Tardive dyskinesia in schizophrenic outpatients" (*Singapore Annals of Academic Medicine*)—but omitting numerous references to controlled studies of the use of ECT in nonmelancholic depression, mania, catatonia, and schizophrenia that have appeared in major world journals.

Not surprisingly, in view of the professional backgrounds of its members, the committee blindly stumbled past the most important references on the subject. Consider for a moment the exclusion of nonmelancholic major depression as an approved indication. The FDA report cited only five references in support of this limitation—four published between 1953 and 1965—and ignored every single random-assignment, double-blind, sham ECT-controlled study of the modern era that had demonstrated the efficacy of ECT in nonmelancholic depressives.

Moreover, the FDA's own summary of data in support of the proposed reclassification relied heavily on Avery and Winokur's (1977) study to support the claim that ECT exerts more potent anti-depressant effects than tricyclic antidepressants. That study, however, employed only a Feighner "probable" diagnosis of depression—that is, at least four depressive symptoms—which is far less restrictive than DSM-III-R requirements for a major depressive episode with melancholia. By neglecting these studies, the FDA reached the untenable conclusion that ECT devices are indicated for one type of major depressive illness (with melancholia), but not for the same type without melancholia. The FDA review of the indications for ECT other conditions, particularly mania and catatonia, is similarly deficient.

The issue remains unsettled at the time of this writing, awaiting final action by the FDA after it has digested the myriad responses to its invitation to comment on the published rule. In the event that the proposed rule becomes law, however, what might be the risk incurred by a physician who administered ECT to a patient with a diagnosis other than melancholia? It should be no more than that of prescribing a medication for an indication not recognized by the FDA in its review of manufacturers' pharmaceutical package inserts. The FDA does not yet regulate or "approve" medical practice; it is empowered only to regulate the classification and labeling of drugs and devices in inter-state commerce, and its historical role has been to limit advertising claims. Technically, if a physician prescribes a treatment for an indication not recognized by the FDA, and his patient claims a bad result and sues, the physician may have a harder time defending his choice of treatment than would otherwise be the case. However, physicians who limit themselves to administering treatments only for FDA-recognized indications by no means spare themselves the risk of malpractice litigation, because the majority of complaints concern treatments that fall in the latter category.

Patients' Rights

Frankel (1982) pointed out that the introduction of civil rights concerns into the mental health controversy over the medicolegal and ethical aspects of ECT has transformed "what might have been a narrow medical debate into a political challenge involving litigation and legislation, while jurists and legislators largely unfamiliar with ECT have been drawn into the debate."

Although there is understandably great interest and concern over the issue of procedural constraints on civil commitment (e.g., Stone, 1977; APA, 1978; Frankel, 1982), this is a problem that does not directly impinge on the administration of ECT, which comes into play only after a patient's legal status has been determined. At this point, there are two major ethical and legal concerns: The competency of a patient to consent to treatment and the components of valid informed consent.

Competency

The general issue of legal competency is enormously complex and far beyond the scope of this volume. Roth et al. (1977), from the Law and Psychiatry Program at Western Psychiatric Institute, have pointed out the dearth of legal guidance on the question of competency to consent to medical treatments. They note that a person may at the same time be considered competent for some legal purposes and incompetent for others; a person is not judged incompetent merely because of the presence of mental illness; the consent to treatment of an incompetent person does not validly authorize a physician to perform such treatment; and a physician who does not take reasonable steps to obtain legal authorization for treating an incompetent patient who refuses treatment may be held liable. These authors agree that, although there is no single valid test for competency,

> It has been our experience that competency is presumed so long as the patient modulates his or her behavior, talks in a comprehensible way, remembers what he or she is told, dresses and acts so as to appear to be in meaningful communication with the environment, and has not been declared legally incompetent.

The ability of a patient to understand the risks, benefits, and alternatives to treatment (including no treatment at all), however, is increasingly becoming the commonly applied standard of competence for consenting to ECT. Interestingly, although the critical element of this "test" of competence is the patient's ability to comprehend the elements that the law presumes to be a part of treatment decision-making, such decision making need not be rational to be legally acceptable. This is exemplified by the patient of Roth et al. (1977) who fully understood the nature of the ECT that was being offered to her, but accepted it because she hoped it would kill her.

The right to refuse treatment is, of course, implicit in the concept of competency. Even committed psychotic patients who are deemed by the law to require continued involuntary psychiatric hospitalization and treatment may refuse ECT, as shown by *N.Y. City Health and Hospitals Corp. vs. Stein*. Paula Stein had been committed to Bellevue Hospital by court order to receive whatever course of treatment the psychiatric staff deemed advisable, including ECT, regardless of her consent and without the necessity of prior judicial approval. Because of a recently introduced state mental hygiene law, however, the hospital nevertheless attempted to obtain the patient's consent; when this was not forthcoming, the hospital petitioned the court to authorize treatment. In a landmark decision, the court denied the petition, concluding that although

> she is sufficiently mentally ill to require further retention . . . that determination does not imply that she lacks the mental capacity to knowingly consent or withhold her consent to electroshock therapy . . . It does not matter whether this court would agree with her judgement; it is enough that she is capable of making a decision, however unfortunate that decision may prove to be.

Informed Consent

The criterion of the ability of the patient to understand the nature of the treatment being offered is, of course, fully consistent with the doctrine of informed consent (Meisel et al., 1977). One of the two 1960 landmark cases of the informed consent doctrine, *Mitchell v. Robinson*, involved a psychiatric patient who had sustained spinal fractures as a result of ECT. Even though the patient's consent had been obtained and the physician was not deemed negligent in the performance of the procedure, the court nevertheless ruled the consent invalid (and the physician liable) because he had not adequately informed the patient beforehand of the hazards of treatment.

Meisel et al. (1977) pointed out that in order for consent to treatment to be valid, the patient must be able to act voluntarily; must be provided with a particular amount of information concerning the treatment (specifically, its risks, benefits, and alternatives); must have the capacity to understand the information provided (that is, the patient must be competent); and must actually make a decision regarding the treatment (although consent may sometimes be implied by the patient's passive acceptance of the treatment).

It was apparent from the testimony from the floor at the National Institute of Mental Health Consensus Development Conference that the anti-ECT sentiment derived almost entirely from two kinds of patients: Those who had received involuntary ECT and those who had received ECT voluntarily but without sufficient warning about the possibility of persistent memory impairment. Psychiatrists who wish to continue having ECT available to them as a therapeutic modality should therefore do three things: (1) discontinue the use of sine-wave devices in favor of those administering a brief-pulse, square-wave stimulus; (2) refrain from giving involuntary ECT except under court order; and (3) carefully inform potential ECT candidates and their families about the possibility, however infrequent, of permanent memory loss after ECT, especially with sine-wave bilateral electrode placement. Moreover, all patients should be started on substantially suprathreshold unilateral ECT unless their clinical condition is so severe as to warrant bilateral ECT at the outset (Abrams and Fink, 1984; American Psychiatric Association, 1990). Following these simple guidelines will help defuse the ECT controversy and ensure the continued availability of ECT for the many patients who are likely to benefit from no other form of treatment.

When obtaining consent for ECT, the physician should present the advantages and disadvantages of the proposed treatment in sufficient detail to permit the patient a truly informed choice, without either exaggerating the potential benefits (e.g., promising favorable results) or unduly alarming the patient with a litany of every conceivable risk, no matter how remote. A good relationship with both patient and family is essential in this process, which is ultimately based on personal trust. Of particular help are videotapes that have recently become available that portray the rationale and procedures of ECT in a straightforward and unbiased fashion (Baxter and Liston, 1986; Frankel, 1986; Ries, 1987). A clearly written, concise consent form is also required, one that can be readily understood by patients who have only a limited ability to focus their attention. The example in the Appendix modified from Abrams and Swartz (1991) can be adapted to suit the needs of a particular physician or institution.

Ethical Aspects of ECT

Ottosson (1992, 1995) has reviewed the principles of biomedical ethics as they apply to ECT. Autonomy, beneficence, nonmaleficence, and justice are the basic concepts of biomedical ethics. With regard to ECT, the principle of respect for individual autonomy is satisfied by adherence to the doctrine of informed consent as presented above; the principle of beneficence is satisfied by the results of the studies of ECT versus sham ECT, and ECT versus drug therapy (Chapter 2); the principle of nonmaleficence is satisfied by the results of the studies of ECT and brain damage (Chapter 4), ECT in the high-risk patient (Chapter 5), and the memory and cognitive effects of ECT (Chapter 10). The principle of justice is more difficult to apply with regard to ECT as it concerns, among other things, effects on society—for example, whether a procedure judged as ethically right for one person has negative consequences for others (Reiter-Theil, 1992). Setting this somewhat murky principle aside, then, it is crystal-clear that ECT as a procedure is ethical when administered with informed consent—but is compulsory ECT ever ethical?

This raises the issue of paternalism and relates to questions of competence, guardianship, and judicial order—that is, whether society is justified in treating patients against their will for their own good or the good of others. This question has historically been answered in the affirmative for other medical procedures (e.g., the forced medical isolation of lepers, the quarantine for smallpox) and other psychiatric therapies (e.g., involuntary commitment), and the above discussion of the principles of beneficence and nonmaleficence shows that there is no objective reason to view compulsory ECT differently. Indeed, the vast majority of requests made by psychiatrists to administer involuntary ECT are approved by the courts (Srinivasaraghavan and Abrams, 1996), emphatically demonstrating that society views such a procedure as appropriate.

In my view, a far more important question is whether it is ethical to withhold ECT from a patient who wants it and might benefit from it, as daily occurs in the hundreds of state and other hospitals in the United States that do not offer this form of therapy. If such hospitals do not have an effective referral procedure for sending the patient elsewhere to receive ECT, then they are in the clearly unethical position of refusing to administer a therapy of demonstrated efficacy to a patient who requests it and whose illness might benefit from it alone.

Malpractice Litigation

Slawson and Guggenheim (1984) reviewed the total malpractice experience of the American Psychiatric Association (APA) professional insurance program from 1974 to 1978 and found that ECT accounted for only 15 out of 71,788 claims (0.02%) and only 0.0051% of the loss ($45,000 out of $876 million), an experience that led to reduction, and then elimination, of the program's ECT surcharge. In a more focused review of the Association's subsequent ECT malpractice experience to 1983, Slawson (1985) found only 16 cases that related to ECT: 15 were settled out of court—8 in favor of the psychiatrist, 7 in favor of the patient—and the only case that went to trial was won by the psychiatrist. Moreover, of the 7 cases settled in favor of the patient, 4 involved amounts that averaged only $1000 (two of which were payment of dental bills).

The three cases that required larger settlements—averaging $110,000—included two claims of wrongful death (one in which a psychiatrist administered the anesthesia and failed to resuscitate the patient when he developed laryngospasm), and one of failure to diagnose cancer—the patient improved with ECT but was found a year later to have carcinoma of the tail of the pancreas.

This unusually favorable ECT malpractice experience was confirmed in subsequent reviews (Slawson, 1989, 1991) of the APA's liability program during the years 1984 through 1990, after it had switched from commercial coverage to managing its own claims. During that interval there were just 6 malpractice claims involving ECT, only 2 of which were lawsuits, and the only payment to date had been for the dental bill of two patients who claimed they had sustained dental damage during ECT. No claims involving ECT went to trial.

Dr. Slawson's reviews affirm the generally small liability incurred by physicians who administer ECT, although only about 60% of American psychiatrists are insured through the APA. I am acquainted as an expert witness with 7 additional ECT-related cases during and since the period most recently reviewed by Slawson. Of the three cases tried, the jury found for the psychiatrist in two, and the third was settled in favor of the plaintiff after the trial ended in a hung jury. The two trial cases won by the psychiatrist are instructive (Abrams, 1989a) and demonstrate that juries are more impressed by facts than emotional claims of plaintiffs and their expert witnesses.

In the first case, a 32-year-old housewife claimed that a course of 6 bilateral, brief-pulse ECT received 2 years earlier for an episode of major depression had caused her to suffer brain damage with permanent memory loss. In support of her claim, the plaintiff presented the expert opinions of a clinical psychologist, who testified that the results of neuropsychological testing—primarily the Luria-Nebraska battery—demonstrated recently acquired brain damage, and a neurologist, who testified that an MRI performed a year after ECT showed cortical atrophy, which he attributed to ECT-induced bitemporal brain hemorrhages. The defense impeached the reliability and validity of the Luria-Nebraska battery as a diagnostic test for recently acquired brain damage and cited the data from Duke University (Coffey et al., 1986) that failed to show any deleterious effects of ECT on MRIs obtained before and after ECT. Trial testimony took 5 days, and the jury deliberated 2 hours before finding for the defendant psychiatrist.

In the second case, a 78-year-old retired architect claimed that a course of 7 bilateral sine-wave ECTs received for the treatment of major depression had caused him to suffer brain damage and permanent memory loss and had also induced a severe and totally disabling progression of his preexisting Parkinson's disease. In support of his claim, the plaintiff presented the expert opinion of Dr. John Friedberg, who held that ECT had been contraindicated because of the preexisting diagnosis of Parkinson's disease, especially in view of the fact that the patient had been taking warfarin at the time ECT was given. Dr. Friedberg further opined that the plaintiff had suffered a stroke during ECT, which was the result of the combined effects of warfarin and the induced seizure, leaving him with a permanent organic mental syndrome. The defense cited numerous case reports and review articles—many published in the journal *Convulsive Therapy*—demonstrating the safety and even advisability of administering ECT to depressed patients with Parkinson's disease, as well as the safety of ECT in patients receiving anticoagulant therapy, including warfarin. The defense also presented the results of its own testing of the plaintiff, which demonstrated normal intellectual functioning on the Wechsler Memory Scale and the Mini-Mental State Examination. Trial testimony took 5 days; the jury deliberated less than an hour before finding for the defendant psychiatrist.

In both cases I was impressed that the expert witnesses for the plaintiff were ill-prepared to substantiate their emotionally based claims under cross-examination—probably because there is simply no convincing data in the literature to support the claim that ECT causes either brain damage or permanent memory loss. Dr. Slawson's reviews and my own experience suggest that the exceedingly small number of

ECT malpractice cases that go to trial are usually returned in favor of the psychiatrist; in fact, I am aware of no case won by the plaintiff since 1972, the beginning year of Slawson and Guggenheim's (1984) first review. It is therefore a mistake for the psychiatrist to settle out of court when the facts are in his favor, as they generally are. In this context, it is worth noting that many malpractice policies prevent the insurer from settling out of court without the insured's agreement.

My experience with these and several additional cases has led me to identify the following key elements as common to many suits:

1. The plaintiff claims ECT-induced brain damage with resulting permanent memory loss and social and economic disability, although objective neuropsychological and memory testing reveals normal to superior functioning.
2. The doctor is charged with
    a. improper diagnosis
    b. failing to document a valid indication for ECT
    c. ignoring concurrent medical conditions
    d. rushing to treatment
    e. failing to obtain informed consent
    f. failing to advise the patient of the possibility of long-term memory loss
    g. improperly administering or documenting treatments
3. The expert witnesses for the plaintiff may include Drs. Peter Breggin (psychiatrist) or John Friedberg (neurologist), both of whom have authored books and articles that are highly critical of ECT (Friedberg, 1976, 1977; Breggin, 1979, 1980). Dr. Breggin has also appeared on virulently anti-ECT talk shows (e.g., the Oprah Winfrey show of 22 April 1987) in tandem with Dennis Clarke, president of the Scientology-funded Citizen's Commission on Human Rights.

Both Dr. Friedberg and Dr. Breggin have had the opportunity to present their views at ECT conferences convened by the APA or the National Institute of Mental Health. Dr. Friedberg presented his view of the evidence for ECT-induced neuropathology at the annual meeting of the APA in 1976, during a symposium held in parallel with an ongoing fact-finding mission of the APA Task Force on ECT. His paper (Friedberg, 1977) concluded with the statement that "it is well to reaffirm the individual's right to pursue happiness through brain damage if he or she so chooses," but that doctors should ask themselves whether they should be offering it. Dr. Fred Frankel, chairman of the session (and of the first APA Task Force on ECT) characterized Dr. Friedberg's data as "carelessly culled from the literature and frequently reported inaccurately," and his presentation as inaccurate, indiscriminate, inconsistent and contradictory (Frankel, 1977).

Dr. Breggin is equally guilty of misrepresenting his sources. For example, in his review of the study of Globus et al. (1943) of whether ECS induced neuropathological changes in animals, Dr. Breggin claims that:

> Globus et al found extreme, permanent pathological changes in every single one of their animals, including 'ghost' cells and other signs of dead and dying cells throughout the brain. (Breggin, 1979)

In fact, Globus et al. (1943) found precisely the opposite:

> Under high magnification (fig. 2A) there are no pathologic alterations visible in the nerve cells. These cells are of the usual form and display a normal amount of tigroid substance. Occasionally there is a cell in which the tigroid substance is not very prominent, but this is probably due to the thinness of the section of these cells in the slide. For similar reasons, an occasional cell shows a faint outline of the cell body, often assuming the character of a ghost cell. But when the aforementioned features are compared with those found in a section obtained from a corresponding area of the brain of a normal dog (fig. 2B) the occasional cellular pseudo-defects will be found to be as common in the control as in the experimental animal. (Globus et al., 1943)

Two reviewers of his book (Breggin, 1979) have characterized it as follows:

> ... personal opinions are presented as if they were scholarly deliberations. In fact, most scientific research concerning ECT contradicts Breggin's hypotheses about the efficacy and adverse effects of the treatment. Breggin repeatedly ignores considerable recent literature on unilateral ECT, as well as low-energy stimulation, both of which have dramatically reduced the side-effect of memory loss. ... Dr. Breggin's arguments fail because he uses supporting data uncritically and inaccurately. (Mandel, 1980)

and,

> ... both quantitatively and qualitatively, factual inaccuracies and notable absences ensure an exceedingly biased presentation. (Weiner, 1980)

With full knowledge of Dr. Breggin's propensity for misrepresenting the facts about ECT, however, the Planning Committee for the 1985 National Institutes of Health Consensus Conference on ECT (of which I was a member) nevertheless invited him to present his opinions on the neuropathology and cognitive dysfunction of ECT to a panel representing psychiatry, psychology, neurology, psychopharmacology, epidemiology, law, and the general public. The panel listened politely to Dr. Breggin's presentation—which largely reprised Dr. Friedberg's of 8 years earlier—but gave it no weight in its final report (National Institutes of Health, 1985), which concluded that:

> . . . objective [neuropsychological] tests have not firmly established persistent or permanent [memory] deficits for a more extensive period [than a few weeks surrounding the treatment] . . .

and that

> In studies that have been controlled for fixation artifacts, hypoxia, and other methodological problems, neuronal cell death has not been detected.

Recent judicial decisions have effectively neutralized both the value of Dr. Breggin's testimony to plaintiffs' lawyers and his undue influence on the public's view of the therapeutic roles of ECT and psychopharmacology (Abrams, 1995). Dr. Breggin's credentials and opinions as an expert medical witness were scathingly rejected by the court in two separate and unrelated lawsuits, one in which the plaintiff claimed damages from ECT, and another in which the plaintiff claimed damages from a psychopharmacologic agent, Halcion.

In the first case, involving ECT (*Lightner vs. Alessi*), I served earlier on as an expert witness for the defendant but was unable to appear at the trial because I was out of the country. Judge Hilary Kaplan in the Circuit Court for Baltimore City issued a 17-page ruling, on 22 February 1995, to strike Dr. Breggin's testimony from the record for the following reasons (excerpted):

> Dr. Breggin was not in a hospital setting for 30 years, he never saw this patient . . . This is what I call telephone psychiatry, not face-to-face. . . . Now I chose to call Breggin's testimony a house of cards, because he selects those pieces of bricks and mortar that he chooses to believe, and excludes those which he chooses not to believe. . . . The factual basis of Breggin's opinions in this case are a number of examples that are either erroneous or he has selective memory,

or there are no factual basis for those. . . . It is okay to differ with mainstream medicine, I have no problem with that. That is not the issue here. But some [of Breggin's] opinions are just incredible. . . . This witness was unprepared. This witness was not grounded in the facts of this case, did not know this chart, not familiar with those items which he believes—which I believe he testified to. . . . The court believes not only is this gentleman [Breggin] unqualified to render the opinions that he did, I believe that his bias in this case is blinding. It is not just a bias that one sees in a normal case. It is a blinding bias that permeated two and a half days of testimony in this courtroom. . . . The court believes that this witness [Breggin] does not have sufficient familiarity with the subject matter in this case to express an opinion, and that opinion has no rational basis in fact. . . . So, reluctantly . . . the court is going to strike the testimony of Dr. Breggin, finding that it has no rational basis, and that it is both biased and lacks the underpinnings to express the opinions that are expressed.

In the second case (*The Estates of Lam v. Upjohn Co.*), U.S. Magistrate Judge Crigler of the U.S. District Court, Western District of Virginia, rendered the opinion on 20 March 1995, that:

The evidence of Peter Breggin as purported expert, fails nearly all particulars under the standard set forth in Daubert and its progeny. The record supports defendant's assertions that: 1) Breggin stands alone in his theory that Halcion causes suicidal or homicidal behavior; 2) his causation theories have not been subjected to peer review; 3) the data principally is anecdotal; and 4) his methodology essentially is an estimate incapable of producing a testable rate of error. As to his testimony regarding the warning on the Halcion package, Breggin has conducted no original research, has performed no personal re-analysis of the work of others, has prescribed Halcion only once since 1983, has no academic training or regulatory experience and has never participated in any FDA-related proceedings addressing what constitutes an adequate warning. Simply put, the court believes that Dr. Breggin's opinions do not rise to the level of an opinion based on "good science." The motion to exclude his testimony as an expert witness should be granted.

The Risk of Litigation

In my view, the prudent physician who gives ECT can best protect himself against even the small risk of a malpractice suit—and position himself to prevail in the unlikely event that one is filed—by adhering to the following few simple tenets of good medical practice.

1. Always obtain explicit, fully informed, written consent for ECT. Give your patient an ECT information pamphlet to read and note this in the chart. If more information is requested, have the patient view a videotape on ECT and note this in the chart as well. Use the sample consent form in the Appendix, or any other that includes a reasonably complete presentation of the risks and potential benefits of ECT, including mention of bilateral compared with unilateral ECT. All of the main risks of ECT—including the possibility of persistent memory dysfunction—should be written into the form, rather than simply being discussed with the patient. If your hospital uses only a general consent form that omits specific language covering the details of ECT, have the patient sign your own form as well. Have someone reliable physically present during your explanation of this material to sign the consent form as a witness. Write everything you tell the patient about ECT in the chart, along with the patient's queries and your responses. If during the treatment course the patient expresses doubts or fears about receiving further ECT, do not proceed with treatment until and unless you have alleviated these apprehensions and documented your discussion and the patient's acquiescence in the chart.

2. Explain your decision to recommend ECT by recording each of its clinical indications in the chart. Do not simply assert that the patient has "melancholia," but rather list each of its syndromal elements (e.g., early waking, guilt, anorexia, etc.). Use the authoritative sources of the 1990 APA ECT Task Force recommendations, the journal *Convulsive Therapy*, and this volume to document all supporting evidence for primary or secondary use of ECT as outlined in the report. The primary indications—justifying the use of ECT as the initial treatment of choice—include:
   a. The need for a rapid, definitive treatment response
   b. The opinion that alternative treatments are riskier than ECT
   c. A history of poor drug response or good ECT response
   d. Patient preference

The secondary indications—justifying use of ECT after another treatment—include:
   a. Treatment failure (e.g., drug therapy resistance)
   b. Adverse effects of other treatments
   c. Deterioration of patient while receiving other treatments

3. If the indication for ECT is atypical or unclear, obtain a second opinion from a consultant who is not associated with your practice.
4. Attend at least one educational course on ECT each year, own the 1990 APA ECT Task Force Report, read at least one up-to-date text that includes a full description of the principles and practice of ECT, and subscribe to and read the *American Journal of Psychiatry* and *Convulsive Therapy*.
5. Document carefully the details of each ECT treatment session, including drugs and dosages given, stimulus parameters, treatment electrode placement, oxygenation, and seizure monitoring method and duration.
6. Avoid giving ECT to patients with pronounced histrionic personality traits, dysthymia, or hypochondriasis, and especially those who frequently express anger and resentment over alleged misdiagnosis or mistreatment by previous physicians, no matter how highly they praise your skills in comparison. Such patients rarely respond favorably to ECT.
7. Read the nursing notes and document each instance of clinical improvement as it occurs. Regularly examine and record the patient's cognitive status. Most importantly, write legibly while imagining each note being read aloud to the jury by a plaintiff's attorney.

Appendix: Consent for Electroconvulsive Therapy

Information: ECT, previously known as shock therapy, is a method for treating certain mental or emotional conditions by stimulating the brain electrically in order to produce a convulsive seizure. The procedure is carried out by doctors and nurses while the patient is fully asleep under general anesthesia.

Description of the Procedure: While the patient is lying on a stretcher, a needle is placed in a vein and an anesthetic medication is injected. After the patient is asleep, a muscle-relaxing medication is then given through the same needle, and the patient is given pure oxygen through a mask. When the patient's muscles are relaxed, an electrical stimulus is briefly applied to the scalp in order to stimulate the brain into a period of intense, rhythmical, electrical activity. This seizure lasts a minute or two and is accompanied by mild contractions of the muscles. When the seizure is over, the patient is taken to a recovery area and observed by trained staff until he awakens, usually in about 20 minutes. ECT is given every other day for about 6 to 12 treatments, although some patients may require more than 12 treatments to reach maximum improvement.

Risks of the Treatment: ECT is among the safest of medical treatments given under general anesthesia. The risk of death or serious injury with ECT is about 1 in 50,000 treatments, much smaller than that reported for childbirth. The extremely rare deaths that do occur are usually due to cardiovascular complications.

Side Effects and Complications: Patients may be confused just after they awaken from ECT; this confusion generally clears up within an hour or so. Memory for recent events may be disturbed, and dates, names of friends, public events, addresses, and telephone numbers may be forgotten. In most patients, this memory difficulty goes away within a few days or weeks, although a very few may continue to experience memory problems for months or years afterwards. Certain treatment techniques prevent or minimize the occurrence of such memory problems (for example, brief-pulse, right unilateral ECT), and your doctor will discuss these options with you. No long-term effects of ECT on intellectual ability (IQ) or memory capacity have been found.

Results of Treatment: Although many patients experience significant improvement after a course of ECT, no specific treatment results can be promised. As is true with all medical treatments, some patients will recover quickly, some slowly, and a few might not recover at all. Even when recovery is complete, relapse is still possible. Medication therapy is often prescribed after a course of ECT in order to prevent such relapses.

Availability of Alternative Treatments: Medications may be available to treat your particular condition, and it is possible that some of them might work as well as, or better than, ECT. The advantages and disadvantages of medication therapy will be discussed with you by your doctor.

Right to Withdraw Consent: Even though a patient voluntarily signs an agreement to receive ECT, he may withdraw his consent at any time, even before the first treatment is given. Withdrawal of consent for ECT does not in any way prejudice the patient's continued treatment with the best alternative methods available.

Risks of Not Having Electroconvulsive Therapy as Recommended: It is possible that ECT may be more effective for your condition than any available medications and that if you choose not to accept your doctor's recommendation to have ECT, you might experience a longer or more severe period of illness and disability. Medication therapy has its own risks and complications and is not generally safer than ECT.

I, _____ have read the above description of the ECT treatment that has been recommended to me, and it has also been explained to me by _____ , who has answered any questions I had. I agree to have the treatments and understand that Dr. _____ will be in charge of administering the treatments.

Patient signature _____ Date _____

Witness signature _____ Date _____

References

Abbott RJ, Loizou LA. (1986) Neuroleptic malignant syndrome. *Br J Psychiatry 148*:47–51.

Abiuso P, Dunkelman R, Proper M. (1978) Electroconvulsive therapy in patients with pacemakers. *JAMA 240*:2459–60.

Abramczuk JA, Rose NM. (1979) Pre-anaesthetic assessment and the prevention of post-ECT morbidity. *Br J Psychiatry 134*:582–7.

Abrams R. (1967) Daily administration of unilateral ECT. *Am J Psychiatry 124*:384–86.

Abrams R. (1972) Recent clinical studies of ECT. *Seminars in Psychiatry 4*:3–12.

Abrams R. (1975) Drugs in combination with ECT. In: M Greenblatt, ed. *Drugs in Combination with Other Therapies*. New York: Grune and Stratton. pp. 157–64.

Abrams R. (1982a) Clinical prediction of ECT response in depressed patients. *Psychopharmacol Bull 18*:73–5.

Abrams R. (1982b) ECT and tricyclic antidepressants in the treatment of endogenous depression. *Psychopharmacol Bull 18*:48–50.

Abrams R. (1986a) Is unilateral electroconvulsive therapy really the treatment of choice in endogenous depression? *Ann NY Acad Sci 462*: 50–5.

Abrams R. (1986b) A hypothesis to explain divergent findings among studies comparing the efficacy of unilateral and bilateral ECT in depression. *Convuls Ther 2*:253–7.

Abrams R. (1987) ECT in schizophrenia. *Convuls Ther 3*:169–70.

Abrams R. (1988) Interview with Lothar Kalinowsky. *Convuls Ther 4*:24–39.

Abrams R. (1989a) Malpractice litigation and ECT [letter]. *Convuls Ther 5*: 365–7.

Abrams R. (1989b) ECT for Parkinson's disease [editorial]. *Am J Psychiatry 146*:1391–3.

Abrams R. (1990) Termination of ECT-induced prolonged seizures [letter]. *Convuls Ther 6*:54–8.

Abrams R. (1991a) Seizure generalization and the efficacy of unilateral Electroconvulsive Therapy. *Convuls Ther* 7:213–17.

Abrams R. (1991b) The FDA proposal to reclassify ECT devices [editorial]. *Convuls Ther* 7:1–4.

Abrams R. (1992) *Electroconvulsive Therapy*. New York: Oxford University Press.

Abrams R. (1994) Stimulus parameters and efficacy of ECT [commentary]. *Convuls Ther* 10:124–8.

Abrams R. (1995) ECT malpractice issues. *Convuls Ther* 11:286–87.

Abrams R. (1996) ECT stimulus parameters as determinants of seizure quality. *Psychiatric Annals* 26:701–4.

Abrams R, Essman WB, eds. (1982) *Electroconvulsive Therapy: Biological Foundations and Clinical Applications*. New York: Spectrum Publications.

Abrams R, Fink M. (1969) *Convulsive Therapy: Methods and Applications*. New York: New York Medical College.

Abrams R, Fink M. (1972) Clinical experiences with multiple electroconvulsive treatments. *Compr Psychiatry* 13:115–22.

Abrams R, Fink M. (1984) The present status of unilateral ECT: some recommendations [editorial]. *J Affect Disord* 7:245–7.

Abrams R, Swartz CM. (1985a) ECT and prolactin release: relation to treatment response in melancholia. *Convuls Ther* 1:38–42.

Abrams R, Swartz CM. (1985b) ECT and prolactin release: effects of stimulus parameters. *Convuls Ther* 1:115–9.

Abrams R, Swartz CM. (1985c) *ECT Instruction Manual*. Lake Bluff, IL: Somatics Inc.

Abrams R, Swartz CM. (1989) Electroconvulsive therapy apparatus and method for automatic monitoring of patient seizures [patent]. U.S. patent 4,878,498.

Abrams R, Swartz CM. (1991) Consent for electroconvulsive therapy. In: R Abrams, CM Swartz, eds. *The Technique of ECT: Documentation and Forms*. Lake Bluff IL: Somatics Inc. pp. 2–3.

Abrams R, Swartz CM. (1997) Convulsive therapy apparatus to stimulate and monitor the extent of the therapeutic value of the treatment. U.S. patent applied for.

Abrams R, Swartz CM, Vedak C. (1989) Antidepressant effects of right versus left unilateral ECT and the lateralization theory of ECT action. *Am J Psychiatry* 146:1190–2.

Abrams R, Taylor MA. (1973) Anterior bifrontal ECT: a clinical trial. *Br J Psychiatry* 122:587–90.

Abrams R, Taylor MA. (1974) Unipolar and bipolar depressive illness: phenomenology and response to electroconvulsive therapy. *Arch Gen Psychiatry* 30:320–1.

Abrams R, Taylor MA. (1976a) Catatonia: a prospective study. *Arch Gen Psychiatry* 33:579–81.

Abrams R, Taylor MA. (1976b) Diencephalic stimulation and the effects of ECT in endogenous depression. *Br J Psychiatry 129*:482–5.

Abrams R, Taylor MA. (1976c) Mania and schizo-affective disorder, manic type: A comparison. *Am J Psychiatry 133*:1445–7.

Abrams R, Taylor MA. (1979) Differential EEG patterns in affective disorder and schizophrenia. *Arch Gen Psychiatry 36*:1355–8.

Abrams R, Taylor MA. (1981) Importance of schizophrenic symptoms in the diagnosis of mania. *Am J Psychiatry 138*:658–61.

Abrams R, Taylor MA. (1985) A prospective follow-up study of cognitive functions after ECT. *Convuls Ther 1*:4–9.

Abrams R, Vedak C. (1991) Prediction of ECT response in melancholia. *Convuls Ther 7*:81–4.

Abrams R, Volavka J. (1982) Electroencephalographic effects of convulsive therapy. In: R Abrams, WB Essman, eds. *Electroconvulsive Therapy: Biological Foundations and Clinical Applications.* New York: Spectrum Publications. pp. 157–67.

Abrams R, Volavka J, Dornbush R, Roubicek J, Fink M. (1970) Lateralized EEG changes after unilateral and bilateral electroconvulsive therapy. *Dis Nerv Syst 31*:28–33.

Abrams R, Fink M, Dornbush R, Feldstein S, Volavka J, Roubicek J. (1972) Unilateral and bilateral ECT: effects on depression, memory, and the electroencephalogram. *Arch Gen Psychiatry 27*:88–91.

Abrams R, Volavka J, Fink M. (1973) EEG seizure patterns during multiple unilateral and bilateral ECT. *Compr Psychiatry 14*:25–8.

Abrams R, Taylor MA, Faber R, Ts'o T, Williams R, Almy G. (1983) Bilateral versus unilateral ECT: efficacy in melancholia. *Am J Psychiatry 140*: 463–5.

Abrams R, Taylor MA, Volavka J. (1987) ECT-induced EEG asymmetry and therapeutic response in melancholia: relation to treatment electrode placement. *Am J Psychiatry 144*:327–9.

Abrams R, Swartz CM, Vedak C. (1991) Antidepressant effects of high-dose right unilateral electroconvulsive therapy. *Arch Gen Psychiatry 48*:746–8.

Abrams R, Volavka J, Schrift M. (1992) Brief pulse ECT in melancholia: EEG and clinical effects. *J Nerv Ment Dis 180*:55–7.

Accornero F. (1988) An eyewitness account of the discovery of electroshock. *Convuls Ther 4*:40–9.

Acevedo AG, Smith JK. (1988) Adverse reaction to use of caffeine in ECT. *Am J Psychiatry 145*:529–30.

Ackermann RF, Engel J, Jr, Baxter L. (1986) Positron emission tomography and autoradiographic studies of glucose utilization following electroconvulsive seizures in humans and rats. *Ann N Y Acad Sci 462*: 263–9.

Addersley DJ, Hamilton M. (1953) Use of succinylcholine in ECT. *Br Med J 1*:195–7.

Addonizio G, Susman V. (1986) Neuroleptic malignant syndrome and use of anesthetic agents. *Am J Psychiatry 143*:127–8.

Adityanjee, Jayaswal SK, Chan TM, Subramaniam M. (1990) Temporary remission of tardive dystonia following electroconvulsive therapy. *Br J Psychiatry 156*:433–5.

Ahlskog JE, Kelly PJ, van Heerden JA, Stoddard SL, Tyce GM, Windebank AJ, Bailey PA, Bell GN, Blexrud MD, Charmichael SW. (1990) Adrenal medullary transplantation into the brain for treatment of Parkinson's disease: clinical outcome and neurochemical studies. *Mayo Clin Proc 65*:305–28.

Albala AA, Greden JF, Tarika J, Carroll BJ. (1981) Changes in serial dexamethasone suppression tests among unipolar depressives receiving electroconvulsive treatment. *Biol Psychiatry 16*:551–60.

Alexander RC, Salomon M, Ionescu-Pioggia M, Cole J. (1988) Convulsive therapy in the treatment of mania: McLean Hospital 1973–1986. *Convuls Ther 4*:115–25.

Alexopoulos GS, Frances RJ. (1980) ECT and cardiac patients with pacemakers. *Am J Psychiatry 137*:1111–2.

Alexopoulos GS, Inturrisi CE, Lipman R, Frances R, Haycox J, Dougherty JR, Jr, Rossier J. (1983) Plasma immunoreactive β-endorphin levels in depression: effect of electroconvulsive therapy. *Arch Gen Psychiatry 40*:181–83.

Alexopoulos GS, Shamoian CJ, Lucas J, Weiser N, Berger H. (1984a) Medical problems of geriatric psychiatric patients and younger controls during electroconvulsive therapy. *J Am Geriatr Soc 32*:651–54.

Alexopoulos GS, Young RC, Shamoian CA. (1984b) Unilateral electroconvulsive therapy: An open clinical comparison of two electrode placements. *Biol Psychiatry 19*:783–7.

Alger I. (1991) History of modern psychiatry, and modern application of electroconvulsive treatment. *Hospital and Community Psychiatry 42*: 355–6.

Allen RE, Pitts FN, Jr. (1978) ECT for depressed patients with lupus erythematosus. *Am J Psychiatry 135*:367–8.

Allman P, Hawton K. (1987) ECT for post-stroke depression: beta blockade to modify rise in blood pressure. *Convuls Ther 3*:218–21.

Almansi R, Impastato DJ. (1940) Electrically induced convulsions in the treatment of mental diseases. *NY State J Medicine 40*:1315–16.

Alpers BJ and Hughes J (1942) Changes in the brain after electrically induced convulsions in cats. *Arch Neurol Psychiatry 47*:385–398.

American Psychiatric Association Task Force on ECT. (1978) Electroconvulsive Therapy: Task Force Report No. 14. Washington, DC: American Psychiatric Association.

American Psychiatric Association Task Force on Electroconvulsive Therapy. (1990) The Practice of Electroconvulsive Therapy: Recommendations for Treatment, Training, and Privileging. Washington, DC: American Psychiatric Association.

Ames D, Burrows G, Davies B, Maguire K, Norman T. (1984) A study of the dexamethasone suppression test in hospitalized depressed patients. *Br J Psychiatry 144*:311–3.

Ananth J, Samra D, Kolivakis T. (1979) Amelioration of drug-induced Parkinsonism by ECT. *Am J Psychiatry 136*:1094.

Andersen K, Balldin J, Gottfries CG, Granerus AK, Modigh K, Svennerholm L, Wallin A. (1987) A double-blind evaluation of electroconvulsive therapy in Parkinson's disease with "on-off" phenomena. *Acta Neurol Scand 76*:191–9.

Andrade C, Gangadhar BN, Subbakrishna DK, Channabasavanna SM, Pradhan N. (1988a) A double-blind comparison of sinusoidal wave and brief-pulse electroconvulsive therapy in endogenous depression. *Convuls Ther 4*:297–305.

Andrade C, Gangadhar BN, Swaminanth G, Channabasavanna SM. (1988b) Predicting the outcome of endogenous depression following electroconvulsive therapy. *Convuls Ther 4*:169–74.

Andrade C, Gangadhar BN, Swaminath G, Channabasavana SM. (1988c) Mania as a side effect of electroconvulsive therapy. *Convuls Ther 4*: 81–3.

Andrade C, Gangadhar BN, Channabasavana SM. (1990) Further characterization of mania as a side effect of ECT. *Convuls Ther 6*:318–9.

Annett M, Hudson PT, Turner A. (1974) Effects of right and left unilateral ECT on naming and visual discrimination analysed in relation to handedness. *Br J Psychiatry 124*:260–4.

Anton AH, Uy DS, Redderson CL. (1977) Autonomic blockade and the cardiovascular and catecholamine response to electroshock. *Anesth Analg 56*:46–54.

Aperia B. (1986) Hormone pattern and post-treatment attitudes in patients with major depressive disorder given electroconvulsive therapy. *Acta Psychiatr Scand 73*:271–4.

Aperia B, Thoren M, Wetterberg L. (1985) Prolactin and thyrotropin in serum during electroconvulsive therapy in patients with major depressive illness. *Acta Psychiatr Scand 72*:302–8.

Arana GW, Baldessarini RJ, Ornsteen M. (1985) The dexamethasone suppression test for diagnosis and prognosis in psychiatry. Commentary and review. *Arch Gen Psychiatry 42*:1193–204.

Arato M, Erdos A, Kurcz M, Vermes I, Fekete M. (1980) Studies on the prolactin response induced by electroconvulsive therapy in schizophrenics. *Acta Psychiatry Scand 61*:239–44

Ashton R, Hess N. (1976) Amnesia for random shapes following unilateral and bilateral electronvulsive shock therapy. *Percept Mot Skills 42*:669–70.

Asnis G. (1977) Parkinson's disease, depression, and ECT: A review and case study. *Am J Psychiatry 134*:191–95.

Asnis GM, Leopold MA. (1978) A single-blind study of ECT in patients with tardive dyskinesia. *Am J Psychiatry 135*:1235–7.

Asnis GM, Fink M, Saferstein S. (1978) ECT in metropolitan New York hospitals: a survey of practice, 1975–1976. *Am J Psychiatry 135*: 479–82.

Atre-Vaidya N, Jampala VC. (1978) Electroconvulsive therapy in parkinsonism with affective disorder. *Br J Psychiatry 152*:55–8.

Avery D, Lubrano A. (1979) Depression treated with imipramine and ECT: the DeCarolis study reconsidered. *Am J Psychiatry 136*:559–62.

Avery D, Winokur G. (1976) Mortality in depressed patients treated with electroconvulsive therapy and antidepressants. *Arch Gen Psychiatry 33*: 1029–37.

Avery D, Winokur G. (1977) The efficacy of electroconvulsive therapy and antidepressants in depression. *Biol Psychiatry 12*:507–23.

Avramov MN, Husain MM, White PF. (1995) The comparative effects of methohexital, propofol, and etomidate for electroconvulsive therapy. *Anesth Analg 81*:596–602.

Babigian HM, Guttmacher LB. (1984) Epidemiologic considerations in electroconvulsive therapy. *Arch Gen Psychiatry 41*:246–53.

Babington RG, Wedeking PW. (1975) Blockade of tardive seizures in rats by electroconvulsive shock. *Brain Res 88*:141–44.

Bagadia VN, Abhyankar RR, Doshi J, Pradhan PV, Shah LP. (1983) A double blind controlled study of ECT vs chlorpromazine in schizophrenia. *J Assoc Physicians India 31*:637–40.

Bailey J, Coppen A. (1976) A comparison between the Hamilton rating scale and the Beck depression inventory in the measurement of depression. *Br J Psychiatry 128*:486–9.

Bajc M, Medved V, Basic M, Topuzovik N, Babic D, Ivancevic D. (1989) Acute effect of electroconvulsive therapy on brain perfusion assessed by Tc99m-hexamethylpropyleneamineoxim and single photon emission computed tomography. *Acta Psychiatr Scand 80*:421–6.

Balldin, J. (1982) Factors influencing prolactin release induced by electroconvulsive therapy. *Acta Psychiatr Scand 65*:365–9.

Balldin J, Berggren U, Lindstedt G, Modigh K. (1992) Neuroendocrine evidence for decreased function of alpha2-adrenergic receptor after electroconvulsive therapy. *Psychiatry Res 41*:257–65.

Balldin J, Bolle P, Eden S, Eriksson E, Modigh K. (1980a) Effects of electroconvulsive treatment on growth hormone secretion induced by monoamine receptor agonists in reserpine-pretreated rats. *Psychoneuroendocrinology 5*:329–37.

Balldin J, Eden S, Granerus AK, Modigh K, Svanborg A, Walinder J, Wallin, M. (1980b) Electroconvulsive therapy in Parkinson's syndrome with "on-off" phenomenon. *J Neural Transm 47*:11–21.

Balldin J, Granerus AK, Lindstedt G, Modigh K, Walinder J. (1981) Predictors for improvement after electroconvulsive therapy in parkinsonian patients with on-off symptoms. *J Neural Transm 52*:199–211.

Balldin J, Granerus AK, Lindstedt G, Modigh K, Walinder J. (1982) Neuroendocrine evidence for increased responsiveness of dopamine receptors in humans following electroconvulsive therapy. *Psychopharmacology 76*:371–6.

Barbour GL, Blumenkrantz MJ. (1978) Videotape aids informed consent decision. *JAMA 240*:2741–42.

Barker JC, Baker AA. (1959) Deaths associated with electroplexy. *Journal of Mental Science 105*:339–48.

Barton JL. (1977) ECT in depression: the evidence of controlled studies. *Biol Psychiatry 12*:687–95.

Barton JL, Mehta S, Snaith RP. (1973) The prophylactic value of extra ECT in depressive illness. *Acta Psychiatr Scand 49*:386–92.

Bates WJ, Smeltzer DJ. (1982) Electroconvulsive treatment of psychotic self-injurious behavior in a patient with severe mental retardation. *Am J Psychiatry 139*:1355–6.

Baxter LR, Jr, Liston EH. (1986) Informed ECT for patients and families with Dr. Max Fink [videotape review]. *Convuls Ther 2*:301–3.

Baxter LR, Roy-Byrne P, Liston EH, Fairbanks L. (1986) Informing patients about electroconvulsive therapy: effects of a videotape presentation. *Convuls Ther 2*:25–29.

Bayles S, Busse EW, Ebaugh FG. (1950) Square waves (BST) versus sine waves in electroconvulsive therapy. *Am J Psychiatry 107*:34–41.

Beale MD, Kellner CH, Pritchett JT, Bernstein HJ, Burns CM, Knapp R. (1994) Stimulus dose-titration in ECT: a 2-year clinical experience. *Convuls Ther 10*:171–76.

Bean GJ, Marchese V, Martin BA. (1991) Electric stimulus energy and the clinical response to electroconvulsive therapy. *Can J Psychiatry 36*: 637–44.

Behar R. (1991) The thriving cult of greed and power [Cover Story]. *Time* May 6. pp. 50–57.

Bellett S, Kershbaum A, Furst W. (1941) The electrocardiogram during electric shock treatment of mental disorders. *American Journal of Mental Science 201*:167–76.

Benbow SM. (1987) The use of electroconvulsive therapy in old age psychiatry. *International Journal of Geriatric Psychiatry 2*:25–30.

Benbow SM. (1988) ECT for depression in dementia. *Br J Psychiatry 152*: 859.

Bennett AE. (1983) Electroshock and Berkeley. *Biol Psychiatry 18*:609–10.

Berens ES, Yesavage JA, Leirer VO. (1982) A comparison of multiple and single electroconvulsive therapy. *J Clin Psychiatry 43*:126–8.

Berent S, Cohen BD, Silverman A. (1975) Changes in verbal and nonverbal learning following a single left or right unilateral electroconvulsive treatment. *Biol Psychiatry 10*:95–100.

Berg S, Gabriel AR, Impastato DJ. (1959) Comparative evaluation of the safety of chlorpromazine and reserpine used in conjunction with ECT. *J Neuropsychiatry 1*:104–7.

Bergman PS, Gabriel AR, Impastato DJ, Wortis SB. (1952) EEG changes following ECT with the Reiter apparatus. *Confinia Neurologica 12*: 347–51.

Bergsholm P, Gran L, Bleie H. (1984) Seizure duration in unilateral electroconvulsive therapy. The effect of hypocapnia induced by hyperventilation and the effect of ventilation with oxygen. *Acta Psychiatr Scand 69*:121–8.

Bergsholm P, Larsen JL, Rosendahl K, Holsten F. (1989) Electroconvulsive therapy and cerebral computed tomography. A prospective study. *Acta Psychiatr Scand 80*:566–72.

Berne RM, Levy MN. (1981) *Cardiovascular Physiology*. St. Louis: C.V. Mosby. pp 145–178.

Berson SA, Yalow RS. (1968) Radioimmunoassay of ACTH in plasma. *J Clin Invest 47*:2725–51.

Bertagnoli MW, Borchardt CM. (1990) A review of ECT for children and adolescents. *J Am Acad Child Adolesc Psychiatry 2*:302–7.

Bidder TG, Strain JJ. (1970) Modifications of electroconvulsive therapy. *Comprehensive Psychiatry 11*:507–17.

Bidder TG, Strain JJ, Brunschwig L. (1970) Bilateral and unilateral ECT: follow-up study and critique. *Am J Psychiatry 127*:737–45.

Bini L. (1938) Experimental researches on epileptic attacks induced by the electric current. *Am J Psychiatry (suppl) 94*:172–4.

Bini L. (1995) Professor Bini's notes on the first electro-shock experiment. *Convuls Ther 11*:260–62.

Birkett DP. (1988) ECT in parkinsonism with affective disorder [letter]. *Br J Psychiatry 152*:712.

Blachly P, Gowing D. (1966) Multiple monitored electroconvulsive treatment. *Compr Psychiatry 7*:100–9.

Blachly PH, Semler HJ. (1967) Electroconvulsive therapy of three patients with aortic valve prostheses. *Am J Psychiatry 124*:233–6.

Black DW, Wilcox JA, Stewart M. (1985) The use of ECT in children: case report. *J Clin Psychiatry 46:*98–9.

Black DW, Winokur G, Nasrallah H. (1987) Treatment of mania: a naturalistic study of electroconvulsive therapy versus lithium in 438 patients. *J Clin Psychiatry 48*:132–9.

Black DW, Winokur G, Hulbert J, Nasrallah A. (1988) Predictors of immediate response in the treatment of mania: the importance of co-morbidity. *Biol Psychiatry 24*:191–8.

Blaurock MF, Lorimer FM, Segal MM, Gibbs FA. (1950) Focal electroencephalographic changes in unilateral electric convulsive therapy. *Arch Neurol Psychiatry 64*:220–6.

Bodley PO, Fenwick PBC. (1966) The effect of electroconvulsive therapy on patients with essential hypertension. *Br J Psychiatry 112*:1241–9.

Boey WK, Lai FO. (1990) Comparison of propofol and thiopentone as anaesthetic agents for electroconvulsive therapy. *Anaesthesia 45*:623–8.

Bolwig TG. (1984) The influence of electrically-induced seizures on deep brain structures. In: B Lerer, RD Weiner, RH Belmaker, eds. *ECT: Basic Mechanisms*. London: John Libbey. pp. 132–8.

Bolwig T. (1987) Training in convulsive therapy in Denmark. *Convuls Ther* 3:156–57.

Bolwig T. (1988) Blood-brain barrier studies with special reference to epileptic seizures. *Acta Psychiatr Scand Suppl 345*:15–20.

Bolwig TG, Hertz MM, Holm-Jensen J. (1977) Blood-brain barrier during electroshock seizures in the rat. *Eur J Clin Invest 7*:95–100.

Bouckoms AJ, Welch CA, Drop L, Dao T, Kolton K. (1989) Atropine in electroconvulsive therapy. *Convuls Ther 5*:48–55.

Bourne H. (1954) Convulsion dependence. *Lancet 2*:1193–6.

Bourne H. (1956) Convulsion dependence and rational convulsion therapy. *Journal of the Indian Medical Profession 3*:1–6.

Boyd DA, Brown DW. (1948) Electroconvulsive therapy in mental disorders associated with childbearing. *Journal of Missouri Medicine 45*: 573–9.

Braasch ER, Demaso DR. (1980) Effect of electroconvulsive therapy on serum isoenzymes. *Am J Psychiatry 137*:625–6.

Bracha S, Hess JP. (1956) Death occurring during combined reserpine-electroshock treatment. *Am J Psychiatry 113*:257.

Brandon S. (1981) The history of shock treatment. In: RL Palmer, ed. *Electroconvulsive Therapy: An Appraisal*. Oxford: Oxford University Press. pp. 3–10.

Brandon S, Cowley P, McDonald C, Neville P, Palmer R, Wellstood-Eason S. (1984) Electroconvulsive therapy: results in depressive illness from the Leicestershire trial. *Br Med J 288*:22–25.

Brandon S, Cowley P, McDonald C, Neville P, Palmer R, Wellstood-Easton S. (1985) Leicester ECT trial. Results in schizophrenia. *Br J Psychiatry 146*:177–83.

Breggin PR. (1979) *Electroshock: Its Brain-Disabling Effects*. New York: Springer.

Breggin PR. (1980) Electroconvulsive therapy for depression [letter]. *N Engl J Med 303*:1305–6.

Bridenbaugh RH, Drake FR, O'Regan TJ. (1972) Multiple monitored electroconvulsive treatment of schizophrenia. *Compr Psychiatry 13*:9–17.

Brill NQ, Crumpton E, Eiduson S, Grayson HM, Hellman LI, Richards RA. (1959) Relative effectiveness of various components of electroconvulsive therapy. *Archives of Neurology and Psychiatry 81*:627–35.

Brockman RJ, Brockman JC, Jacobsohn N, Gleser GC, Ulett GA. (1956) Changes in convulsive threshold as related to type of treatment. *Confinia Neurologica 16*:97–104.

Brodersen P, Paulson OB, Bolwig TG, Rogon ZE, Rafaelsen OJ, Lassen NA. (1973) Cerebral hyperemia in electrically induced epileptic seizures. *Arch Neurol 28*:334–8.

Bross R. (1957) Near fatality with combined ECT and reserpine. *Am J Psychiatry 113*:933.

Brown GL. (1975) Parkinsonism, depression, and ECT. *Am J Psychiatry 132*: 1084.

Brown GL, Wilson WP, Green RL, Jr. (1973) Mental aspects of Parkinsonism and their management. In: SJ Bern, ed. *Parkinson's Disease—Rigidity, Akinesia, Behavior. vol. 2; Selected Communications on Topic.* Toronto: Hans Huber. pp. 265–78.

Brumback RA. (1983) EEG monitoring of ECT. *Br J Psychiatry 142*: 104–5.

Brumback RA. (1987) EEG monitoring. *Convuls Ther 3*:151–7.

Brunschwig L, Strain JJ, Bidder TG. (1971) Issues in the assessment of post-ECT memory changes. *Br J Psychiatry 119*:73–4.

Buckholtz NS, Davies AO, Rudorfer MV, Golden RN, Potter WZ. (1988) Lymphocyte beta adrenergic receptor function versus catecholamines in depression. *Biol Psychiatry 24*:451–7.

Burke WJ, Peterson J, Rubin EH. (1988) Electroconvulsive therapy in the treatment of combined depression and Parkinson's disease. *Psychosomatics 29*:341–6.

Burke WJ, Rubin EH, Zorumski CF, Wetzel RD. (1987) The safety of ECT in geriatric psychiatry. *J Amer Geriatric Society 35*:516–21.

Burke WJ, Rutherford JL, Zorumski CF, Reich T. (1985) Electroconvulsive therapy and the elderly. *Compr Psychiatry 26*:480–86.

Burrows SG. (1828) *Commentaries on the Causes, Forms, Symptoms and Treatment, Moral and Medical, of Insanity.* London: T&G Underwood, pp. 656–57. [as cited in Sandford, 1966]

Burton TM. (1991) Medical flap. *The Wall Street Journal*, April 19.

Calev A, Ben-Tzvi E, Shapira B, Drexler H, Carasso R, Lerer B. (1989) Distinct memory impairments following electroconvulsive therapy and imipramine. *Psychol Med 19*:111–9.

Calev A, Drexler H, Tubi N, Nigal D, Shapira B, Kugelmass S, Lerer B. (1991a) Atropine and cognitive performance after electroconvulsive therapy. *Convuls Ther 7*:92–8.

Calev A, Cohen R, Tubi N, Nigal D, Shapira B, Kugelmass, S, Lerer B. (1991b) Disorientation and bilateral moderately suprathreshold ECT. *Convuls Ther 7*:99–110.

Calev A, Fink M, Petrides G, Francis A, Fochtmann L. (1993) Caffeine pretreatment enhances clinical efficacy and reduces cognitive effects of electroconvulsive therapy. *Convuls Ther 9*:95–100.

Calloway SP, Dolan RJ, Jacoby RJ, Levy R. (1981) ECT and cerebral atrophy. A computed tomographic study. *Acta Psychiatr Scand 64*:442–5.

Cammermeyer J. (1961) The importance of avoiding "dark" neurons in experimental neuropathology. *Acta Neuropathol 1*:245–70.

Cammermeyer J. (1972) Nonspecific changes of the central nervous system in normal and experimental material. In GH Bourne, ed. *The Struc-*

ture and Function of Nervous Tissue, vol. VI. New York: Academic Press.

Campbell D. (1960) The psychological effects of cerebral electroshock. In: HJ Eysenck, ed. *Handbook of Abnormal Psychology: An Experimental Approach*. London: Pitnam. pp. 611–33.

Cannicott SM (1962) Unilateral electro-convulsive therapy. *Postgrad Med J 38*:451–9.

Cannicott SM, Waggoner RW. (1967) Unilateral and bilateral electroconvulsive therapy. *Arch Gen Psychiatry 16*:229–32.

Cantor C. (1986) Carbamazepine and ECT: a paradoxical combination. *J Clin Psychiatry 47*:276–7.

Caplan G. (1946) Electrical convulsion therapy in the treatment of epilepsy. *J Ment Sci 92*:784.

Cardno AG, Simpson CJ. (1991) Electroconvulsive therapy in Paget's disease and hydrocephalus. *Convuls Ther 7*:48–51.

Carl C, Engelhardt W, Teichmann G, Fuchs G. (1988) Open comparative study with treatment-refractory depressed patients: Electroconvulsive therapy–anesthetic therapy with isoflurane (preliminary report). *Pharmacopsychiatry 21*:432–33.

Carlson GA, Goodwin FR. (1973) The stages of mania. *Arch Gen Psychiatry 28*:221–8.

Carney MV, Sheffield BF. (1973) Electroconvulsion therapy and the diencephalon. *Lancet 1*:1505–6.

Carney MW, Sheffield BF. (1972) Depression and Newcastle scales. Their relationship to Hamilton's scale. *Br J Psychiatry 121*:35–40.

Carney MWP, Sheffield BF. (1974) The effects of pulse ECT in neurotic and endogenous depression. *Br J Psychiatry 125*:91–4.

Carney MWP, Roth M, Garside RF. (1965) The diagnosis of depressive syndromes and the prediction of E.C.T. response. *Br J Psychiatry 111*: 659–74.

Carr V, Dorrington C, Schader G, Wale J. (1983) The use of ECT in childhood bipolar disorder. *Br J Psychiatry 143*:411–5.

Carroll BJ, Feinberg M, Smouse PE, Rawson SG, Greden JF. (1981) The Carroll rating scale for depression I. Development, reliability and validation. *Br J Psychiatry 138*:194–200.

Carter C. (1977) Neurological considerations with ECT. *Convulsive Therapy Bulletin and Tardive Dyskinesia Notes 2*:6–19.

Casey DA (1987) Electroconvulsive therapy in the neuroleptic malignant syndrome. *Convuls Ther 3*:278–83.

Casey DA. (1991) Electroconvulsive therapy and Friedrich's ataxia. *Convuls Ther 7*:45–7.

Castelli I, Steiner LA, Kaufmann MA, Alfille PH, Schouten R, Welch CA, Drop LJ. (1995) Comparative effects of esmolol and labetalol to attenuate hyperdynamic states after electroconvulsive therapy. *Anesth Analg 80*:557–61.

Cerletti U. (1940) L'Elettroshock. *Rivista Sperimentale Freniatria 64*: 209–310.

Cerletti U. (1950) Old and new information about electroshock. *Am J Psychiatry 107*:87–94.

Cerletti U. (1956) Electroshock therapy. In: F Marti-Ibanez, AM Sackler, RR Sackler, eds. *The Great Physiodynamic Therapies in Psychiatry*. New York: Hoeber-Harper. pp. 91–120.

Cerletti U, Bini L. (1938) Un nuevo metodo di shockterapie "L'elettroshock." *Bollettino Accademia Medica Roma 64*:136–8.

Chacko RC, Root L. (1983) ECT and tardive dyskinesia: two cases and a review. *J Clin Psychiatry 44*:265–6.

Chapman AH. (1961) Aortic dacron graft surgery and electroshock: Report of a case. *Am J Psychiatry 117*:937.

Charatan FB, Oldham AJ. (1954) Electroconvulsive treatment in pregnancy. *Journal of Obstetrics and Gynecology of the British Empire 61*: 665–7.

Charney DS, Nelson JC. (1981) Delusional and nondelusional unipolar depression: further evidence for distinct subtypes. *Am J Psychiatry 138*: 328–333.

Chater SN, Simpson KH. (1988) Effect of passive hyperventilation on seizure duration in patients undergoing electroconvulsive therapy. *Br J Anaesth 60*:70–3.

Chatrian GE, Petersen MC. (1960) The convulsive patterns provoked by Indoklon, Metrazol and electroshock: Some depth electrographic observations in human patients. *Electroencephalogr Clin Neurophysiol 12*: 715–25.

Checkley SA, Meldrum BS, McWilliam JR. (1984) Mechanism of action of ECT: neuroendocrine studies. In: B Lerer, RD Weiner, RH Belmaker, eds. *ECT: Basic Mechanisms*. London: John Libbey. pp. 101–106.

Chen JJ, Velamati S, Stewart C. (1990) Detection of prolonged seizure by audible EEG. *Convuls Ther 6*:248–50.

Christie JE, Whalley LJ, Brown NS, Dick H. (1982) Effect of ECT on the neuroendocrine response to apomorphine in severely depressed patients. *Br J Psychiatry 140*:268–73.

Cinca J, Evangelista A, Montoyo J, Barutell C, Figueras J, Valle V, Rius J, Soler-Soler J. (1985) Electrophysiologic effects of unilateral right and left stellate ganglion block on the human heart. *Am Heart J 109*: 46–54.

Ciraulo D, Lind L, Salzman C, Pilon R, Elkins R. (1978) Sodium nitroprusside treatment of ECT-induced blood pressure elevations. *Am J Psychiatry 135*:1105–6.

Cizlado BC, Wheaton A. (1995) Case study: ECT treatment of a young girl with catatonia. *J Am Acad Child Adolesc Psychiatry 34*:332–35.

Clement AJ. (1962) Atropine premedication for electroconvulsive therapy. *Br Med J i*:228–9.

Clinical Research Centre Division of Psychiatry. (1984) The Northwick Park

ECT trial: Predictors of response to real and simulated ECT. *Br J Psychiatry 144*:227–37.

Clyma EA. (1975) Unilateral electroconvulsive therapy: how to determine which hemisphere is dominant. *Br J Psychiatry 126*:372–9.

Coffey CE, Weiner RD, Hinkle PE, Cress M, Daughtry G, Wilson WH. (1987a) Augmentation of ECT seizures with caffeine. *Biol Psychiatry 22*:637–49.

Coffey CE, Weiner RD, McCall WV, Heinz ER. (1987b) Electroconvulsive therapy in multiple sclerosis: A magnetic resonance imaging study of the brain. *Convuls Ther 3*:137–44.

Coffey CE, McCall WV, Hoelscher TJ, Carroll BJ, Hinkle PE, Saunders WB, Erwin CW, Marsh GR, Weiner RD. (1988a) Effects of ECT on poly-somnographic sleep: a prospective investigation. *Convuls Ther 4*: 269–79.

Coffey CE, Figiel GS, Djang WT, Cress M, Saunders WB, Weiner RD. (1988b) Leukoencephalopathy in elderly depressed patients referred for ECT. *Biol Psychiatry 24*:143–61.

Coffey CE, Figiel GS, Djang WT, Sullivan DC, Herfkens RJ, Weiner RD. (1988c) Effects of ECT on brain structure: a pilot prospective magnetic resonance imaging study. *Am J Psychiatry 145*:701–6.

Coffey CE, Figiel GS, Djang WT, Weiner RD. (1990a) Subcortical hyperin-tensity on magnetic resonance imaging: a comparison of normal and depressed subjects. *Am J Psychiatry 45*:187–9.

Coffey CE, Figiel GS, Weiner RD, Saunders WB. (1990b) Caffeine augmen-tation of ECT. *Am J Psychiatry 147*:579–85.

Coffey CE, Weiner RD, Djang WT, Figiel GS, Soady SAR, Patterson LJ, Holt PD, Spritser CE, Wilkinson WE. (1991) Brain anatomic effects of ECT: a prospective magnetic resonance imaging study. *Arch Gen Psy-chiatry 48*:1013–21.

Coffey CE, Lucke J, Weiner RD, Krystal AD, Aque M. (1995a) Seizure threshold in electroconvulsive therapy: I. Initial seizure threshold. *Biol Psychiatry 37*:713–20.

Coffey CE, Lucke J, Weiner RD, Krystal AD, Aque M. (1995b) Seizure threshold in electroconvulsive therapy (ECT) II. The anticonvulsant effect of ECT. *Biol Psychiatry 37*:777–888.

Cohen BD, Noblin CD, Silverman AJ, Penick SB. (1968) Functional asym-metry of the human brain. *Science 162*:475–7.

Colenda CC, McCall WV. (1996) A statistical model predicting the seizure threshold for right unilateral ECT in 106 patients. *Convuls Ther 12*: 3–12.

Cooper AJ, Moir AT, Guldberg HC. (1968) The effect of electroconvulsive shock on the cerebral metabolism of dopamine and 5-hydroxytryptam-ine. *J Pharm Pharmacol 20*:729–30.

Cooper AJ, Finlayson R, Velamoor VR, Magnus RV, Cernovsky Z. (1989) Effects of ECT on prolactin, LH, FSH and testosterone in males with major depressive illness. *Can J Psychiatry 34*:814–7.

Cooper SJ, Leahey W, Green DF, King DJ. (1988) The effect of electroconvulsive therapy on CSF amine metabolites in schizophrenic patients. *Br J Psychiatry 152*:59–63.

Coppen A, Rao VA, Bishop M, Abou-Saleh MT, Wood K. (1980a) Neuroendocrine studies in affective disorders. Part 1. Plasma prolactin response to thyrotropin-releasing hormone in affective disorders: effect of ECT. *J Affect Disord 2*:311–5.

Coppen A, Rao VA, Bishop M, Abou-Saleh MT, Wood K. (1980b) Neuroendocrine studies in affective disorders. Part 2. Plasma thyroid-stimulating hormone response to thyrotropin-releasing hormone in affective disorders: effect of ECT. *J Affect Disord 2*:317–20.

Coppen A, Abou-Saleh MT, Milln P, Bailey J, Metcalfe M, Burns BH, Armond A. (1981) Lithium continuation therapy following electroconvulsive therapy. *Br J Psychiatry 139*:284–7.

Coppen A, Milln P, Harwood J, Wood K. (1985) Does the dexamethasone suppression test predict antidepressant treatment success? *Br J Psychiatry 146*:294–6.

Coryell W. (1978) Intrapatient responses to ECT and tricyclic antidepressants. *Am J Psychiatry 135*:1108–10.

Coryell W. (1982) Hypothalamic-pituitary-adrenal axis abnormality and ECT response. *Psychiatr Res 6*:283–91.

Coryell W, Zimmerman M. (1983) The dexamethasone suppression test and ECT outcome: a six-month follow-up. *Biol Psychiatry 18*:21–7.

Coryell W, Zimmerman M. (1984) Outcome following ECT for primary unipolar depression: a test of newly proposed response predictors. *Am J Psychiatry 141*:862–7.

Coryell W, Pfohl B, Zimmerman M. (1985) Outcome following electroconvulsive therapy: A comparison of primary and secondary depression. *Convuls Ther 1*:10–4.

Costain DW, Cowen PJ. (1982) ECT and the growth hormone response to apomorphine [letter]. *Br J Psychiatry 141*:213.

Costain DW, Cowen PJ, Gelder MG, Grahame-Smith DG. (1982) Electroconvulsive therapy and the brain: evidence for increased dopamine-mediated responses. *Lancet 2*:400–4.

Costello CG, Belton GP, Abra JC, Dunn BE. (1970) The amnesic and therapeutic effects of bilateral and unilateral ECT. *Br J Psychiatry 116*:69–78.

Coull DC, Crooks J, Dingwall-Fordyce I, Scott AM, Weir RD. (1970) Amitriptyline and cardiac disease: Risk of sudden death identified by monitoring system. *Lancet 2*:590–1.

Couture LJ, Thomas DR, Lippman SB, Edmonds HL, Lucas LF. (1988a) Monitoring seizure duration in patients undergoing electroconvulsive therapy. *Anesth Analg 67*:S42.

Couture LJ, Lucas LF, Lippmann SB, Shaltout T, Paloheimo MPJ, Edmonds HL, Jr. (1988b) Monitoring seizure duration during electroconvulsive therapy. *Convuls Ther 4*:206–14.

Cowen PJ, Braddock LE, Gosden B. (1984) The effect of amitriptyline treatment on the growth hormone response to apomorphine. *Psychopharmacology 83*:378–9.

Cronholm B. (1969) Post-ECT amnesias. In: GA Talland, N Waugh, eds. *The Pathology of Memory.* New York: Academic Press. pp. 81–89.

Cronholm B, Blomquist C. (1959) Memory disturbances after electroconvulsive therapy: II. Conditions one week after a series of treatments. *Acta Psychiatr Scand 32*:18–25.

Cronholm B, Lagergren A. (1959) Memory disturbances after electroconvulsive therapy. *Acta Psychiatr Scand 34*:283–310.

Cronholm B, Molander L. (1957) Memory disturbances after electroconvulsive therapy: I. Conditions six hours after electroshock treatment. *Acta Psychiatr Scand 32*:280–306.

Cronholm B, Molander L. (1961) Memory disturbances after electroconvulsive therapy. IV. Influence of an interpolated electroconvulsive shock on retention of memory material. *Acta Psychiatr Scand 36*:83–90.

Cronholm B, Molander L. (1964) Memory disturbances after electroconvulsive therapy. V. Conditions one month after a series of treatments. *Acta Psychiatr Scand 40*:212–6.

Cronholm B, Ottosson J-O. (1960) Experimental studies of the therapeutic action of electroconvulsive therapy in endogenous depression. *Acta Psychiatrica et Neurologica Scandinavica 35*:69–102.

Cronholm B, Ottosson J-O. (1961a) Memory functions in endogenous depression before and after electroconvulsive therapy. *Arch Gen Psychiatry 5*:193–9.

Cronholm B, Ottosson J-O. (1961b) "Countershock" in electroconvulsive therapy. Influence on retrograde amnesia. *Arch Gen Psychiatry 4*:254–8.

Cronholm B, Ottosson J-O. (1963a) The experience of memory function after electroconvulsive therapy. *Br J Psychiatry 109*:251–8.

Cronholm B, Ottosson J-O. (1963b) Ultrabrief stimulus technique in electroconvulsive therapy. I. Influence on retrograde amnesia of treatments with the Elther ES electroshock apparatus, Siemens Konvulsator III and of lidocaine-modified treatment. *J Nerv Ment Dis 137*:117–23.

Cronin D, Bodley P, Potts L, Mather MD, Gardner RK, Tobin JC. (1970) Unilateral and bilateral ECT: a study of memory disturbance and relief from depression. *J Neurol Neurosurg Psychiatry 33*:705–11.

Cropper CFJ, Hughes M. (1964) Cardiac arrest (with apnoea) after E.C.T. *Br J Psychiatry 110*:222–5.

Crow TJ, Johnstone EC. (1986) Controlled trials of electroconvulsive therapy. *Ann N Y Acad Sci 462*:12–29.

Crowe RR. (1984) Current concepts. Electroconvulsive therapy—a current perspective. *N Engl J Med 311*:163–7.

Cuche J-L, Brochier P, Klioua N, Poirier M-F, Cuche H, Benimould M, Loo H, Safer M. (1990) Conjugated catecholamines in human plasma: where are they coming from? *J Lab Clin Med 116*:681–6.

Culver CM, Ferrell RB, Green RM. (1980) ECT and special problems of informed consent. *Am J Psychiatry 137*:586–91.

Dam AM, Dam M. (1986) Quantitative neuropathology in electrically induced generalized convulsions. *Convuls Ther 2*:77–89.

Daniel WF. (1985) ECT-induced hyperactive delirium and brain laterality. *Am J Psychiatry 142*:521–2.

Daniel WF, Crovitz HF. (1983a) Acute memory impairment following electroconvulsive therapy. 1. Effects of electrical stimulus waveform and number of treatments. *Acta Psychiatr Scand 67*:1–7.

Daniel WF, Crovitz HF. (1983b) Acute memory impairment following electroconvulsive therapy. 2. Effects of electrode placement. *Acta Psychiatr Scand 67*:57–68.

Daniel WF, Crovitz HF. (1986) Disorientation during electroconvulsive therapy: Technical, theoretical, and neuropsychological issues. *Ann N Y Acad Sci 462*:293–306.

Daniel WF, Weiner RD, Crovitz HF. (1983) Autobiographical amnesia with ECT: an analysis of the roles of stimulus wave form, electrode placement, stimulus energy, and seizure length. *Biol Psychiatry 18*:121–6.

Daniel WF, Crovitz HF, Weiner RD, Swartzwelder HS, Kahn EM. (1985) ECT-induced amnesia and postictal EEG suppression. *Biol Psychiatry 20*:344–8.

Daniel WF, Crovitz HF, Weiner RD. (1987) Neuropsychological aspects of disorientation. *Cortex 23*:169–87.

Davidson J, McLeod M, Law-Yone B, Linnoila M. (1978) Comparison of electroconvulsive therapy and combined phenelzine-amitriptyline in refractory depression. *Arch Gen Psychiatry 35*:639–44.

Davis JM, Janicak PG, Sakkas P, Gilmore C, Wang Z. (1991) Electroconvulsive therapy in the treatment of the neuroleptic malignant syndrome. *Convuls Ther 7*:111–20.

De Montigny C, Cournoyer G, Morissette R, Langlois R, Caille G. (1983) Lithium carbonate addition in tricyclic antidepressant resistant unipolar depression. *Arch Gen Psychiatry 40*:1327–34.

Deakin JF, Ferrier IN, Crow TJ, Johnstone EC, Lawler P. (1983) Effects of ECT on pituitary hormone release: relationship to seizure, clinical variables and outcome. *Br J Psychiatry 143*:618–24.

Dec GW, Stern TA, Welch C. (1985) The effects of electroconvulsive therapy on serial electrocardiograms and serum cardiac enzyme values: a prospective study of depressed hospitalized inpatients. *JAMA 253*: 2525–29.

Decina P, Malitz S, Sackeim HA, Holzer J, Yudofsky S. (1984) Cardiac arrest during ECT modified by beta-adrenergic blockade. *Am J Psychiatry 141*:298–300.

Decina P, Sackeim HA, Kahn DA, Pierson D, Hopkins N, Malitz S. (1987) Effects of ECT on the TRH stimulation test. *Psychoneuroendocrinology 12*:29–34.

Devanand DP, Dwark AJ, Hutchinson ER, Bolwig TG, Sackeim HA. (1994) Does ECT alter brain structure? *Am J Psychiatry 151*:951–70.

d'Elia G. (1970) Comparison of electroconvulsive therapy with unilateral and bilateral stimulation: II. Therapeutic efficiency in endogenous depression. *Acta Psychiatr Scand Suppl 215*:30–43.

d'Elia G. (1992) Electrode placement and antidepressant efficacy [letter]. *Convuls Ther 8*:294–98.

d'Elia G, Perris C. (1970) Comparison of electroconvulsive therapy with unilateral and bilateral stimulation: I Seizure and post-seizure electroencephalographic pattern. *Acta Psychiatr Scand Suppl 215*:9–29.

d'Elia G, Raotma H. (1975) Is unilateral ECT less effective than bilateral ECT? *Br J Psychiatry 126*:83–9.

d'Elia G, Widepalm K. (1974) Comparison of frontoparietal and temporoparietal unilateral electroconvulsive therapy. *Acta Psychiatr Scand 50*: 225–32.

d'Elia G, Ottosson J-O, Stromgren S. (1983) Present practice of electroconvulsive therapy in Scandinavia. *Arch Gen Psychiatry 40*:577–81.

Deliyiannis S, Eliakim M, Bellet S. (1962) The electrocardiogram during electroconvulsive therapy as studied by radioelectrocardiography. *Am J Cardiol 10*:187–92.

Demuth GW, Rand BS. (1980) Atypical major depression in a patient with severe primary degeneration dementia. *Am J Psychiatry 137*:1609–10.

Dennison S, French RN. (1989) Cardiac problems in ECT. *Am J Psychiatry 146*:939.

Department of Health and Social Security: Health Notice HN(82)18. (1982) *Health Service Management, Psychiatric Services, Electro-convulsive Therapy: Equipment.* London: DHSS Store, Health Publications Unit.

DeQuardo JR, Tandon R. (1988) Concurrent lithium therapy prevents ECT-induced switch to mania. *J Clin Psychiatry 49*:167–8.

DeQuardo JR, Tandon R. (1988) ECT in post-stroke major depression. *Convuls Ther 4*:221–4.

Devanand DP, Decina P, Sackeim HA, Hopkins N, Novacenko H, Malitz S. (1987) Serial dexamethasone suppression tests in initial suppressors and nonsuppresssors treated with electroconvulsive therapy. *Biol Psychiatry 22*:463–72.

Devanand DP, Decina P, Sackeim HA, Prudic J. (1988a) Status epilepticus following ECT in a patient receiving theophylline. *J Clin Psychopharmacology 8*:153.

Devanand DP, Sackeim HA, Decina P, Prudic J. (1988b) The development of mania and organic euphoria during ECT. *J Clin Psychiatry 49*:69–71.

Devanand DP, Bowers MB, Hoffman FJ, Jr, Sackeim HA. (1989a) Acute and subacute effects of ECT on plasma HVA, MHPG, and prolactin. *Biol Psychiatry 26*:408–12.

Devanand DP, Briscoe KM, Sackeim HA. (1989b) Clinical features and predictors of postictal excitement. *Convuls Ther 5*:140–6.

Devanand DP, Verma AK, Tirumalasetti F, Sackeim HA. (1991) Absence of cognitive impairment after more than 100 lifetime ECT treatments. *Am J Psychiatry 148*:929–32.

Dewald PA, Margolis NM, Weiner H. (1954) Vertebral fractures as complications of electroconvulsive therapy. *JAMA 154*:981–4.

di Michele V, Giordano L, de Cataldo S, Sabatini MD, Petruzzi C, Casacchia M, Rossi A. (1992) Electroencephalographic seizure duration in electroconvulsive therapy: a clinical study. *Convuls Ther 8*:258–61.

Dinan TG, Barry S. (1989) A comparison of electroconvulsive therapy with a combined lithium and tricyclic combination among depressed tricyclic nonresponders. *Acta Psychiatr Scand 80*:97–100.

Dodwell D, Goldberg D. (1989) A study of factors associated with response to electroconvulsive therapy in patients with schizophrenic symptoms. *Br J Psychiatry 154*:635–9.

Dored G, Stefansson S, d'Elia G, Kagedal B, Karlberg E, Ekman R. (1990) Corticotropin, cortisol and beta-endorphin responses to the human corticotropin-releasing hormone during melancholia and after unilateral electroconvulsive therapy. *Acta Psychiatr Scand 82*:204–9.

Dornbush RL. (1972) Memory and induced ECT convulsions. *Seminars in Psychiatry 4*:47–54.

Dornbush R, Abrams R, Fink M. (1971) Memory changes after unilateral and bilateral convulsive therapy (ECT). *Br J Psychiatry 119*:75–8.

Dornbush RL, Williams M. (1974) Memory and ECT. In: M Fink, S Kety, J McGaugh, T Williams, eds. *Psychobiology of Convulsive Therapy.* Washington, DC: VH Winston and Sons. pp. 199–205.

Douglas CJ, Schwartz HI. (1982) ECT for depression caused by lupus cerebritis: a case report. *Am J Psychiatry 139*:1631–2.

Douyon R, Serby M, Kluteh K, Rotroseu J. (1989) ECT and Parkinson's disease revisited: A "naturalistic" study. *Am J Psychiatry 146*: 1451–5.

Dressler DM, Folk J. (1975) The treatment of depression with ECT in the presence of brain tumor. *Am J Psychiatry 132*:1320–1.

Drop LJ, Welch CA. (1989) Anesthesia for electroconvulsive therapy in patients with major cardiovascular risk factors. *Convuls Ther 5*:88–101.

Drop LJ, Bouckoms AJ, Welch CA. (1988) Arterial hypertension and multiple cerebral aneurysms in a patient treated with electroconvulsive therapy. *J Clin Psychiatry 49*:280–2.

Dubin WR, Jaffe RL, Roemer RA, Lipschutz L, Spencer M. (1989) Maintenance ECT in coexisting affective and neurologic disorders. *Convuls Ther 5*:162–7.

Dubovsky SL, Gay M, Franks RD, Haddenhorst A. (1985) ECT in the presence of increased intracranial pressure and respiratory failure: case report. *J Clin Psychiatry 46*:489–91.

Dunn CG, Quinlan D. (1978) Indicators of E.C.T. response and non-response in the treatment of depression. *J Clin Psychiatry 39*:620–2.

Durrant BW. (1966) Dental care in electroplexy. *Br J Psychiatry 112*: 1173–6.

Dwyer R, McCaughey W, Lavery J, McCarthy G, Dundee JW. (1988) Comparison of propofol and methohexitone as anaesthetic agents for electroconvulsive therapy. *Anaesthesia 43*:459–62.

Dykes S, Scott AIF, Gow SM, Whalley LJ. (1987) Effects of seizure duration on serum TSH concentration after ECT. *Psychoneuroendocrinology 12*: 477–82.

Dysken M, Evans HM, Chan CH, Davis JM. (1976) Improvement of depression and parkinsonism during ECT: a case study. *Neuropsychobiology 2*:281–6.

Edwards RM, Stoudemire A, Vela MA, Morris R. (1990) Intraocular pressure changes in nonglaucomatous patients undergoing electroconvulsive therapy. *Convuls Ther 6*:209–213.

Ebadi M, Pfeiffer RF, Murrin LC. (1990) Pathogenesis and treatment of neuroleptic malignant syndrome. *Gen Pharmacol 21*:367–86.

Egbert LD, Wolfe S, Melmed RM, Deas TC, Mullin CS, Jr. (1959) Reduction of cardiovascular stress during electroshock therapy by trimethaphan. *Journal of Clinical and Experimental Psychopathology 20*:315–9.

Egbert LD, Wolfe S. (1960) Evaluation of methohexital for premedication in electroshock therapy. *Anesth Analg 39*:416–9.

Eitzman DT, Bach DS, Rubenfire M. (1994) Management of myocardial stunning associated with electroconvulsive therapy guided by hyperventilation echocardiography. *Am Heart J 127*:928–29.

el-Ganzouri AR, Ivankovich AD, Braverman B, McCarthy R. (1985) Monoamine oxidase inhibitors: should they be discontinued preoperatively? *Anesth Analg 64*:592–6.

Elithorn A, Bridges PK, Hodges JR, Jones MT. (1968) Adrenocortical responsiveness during courses of electroconvulsive therapy. *Br J Psychiatry 114*:575–80.

Elliot DL, Linz DH, Kane JA. (1982) Electroconvulsive therapy: Pretreatment medical evaluation. *Arch Intern Med 142*:979–81.

el-Mallakh RS. (1988) Complications of concurrent lithium and electroconvulsive therapy: a review of clinical material and theoretical considerations. *Biol Psychiatry 23*:595–601.

Emrich HM, Holt V, Kissling W, Fischler M, Lapse H, Heinemann H, von Zerssen D, Herz A. (1979) β-endorphin-like immunoreactivity in cerebrospinal fluid and plasma of patients with schizophrenia and other neuropsychiatric disorders. *Pharmakopsychiatrie 12*:269–76.

Endler NS. (1988) The origins of electroconvulsive therapy (ECT). *Convuls Ther 4*:5–23.

Endler NS, Persad E. (1988) *Electroconvulsive Therapy: The Myths and The Realities*. Toronto: Hans Huber.

Engelhardt W, Carl G, Hartung E. (1993) Intra-individual open comparison of burst-suppression-isoflurane-anesthesia versus electroconvulsive therapy in the treatment of severe depression. *Eur J Anaesthesiol 10*: 113–18.

Engle J, Jr. (1984) The use of positron emission tomographic scanning in epilepsy. *Ann Neurol 15*:S180–91.

Engle J, Jr, Duhl DE, Phelps ME. (1982) Patterns of human local cerebral glucose metabolism during epileptic seizures. *Science 218*:64–6.

Enns N, Karvelas L. (1995) Electrical dose titration for electroconvulsive therapy: a comparison with dose prediction methods. *Convuls Ther 11*: 86–93.

Epstein HM, Fagman W, Bruce DL, Abram A. (1975) Intraocular pressure changes during anesthesia for electroshock therapy. *Anesth Analg 54*: 479–81.

Erman MK, Welch CA, Mandel MR. (1979) A comparison of two unilateral ECT electrode placements: efficacy and electrical energy considerations. *Am J Psychiatry 136*:1317–9.

Escalona PR, Coffey CE, Maus-Feldman J. (1991) Electroconvulsive therapy in a depressed patient with an intracranial arachnoid cyst: a brain magnetic resonance imaging study. *Convuls Ther 7*:133–8.

Essig CF. (1969) Frequency of repeated electroconvulsions and the acquisition rate of a tolerance-like response. *Exp Neurol 25*:571–4.

Faber R. Dental fracture during ECT [letter]. (1983) *Am J Psychiatry 140*: 1255–6.

Farah A, McCall WV, Amundson RH. (1996) ECT after cerebral aneurysm repair. *Convuls Ther 12*:165–70.

Farah A, McCall WV. (1993) Electroconvulsive therapy stimulus dosing: a survey of contemporary practices. *Convuls Ther 9*:90–4.

Fear C, Littlejohns CS, Rouse E, McQuail P. (1994) Propofol anaesthesia in electroconvulsive therapy. Reduced seizure duration may not be relevant. *Br J Psychiatry 165*:506–9.

Feldman MJ. (1951) A prognostic scale for shock therapy. *Psychological Monograph* No. 327.

Ferraro A, Roizin L, Helfand M. (1946) Morphologic changes in the brain of monkeys following convulsions electrically induced. *J Neuropath Exper Neurology 5*:285–308.

Ferraro TN, Golden GT, Hare TA. (1990) Repeated electroconvulsive shock selectively alters γ-aminobutyric acid levels in rat brain: effect of electrode placement. *Convuls Ther 6*:199–208.

Fetterman JL. (1942) Electrocoma therapy of the psychoses. *Ann Intern Med 17*:775–789.

Figiel GS, Stoudemire A. (1994) The use of ECT for elderly patients with cardiac disease. *Psychiatric Times*, 13–17 December.

Figiel GS, DeLeo B, Zorumski CF, Baker K, Goewert A, Jarvis M, Smith DS, Mattingly G, Ruwitch J. (1993) Combined use of labetalol and nifedipine in controlling the cardiovascular response from ECT. *J Geriatr Psychiatry Neurol 6*:20–4.

Fink M. (1966) Cholinergic aspects of convulsive therapy. *J Nerv Ment Dis* *142*:475–84.

Fink M. (1979) *Convulsive Therapy: Theory and Practice.* New York: Raven Press.

Fink M. (1983) Missed seizures and the bilateral-unilateral electroconvulsive therapy controversy [letter]. *Am J Psychiatry 140*:198–9.

Fink M. (1984) Meduna and the origins of convulsive therapy. *Am J Psychiatry 141*:1034–41.

Fink M. (1986a) Neuroendocrine predictors of electroconvulsive therapy outcome: dexamethasone suppression test and prolactin release. *Ann N Y Acad Sci 462*:30–6.

Fink M. (1986b) Training in convulsive therapy [editorial]. *Convuls Ther 2*: 227–9.

Fink M. (1987) Douglas Goldman (1906–1986) [obituary]. *Convuls Ther 3*:163.

Fink M. (1988) ECT for Parkinson's Disease? [editorial]. *Convuls Ther 4*: 189–91.

Fink M. (1990) How does convulsive therapy work? *Neuropsychopharmacology 3*:73–82.

Fink M, Johnson L. (1982) Monitoring the duration of electroconvulsive therapy seizures: 'cuff' and EEG methods compared. *Arch Gen Psychiatry 39*:1189–91.

Fink M, Kahn RL. (1957) Relation of EEG delta activity to behavioral response in electroshock: Quantitative serial studies. *Arch Neurol Psychiatry 78*:516–25.

Fink M, Kahn RL. (1961) Behavioral patterns in convulsive therapy. *Arch Gen Psychiatry 5*:30–6.

Fink M, Nemeroff CB. (1989) A neuroendocrine view of ECT. *Convuls Ther 5*:296–304.

Fink M, Ottosson JO. (1980) A theory of convulsive therapy in endogenous depression: significance of hypothalamic functions. *Psychiatr Res 2*: 49–61.

Fink M, Kahn RL, Korin H. (1959a) Relation of tests of altered brain function to behavioral change following induced convulsions. In: L van Bogaert, J Radermaker, eds. *First International Congress of Neurological Sciences.* London: Pergamon Press. pp. 613–619.

Fink M, Kahn RL, Pollack M. (1959b) Psychological factors affecting individual differences in behavioral response to convulsive therapy. *J Nerv Ment Dis 128*:243–8.

Fink M, Kahn RL, Karp E, Pollack M, Green M, Alan B, Lefkowitz HJ. (1961) Inhalant-induced convulsions: Significance for the theory of the convulsive therapy process. *Arch Gen Psychiatry 4*:259–66.

Fink M, Gujavarty K, Greenberg L. (1987) Serial dexamethasone suppression tests and clinical outcome in ECT. *Convuls Ther 3*:111–20.

Finlayson AJ, Vieweg WV, Wilkey WD, Cooper AJ. (1989) Hyponatremic seizure following ECT. *Can J Psychiatry 34*:463–4.

Finner RW. (1954) Duration of convulsion in electric shock therapy. *J Nerv Ment Dis 119*:530–7.

Fisher KA. (1949) Changes in test performance of ambulatory depressed patients undergoing E.C.T. *J Gen Psychol 41*:195–232.

Fisman M. (1988) Intractable depression and pseudodementia: a report of two cases. *Can J Psychiatry 33*:628–30.

Flaherty JA, Naidu J, Dysken M. (1984) ECT, emergent dyskinesia, and depression. *Am J Psychiatry 141*:808–9.

Fleming GWTH, Golla FC, Walter WG. (1939) Electric convulsion therapy of schizophrenia. *Lancet 2*:1353–55.

Fleminger JJ, de Horne DJ, Nair NPV, Nott PN. (1970a) Differential effect of unilateral and bilateral ECT. *Am J Psychiatry 127*:430–6.

Fleminger JJ, Horne DJ, Nott PN. (1980b) Unilateral electroconvulsive therapy and cerebral dominance: Effect of right- and left-sided electrode placement on verbal memory. *J Neurol Neurosurg Psychiatry 33*: 408–11.

Flor-Henry P. (1986) Electroconvulsive therapy and lateralized affective systems. *Ann N Y Acad Sci 462*:389–97.

Fochtmann LJ. (1994a) Animal studies of electroconvulsive therapy: foundations for future research. *Psychopharmacol Bull 30*:321–444.

Fochtmann LJ. (1994b) What do rodents and test tubes teach us about ECT? *Convuls Ther 10*:287–89.

Folstein MF, Folstein SW, McHugh PR. (1975) "Mini Mental State," a practical method of grading the cognitive state of patients for the clinician. *J Psychiatr Res 12*:189–98.

Forssman H. (1955) Follow-up study of 16 children whose mothers were given electric convulsive therapy during gestation. *Acta Psychiatrica et Neurologica Scandinavica 30*:437–41.

Foster MW, Gayle RF. (1955) Dangers in combining reserpine (Serpasil) with electroconvulsive therapy. *JAMA 159*:1520–22.

Foster S, Ries R. (1988) Delayed hypertension with electroconvulsive therapy. *J Nerv Ment Dis 176*:374–6.

Foulds GA. (1952) Temperamental differences in maze performance: II. The effect of distraction and of electroconvulsive therapy on psychomotor retardation. *Br J Psychol 43*:33–41.

Fox HA, Rosen A, Campbell RJ. (1989) Are brief pulse and sine wave ECT equally efficient? *J Clin Psychiatry 50*:432–5.

Frame J. (1984) *An Angel at My Table. An autobiography.* Vol 2. New Zealand: Century Hutchinson.

Frankel FH. (1973) Electro-convulsive therapy in Massachusetts: A task force report. *Massachusetts Journal of Mental Health 3*:3–29.

Frankel FH. (1977) Current perspectives on ECT: a discussion. *Am J Psychiatry 134*:1014–9.

Frankel FH. (1982) Medicolegal and ethical aspects of treatment. In: R Abrams, WB Essman, eds. *Electroconvulsive Therapy: Biological*

Foundations and Clinical Applications. New York: Spectrum Publications. pp. 245–258.

Frankel FH. (1986) *Informed ECT for Health Professionals*, with Dr. Max Fink [videotape review]. *Convuls Ther 2*:303.

Fraser RM, Glass IB. (1980) Unilateral and bilateral ECT in elderly patients. A comparative study. *Acta Psychiatr Scand 62*:13–31.

Frederiksen SO, d'Elia G. (1979) Electroconvulsive therapy in Sweden. *Br J Psychiatry 134*:283–7.

Freeman CPL, Cheshire KE. (1988) Attitude studies on electroconvulsive therapy. *Convuls Ther 2*:31–42.

Freeman CP, Kendell RE. (1980) ECT: I. Patients' experiences and attitudes. *Br J Psychiatry 137*:8–16.

Freeman CPL, Basson JV, Crighton A. (1978) Double-blind controlled trial of electroconvulsive therapy (E.C.T.) and simulated E.C.T. in depressive illness. *Lancet 1*:738–40.

Freeman CP, Weeks D, Kendell RE. (1980) ECT: II: patients who complain. *Br J Psychiatry 137*:17–25.

Freese KJ. (1985) Can patients safely undergo electroconvulsive therapy while receiving monoamine oxidase inhibitors? *Convuls Ther 1*:190–4.

Fricchione GL, Kaufman LD, Gruber BL, Fink M. (1990) Electroconvulsive therapy and cyclophosphamide in combination for severe neuropsychiatric lupus with catatonia. *Am J Med 88*:442–3.

Fried D, Mann JH. (1988) Electroconvulsive treatment of a patient with known intracranial tumor. *Biol Psychiatry 23*:176–80.

Friedberg J. (1976) *Shock Treatment Is Not Good For Your Brain.* San Francisco: Glide Publications.

Friedberg J. (1977) Shock treatment, brain damage, and memory loss: a neurological perspective. *Am J Psychiatry 134*:1010–4.

Friedel RO. (1986) The combined use of neuroleptics and ECT in drug resistant schizophrenic patients. *Psychopharmacol Bull 22*:928–930.

Friedman E. (1942) Unidirectional electrostimulated convulsive therapy. I: The effect of wave form and stimulus characteristics on the convulsive dose. *Am J Psychiatry 99*:218–23.

Friedman E, Wilcox PH. (1942) Electrostimulated convulsive doses in intact humans by means of unidirectional currents. *J Nerv Ment Dis 96*:56–63.

Fromholt P, Christensen AL, Stromgren LS. (1973) The effects of unilateral and bilateral electroconvulsive therapy on memory. *Acta Psychiatr Scand 49*:466–78.

Fromm GH. (1959) Observation on the effects of electroshock treatment in patients with parkinsonism. *Bulletin of Tulane University 18*:71–3.

Funkenstein DH, Greenblatt M, Solomon HC. (1952) An autonomic nervous system test of prognostic significance in relation to electroshock treatment. *Psychosom Med 14*:347–62.

Gaines GY, Rees DI. (1986) Electroconvulsive therapy and anesthetic considerations. *Anesth Analg 65*:1345–56.

Gaitz CM, Essa M. (1991) Propranolol in ECT. *Convuls Ther* 7:60–1.

Gaitz CM, Pokorny AD, Mills M, Jr. (1956) Death following electroconvulsive therapy. *Arch Neurol Psychiatry* 75:493–9.

Galen RS, Gambino SR. (1975) *Beyond Normality: The Predictive Value and Efficiency of Medical Diagnoses.* New York: John Wiley, p. 17.

Galin D. (1974) Implications for psychiatry of left and right cerebral specialization: a neurophysiological context for unconscious processes. *Arch Gen Psychiatry* 31:572–83.

Gallinek A. (1952a) Controversial indications for electric convulsive therapy. *Am J Psychiatry* 109:361–6.

Gallinek A. (1952b) Organic sequelae of electric convulsive therapy including facial and body dysgnosias. *J Nerv Ment Dis* 115:377–93.

Gallinek A, Kalinowsky LB. (1958) Psychiatric aspects of multiple sclerosis. *Dis Nerv Syst* 19:77–80.

Gambill JD, McLean PE. (1983) Suicide after unilateral ECT in a patient previously responsive to bilateral ECT. *Psychiatr Q* 55:279–81.

Gangadhar BN, Kapur RL, Kalyanasundaram S. (1982) Comparison of electroconvulsive therapy with imipramine in endogenous depression: a double blind study. *Br J Psychiatr* 141:367–71.

Gangadhar BN, Lakshmanna G, Subba Krishna DK, Channabasavanna SM. (1985) Impedance measurements during electroconvulsive therapy. *NIMHANS Journal* 3:135–9.

Gassell MM. (1960) Deterioration after electroconvulsive therapy in patients with intracranial meningioma. *Arch Gen Psychiatry* 3:504–6.

Geiduschek J, Cohen SA, Khan A, Cullen BF. (1988) Repeated anesthesia for a patient with neuroleptic malignant syndrome. *Anesthesiology* 68:134–7.

Geoghegan JJ, Stevenson GH. (1949) Prophylactic electroshock. *Am J Psychiatry* 105:494–6.

George MS, Wasserman EM. (1994) Rapid-rate transcranial magnetic stimulation and ECT [editorial]. *Convuls Ther* 10:252–54.

Gerring JP, Shields HM. (1982) The identification and management of patients with a high risk for cardiac arrhythmias during modified ECT. *J Clin Psychiatry* 43:140–3.

Gerst JW, Enderle JD, Staton RD, Barr CE, Brumback RA. (1982) The electroencephalographic pattern during electroconvulsive therapy II. Preliminary analysis of spectral energy. *Clin Electroencephalogr* 13:251–6.

Ghadirian AM, Gianoulakis C, Nair NP. (1988) The effect of electroconvulsive therapy on endorphins in depression. *Biol Psychiatry* 23:459–64.

Gibbons JL, McHugh PR. (1962) Plasma cortisol in depressive illness. *J Psychiatr Res* 1:162–71.

Gibson TC, Leaman DM, Devors J, Lepeschkin EE. (1973) Pacemaker function in relation to electroconvulsive therapy. *Chest* 63:1025–7.

Gilbert DT. (1981) Shock therapy and informed consent. *Illinois Bar Journal* January:272–87.

Gill D, Lambourn J. (1979) Indications for electric convulsion therapy and its use by senior psychiatrists. *Br Med J 1*:1169–71.

Gilmore JH, Isley MR, Evans DL, Kong LS, Ekstrom D, Kafer ER, Golden RN, et al. (1991) The reliability of computer-processed EEG in the determination of ECT seizure duration. *Convuls Ther 7*:166–74.

Glassman A, Kantor SJ, Shostak M. (1975) Depression, delusions and drug response. *Am J Psychiatry 132*:716–9.

Glassman AH, Perel JM, Shostak M, Kantor SJ, Fleiss JL. (1977) Clinical implications of imipramine plasma levels for depressive illness. *Arch Gen Psychiatry 34*:197–204.

Gleiter CE, Nutt DJ. (1989) Chronic electroconvulsive shock and neurotransmitter receptors—an update. *Life Sci 44*:985–1006.

Gleiter CH, Deckert J, Nutt DJ, Marangos PJ. (1989) Electroconvulsive shock (ECS) and the adenosine neuromodulatory system: effect of single and repeated ECS on the adenosine A1 and A2 receptors, adenylate cyclase, and the adenosine uptake site. *J Neurochem 52*:641–6.

Globus JH, van Harreveld A, Wiersma CAG. (1943) The influence of electric current applications on the structure of the brain of dogs. *J Neuropathol Exp Neurol 2*:263–276.

Glynn RJ, Field TS, Rosner B, Hebert PR, et al. (1995) Evidence for a positive linear relation between blood pressure and mortality in elderly people. *Lancet 345*:825–29.

Goetz CG, Olanow W, Koller WC, Penn RD, Cahill D, Morantz R, Stebbins G, Tonner CT, Klawans HL, Shannon KM, Comella CL, Witt T, Cox C, Waxhan M, Gauger L. (1989) Multicenter study of autologous adrenal medullary transplantation to the corpus striatum in patients with advanced Parkinson's disease. *N Engl J Med 320*:337–41.

Golden CJ, Hammeke TA, Purisch AD. (1978) Diagnostic validity of a standardized neuropsychological battery derived from Luria's neuropsychological tests. *J Consult Clin Psychol 46*:1258–65.

Goldman D. (1949) Brief stimulus electric shock therapy. *J Nerv Ment Dis 110*:36–45.

Goldstein MZ, Richardson C. (1988) Meningioma with depression: ECT risk or benefit? *Psychosomatics 29*:349–51.

Goldstein MZ, Jensvold MF.(1989) ECT treatment of an elderly mentally retarded man. *Psychosomatics 30*:104–6.

Gomez J. (1975) Subjective side-effects of ECT. *Br J Psychiatry 127*: 609–11.

Gordon D. (1981) The electrical and radiological aspects of ECT. In: RL Palmer, ed. *Electroconvulsive Therapy: An Appraisal.* Oxford: Oxford University Press. pp. 79–96.

Gordon D. (1982) Electro-convulsive therapy with minimum hazard. *Br J Psychiatry 141*:12–18.

Gosek E, Weller RA. (1988) Improvement of tardive dyskinesia associated with electroconvulsive therapy. *J Nerv Ment Dis 176*:120–2.

Goswami U, Dutta S, Kuruvilla K, Papp E, Perenyi A. (1989) Electroconvulsive therapy in neuroleptic-induced parkinsonism. *Biol Psychiatry 26*: 234–8.

Gottlieb G, Wilson I. (1965) Cerebral dominance: temporary disruption of verbal memory by unilateral electroconvulsive shock treatment. *Journal of Comparative Physiology and Psychology 60*:368–70.

Grahame-Smith DG, Green AR, Costain DW. (1978) Mechanism of the antidepressant action of electroconvulsive therapy. *Lancet 1*:254–7.

Gran L, Bergsholm P, Bleie H. (1984) Seizure duration in unilateral electroconvulsive therapy. A comparison of the anaesthetic agents etomidate and althesin with methohexitone. *Acta Psychiatr Scand 69*:472–83.

Gravenstein JS, Anton AH, Weiner SM, Tetlow AG. (1965) Catecholamine and cardiovascular response to electroconvulsion therapy in man. *Br J Anaesth 37*:833–9.

Graybar G, Goethe J, Levy T, Phillips J, Youngberg J, Smith D. (1983) Transient large upright T-waves on the electrocardiogram during multiple monitored electroconvulsive therapy. *Anesthesiology 59*:467–9.

Green MA. (1957) Significance of individual variability in EEG response to electroshock. *Journal of Hillside Hospital 6*:229–40.

Green MA. (1960) Relation between threshold and duration of seizures and electrographic change during convulsive therapy. *J Nerv Ment Dis 131*: 117–20.

Green R, Woods A. (1955) Effects of modified electro-convulsive therapy on the electrocardiogram. *Br Med J 1*:1503.

Greenbank RK. (1958) Aortic homograft surgery and electroshock: case report. *Am J Psychiatry 115*:469.

Greenberg LB. (1985) Detection of prolonged seizures during electroconvulsive therapy: a comparison of electroencephalogram and cuff monitoring. *Convuls Ther 1*:32–7.

Greenberg LB, Gujavarty K. (1985) The neuroleptic malignant syndrome: review and report of three cases. *Compr Psychiatry 26*: 63–70.

Greenberg LB, Anand A, Roque CT, Grinberg Y. (1986) Electroconvulsive therapy and cerebral venous angioma. *Convuls Ther 2*:197–202.

Greenberg LB, Gage J, Vitkun S, Fink M. (1987) Isoflurane anesthesia therapy: a replacement for ECT in depressive disorders? *Convuls Ther 3*: 269–77.

Greenberg LB, Mofson R, Fink M. (1988) Prospective electroconvulsive therapy in a delusional depressed patient with a frontal meningioma. *Br J Psychiatry 153*:105–7.

Greenblatt M, Grosser GH, Wechsler H. (1964) Differential response of hospitalized depressed patients in somatic therapy. *Am J Psychiatry 120*: 935–43.

Gregory S, Shawcross CR, Gill D. (1985) The Nottingham ECT study. A double-blind comparison of bilateral, unilateral and simulated ECT in depressive illness. *Br J Psychiatry 146*:520–4.

Griffiths EJ, Lorenz RP, Baxter S, Talon NS. (1989) Acute neurohumoral response to electroconvulsive therapy during pregnancy. A case report. *J Reprod Med 4*:907–11.

Grigg JR. (1988) Neuroleptic malignant syndrome and malignant hyperthermia. *Am J Psychiatry 145*:1175.

Grinspoon L, Greenblatt M. (1963) Pharmacotherapy combined with other treatment methods. *Compr Psychiatry 4*:256–62.

Griswold RL. (1958) Plasma adrenaline and noradrenaline in electroshock therapy in man and in rats. *J Appl Physiol 12*:117.

Grogan R, Wagner DR, Sullivan T, Labar D. (1995) *Convuls Ther 11*:51–6.

Grunhaus L. (1991) The technique of ECT [videotape review]. *Convuls Ther 7*:143–4.

Grunhaus L, Pande AC, Haskett RF. (1990) Full and abbreviated courses of maintenance electroconvulsive therapy. *Convuls Ther 6*:130–8.

Gujavarty K, Greenberg LB, Fink M. (1987) Electroconvulsive therapy and neuroleptic medication in therapy-resistant positive-symptom psychosis. *Convuls Ther 3*:185–195.

Guttmacher LB, Cretella H. (1988) Electroconvulsive therapy in one child and three adolescents. *J Clin Psychiatry 4*:20–3.

Guttmacher LB, Greenland P. (1990) Effects of electroconvulsive therapy on the electrocardiogram in geriatric patients with stable cardiovascular diseases. *Convuls Ther 6*:5–12.

Guze BH, Weinman B, Diamond RP. (1987) Use of ECT to treat bipolar depression in a mental retardate with cerebral palsy. *Convuls Ther 3*: 60–4.

Guze BH, Baxter LR, Schwartz JM, Szuba MP, Liston EH. (1991) Electroconvulsive therapy and brain glucose metabolism. *Convuls Ther 7*: 20–7.

Guze BH, Liston EH, Baxter LR Jr, Richeimer SH, Gold ME. (1989) Poor interrater reliablity of MECTA EEG recordings of ECT seizure duration. *J Clin Psychiatry 50*:140–2.

Guze SB. (1967) The occurrence of psychiatric illness in systemic lupus erythematosus. *Am J Psychiatry 123*:1562–70.

Halliday AM, Davison K, Browne MW, Kreeger LC. (1968) A comparison of the effects on depression and memory of bilateral E.C.T. and unilateral E.C.T. to the dominant and non-dominant hemispheres. *Br J Psychiatry 114*:997–1012.

Halsall PJ, Carr CM, Stewart KG. (1988) Propofol reduces seizure duration in patients having anaesthesia for electroconvulsive therapy. *Br J Anaesth 61*:343–4.

Hamilton M. (1960) A rating scale for depression. *J Neurol Neurosurg Psychiatry 23*:56–62.

Hamilton M. (1982) Prediction of the response of depressions to ECT. In: R Abrams, WB Essman, eds. *Electroconvulsive Therapy: Biological Foundations and Clinical Applications.* New York: Spectrum Publications. pp. 113–28.

Hamilton M, White JM. (1960) Factors related to the outcome of depression treated with ECT. *Journal of Mental Science 106*:1031–41.

Hamilton M, Stocker MJ, Spencer CM. (1979) Post-ECT cognitive defect and elevation of blood pressure. *Br J Psychiatry 135*:77–8.

Handforth A. (1982) Postseizure inhibition of kindled seizures by electroconvulsive shock. *Exp Neurol 78*:483–91.

Hardman JB, Morse RM. (1972) Early electroconvulsive treatment of a patient who had artificial aortic and mitral valves. *Am J Psychiatry 128*:895–7.

Harland CC, O'Leary MM, Winters R, Owens J, Hayes B, Melikian V. (1990) Neuroleptic malignant syndrome: a case for electroconvulsive therapy. *Postgrad Med J 66*:49–51.

Harms E. (1956) The origin and early history of electrotherapy and electroshock. *Am J Psychiatry 111*:933–4.

Harper RG, Wiens AN. (1975) Electroconvulsive therapy and memory. *J Nerv Ment Dis 161*:245–54.

Harris JA, Robin AA. (1960) A controlled trial of phenelzine in depressive reactions. *Journal of Mental Science 106*:1432–7.

Harris MJ, Gierz M, Lohr JB. (1989) Recognition and treatment of depression in Alzheimer's disease. *Geriatrics 44*:26–30.

Hartelius H. (1952) Cerebral changes following electrically induced convulsions. An experimental study of cats. *Acta Psychiatry Neurol Scand Suppl 77.*

Hartmann SJ, Saldivia A. (1990) ECT in an elderly patient with skull defects and shrapnel. *Convuls Ther 6*:165–71.

Haskett RF, Zis AP, Albala AA. (1985) Hormone response to repeated electroconvulsive therapy: effects of naloxone. *Biol Psychiatry 20*: 623–33.

Hastings DW. (1961) Circular manic-depressive reaction modified by "prophylactic electroshock." *Am J Psychiatry 118*:258–60.

Hauser WA. (1983) Status epilepticus: frequency, etiology, and neurological sequelae. *Adv Neurol 34*:3–14.

Hay D. (1989) ECT in the medically ill elderly. *Convuls Ther 5*:8–16.

Heath ES, Adams A, Wakeling PLG. (1964) Short courses of ECT and simulated ECT in chronic schizophrenia. *Br J Psychiatry 110*:800–7.

Heilbrunn G, Weil J. (1942) Pathologic changes in the central nervous system in experimental electric shock. *Arch Neurol Psychiatry 47*:918–930.

Hemphill RE. (1940) Studies in certain pathophysiological and psychological phenomena in convulsive therapy. *Journal of Mental Science 86*:799.

Heninger GR, Charney DS, Sternberg DE. (1983) Lithium carbonate augmentation of antidepressant treatment—an effective prescription for treatment of refractory depression. *Arch Gen Psychiatry 40*:1335–42.

Hermann RC, Dorwart RA, Hoover CW, Brody J. (1995) Variation in ECT use in the United States. *Am J Psychiatry 152*:869–75.

Hermesh H, Aizenberg D, Weizman A. (1987) A successful electroconvulsive treatment of neuroleptic malignant syndrome. *Acta Psychiatr Scand 75*:237–79.

Hermesh H, Aizenberg D, Lapidot M, Munitz H. (1988) Risk of malignant hyperthermia among patients with neuroleptic malignant syndrome and their families. *Am J Psychiatry 145*:1431–4.

Herrington RM, Bruce A, Johnstone EC. (1974) Comparative trial of L-tryptophan and E.C.T. in severe depressive illness. *Lancet 2*:731–4.

Heshe J, Roeder E. (1976) Electroconvulsive therapy in Denmark. *Br J Psychiatry 128*:241–5.

Heshe J, Roeder E, Theilgaard A. (1978) Unilateral and bilateral ECT. A psychiatric and psychological study of therapeutic effect and side effects. *Acta Psychiatr Scand Suppl 275*:1–180.

Hickey DR, O'Connor JP, Donati F. (1987) Comparison of atracurium and succinylcholine for electroconvulsive therapy in a patient with atypical plasma cholinesterase. *Can J Anaesthesiology 34*:280–3.

Hickie I, Parsonage B, Parker G. (1990) Prediction of response to electroconvulsive therapy. Preliminary validation of a sign-based typology of depression. *Br J Psychiatry 157*:65–71.

Hicks FG. (1987) ECT modified by atracurium. Case report. *Convuls Ther 3*: 54–9.

Hill GE, Wong KC, Hodges MR. (1976) Potentiation of succinylcholine neuromuscular blockade by lithium carbonate. *Anesthesiology 44*: 439–42.

Hillard JR, Folger R. (1977) Patients' attitudes and attributions to electroconvulsive shock therapy. *J Clin Psychol 33*:855–61.

Hinkle PE, Coffey CE, Weiner RD, Cress M, Christison C. (1987) Use of caffeine to lengthen seizures in ECT. *Am J Psychiatry 144*:1143–8.

Hobson RF. (1953) Prognostic factors in electric convulsive therapy. *J Neurol Neurosurg Psychiatry 16*:275–81.

Hodges JR, Jones M, Elithorn A, Bridges P. (1964) Effect of electroconvulsive therapy on plasma cortisol-levels. *Nature 204*:754–6.

Hoenig J, Chaulk R. (1977) Delirium associated with lithium therapy and electroconvulsive therapy. *Can Med Assoc J 116*:837–8.

Hoffman G, Linkowski P, Kerkhofs M, Desmedt D, Mendlewicz J. (1985) Effects of ECT on sleep and CSF biogenic amines in affective illness. *Psychiatry Res 16*:199–206.

Hofmann P, Gangadhar BN, Probst C, Koinig G, Hatzinger R. (1994) TSH response to TRH and ECT. *J Affect Disord 32*:127–31.

Holcomb HH, Sternberg DE, Heninger GR. (1983) Effects of electroconvulsive therapy on mood, parkinsonism, and tardive dyskinesia in a depressed patient: ECT and dopamine systems. *Biol Psychiatry 18*: 865–73.

Hollender MH, Steckler PP. (1972) Multiple sclerosis and schizophrenia: a case report. *Psychiatr Med 3*:251–7.

Holmberg G. (1953a) The influence of oxygen administration on electrically induced convulsions in man. *Acta Psychiatrica et Neurologica Scandinavica 28*:365–86.

Holmberg G. (1953b) The factor of hypoxemia in electroshock therapy. *Am J Psychiatry 110*:115–8.

Holmberg G. (1954a) Effect on electrically induced convulsions of the number of previous treatments in a series. *Archives of Neurology and Psychiatry 71*:619–23.

Holmberg G. (1954b) Influence of sex and age on convulsions induced by electric shock treatment. *Acta Neurologica et Psychiatrica 71*:619–23.

Holmberg G. (1955) The effect of certain factors on the convulsions in electric shock treatment. *Acta Psychiatrica et Neurologica Scandinavica Suppl 98*:1–19.

Holt WL. (1965) Intensive maintenance EST. A clinical note concerning two unusual cases. *International Journal of Neuropsychiatry 1*:391–4.

Holtzman JL, Finley D, Johnson B, Berry DA, Sirgo MA. (1986) The effects of single-dose atenolol, labetalol, and propranolol on cardiac and vascular function. *Clin Pharmacol Ther 40*:268–273.

Honcke P, Zahle V. (1946) On the correlation between clinical and electroencephalographic observations in patients treated with electro-shock. *Acta Psychiatrica et Neurologica Scandinavica 47*:451–8.

Hood DD, Mecca RS. (1983) Failure to initiate electroconvulsive seizures in a patient pretreated with lidocaine. *Anesthesiology 58*:379–81.

Horan M, Ashton R, Minto J. (1980) Using ECT to study hemispheric specialization for sequential processes. *Br J Psychiatry 137*:119–25.

Hordern A, Holt HF, Burt CG, Gordon WF. (1963) Amitriptyline in depressive cases. *Br J Psychiatry 109*:815–25.

Hordern A, Burt CG, Holt NF. (1965) *Depressive States*. Springfield, IL: Charles C Thomas.

Horne RL, Pettinati HM, Sugerman AA, Varga E. (1985) Comparing bilateral to unilateral electroconvulsive therapy in a randomized study with EEG monitoring. *Arch Gen Psychiatry 42*:1087–92.

Howie MB, Black HA, Zvara D, McSweeney TD, Martin DJ, Coffman JA. (1990) Esmolol reduces autonomic hypersensitivity and length of seizures induced by electroconvulsive therapy. *Anesth Analg 71*:384–8.

Howie MB, Hiestand DC, Zvara DA, Kim PY, McSweeney TD, Coffman JA. (1992) Defining the dose range for esmolol used in electroconvulsive therapy hemodynamic attenuation. *Anesth Analg 75*:805–10.

Hoyle NR, Pratt RT, Thomas DG. (1984) Effect of electroconvulsive therapy on serum myelin basic protein immunoreactivity. *Br Med J 288*: 1110–1.

Hsiao JK, Evans DL. (1984) ECT in a depressed patient after craniotomy. *Am J Psychiatry 141*:442–4.

Huang KC, Lucas LF, Tsueda K, Thomas M, Lippmann SB. (1989) Age-related changes in cardiovascular function associated with electroconvulsive therapy. *Convuls Ther* 5:17–25.

Hughes JR. (1986) ECT during and after the neuroleptic malignant syndrome: case report. *J Clin Psychiatry* 47:42–3.

Hughes J, Wigton R, Jardon F. (1941) Electroencephalographic studies in patients receiving electroshock treatment. *Archives of Neurology and Psychiatry* 46:748–9.

Hughes J, Barraclough BM, Reeve W. (1981) Are patients shocked by ECT? *J Roy Soc Med* 74:283–285.

Hurwitz TD. (1974) Electroconvulsive therapy: a review. *Compr Psychiatry* 15:303–14.

Hussar AE, Pachter M. (1968) Myocardial infarction and fatal coronary insufficiency during electroconvulsive therapy. *JAMA* 204:1004–7.

Huston PE, Strother CH. (1948) The effect of E.C.T. on mental efficiency. *Am J Psychiatry* 104:707.

Husum B, Vester-Andersen T, Buchmann G, Bolwig TG. (1983) Electroconvulsive therapy and intracranial aneurysm. Prevention of blood pressure elevation in a normotensive patient by hydralazine and propranolol. *Anaesthesia* 38:1205–7.

Hyrman V, Palmer LH, Cernik J, Jetelina J. (1985) ECT: The search for the perfect stimulus. *Biol Psychiatry* 20:634–5.

Imlah NW, Ryan E, Harrington JA. (1965) The influence of antidepressant drugs on the response to electroconvulsive therapy and on subsqunt relapse rates. *Neuropsychopharmacology* 4:438–42.

Impastato DJ. (1966) Tendon reflexes as a guide to the safe use of succinylcholine in medicine. *Canadian Psychiatric Association Journal* 11:67–77.

Impastato DJ, Almansi R. (1942) The electrofit in the treatment of mental disease. *J Nerv Ment Dis* 96:395–409.

Impastato DJ, Karliner W. (1966) Control of memory impairment in EST by unilateral stimulation of the non-dominant hemisphere. *Diseases of the Nervous System* 27:182–8.

Impastato DJ, Pacella BL. (1952) Electrically produced unilateral convulsions. *Diseases of the Nervous System* 13:368–9.

Impastato DJ, Berg S, Pacella BL. (1953) Electroshock therapy: focal spread technique. A new form of treatment of psychiatric illness. *Confinia Neurologica* 13:266–70.

Inglis J. (1970) Shock, surgery, and cerebral asymmetry. *Br J Psychiatry* 117:143–8.

Inturrisi CE, Alexopoulos G, Lipman R, Foley K, Rossier J. (1982) beta-Endorphin immunoreactivity in the plasma of psychiatric patients receiving electroconvulsive treatment. *Ann N Y Acad Sci* 398:413–23.

Irving AD, Drayson AM. (1984) Bladder rupture during ECT. *Br J Psychiatry* 144:670.

Isaac RJ. (1990) FDA's shocking treatment of a valuable device. *The Wall Street Journal*, Dec. 5.

Isenberg KE, Dinwiddie SH, Heath AC, et al. (1996) Effect of stimulus parameters on seizure threshold and duration [abstract]. *Convuls Ther* 12:68.

Ives JO, Weaver LA, Williams R. (1976) Portable electromyograph monitoring of unilateral ECT. *Am J Psychiatry* 133:1340–1.

Jaeckle RS, Dilsaver SC. (1986) Covariation of depressive symptoms, parkinsonism, and post-dexamethasone plasma cortisol levels in a bipolar patient: simultaneous response to ECT and lithium carbonate. *Acta Psychiatr Scand* 74:68–72.

Jaffe R, Dubin W, Shoyer B, Roemer R, Sharon D, Lipschutz L. (1990a) Outpatient electroconvulsive therapy: efficacy and safety. *Convuls Ther* 6:231–8.

Jaffe R, Brubaker G, Dubin WR, Roemer R. (1990b) Caffeine-associated cardiac dysrhythmia during ECT: report of three cases. *Convuls Ther* 6: 308–13.

Janakiramaiah N, Channabasavanna SM, Murthy NS. (1982) ECT/chlorpromazine combination versus chlorpromazine alone in acutely schizophrenic patients. *Acta Psychiatr Scand* 66:464–70.

Janicak PG, Davis JM, Gibbons RD, Ericksen S, Chang S, Gallagher P. (1985) Efficacy of ECT: a meta-analysis. *Am J Psychiatry* 142: 297–302.

Janis IL. (1950a) Psychologic effects of electric convulsive treatments (post-treatment amnesias). *J Nerv Ment Dis* 111:359–82.

Janis IL. (1950b) Psychologic effects of electric convulsive treatments (changes in word association reactions). *J Nerv Ment Dis* 111: 383–97.

Jauhar P, Weller M, Hirsch SR. (1979) Electroconvulsive therapy for patient with cardiac pacemaker. *Br Med J* 1:90–1.

Jeffries BF, Kishore PRS, Singh KS, Ghatak NR, Krempa J. (1980) Postoperative computed tomographic changes in the brain. *Radiology* 135: 751–3.

Jensen AV, Becker RF, Windle WF. (1948) Changes in brain structure and memory after intermittent exposure to simulated altitude of 30,000 feet. *Arch Neurol Psychiatry* 60:221–239.

Jephcott G, Kerry RJ. (1974) Lithium: an anesthetic risk. *Br J Anaesth* 46: 389–90.

Jessee SS, Anderson GF. (1983) ECT in the neuroleptic malignant syndrome: case report. *J Clin Psychiatry* 44:186–8.

Johansson F, von Knorring L. (1987) Changes in serum prolactin after electroconvulsive and epileptic seizures. *Eur Arch Psychiatry Neurol Sci* 236:312–8.

Johnson LC, Ulett GA, Johnson M, Sineth K, Sines JO. (1960) Electroconvulsive therapy (with and without atropine). *Arch Gen Psychiatry* 2: 324–36.

Johnstone EC, Deakin JF, Lawler P, Frith CD, Stevens M, McPherson K, et al. (1985) The Northwick Park electroconvulsive therapy trial. *Lancet* 2:1317–20.

Jones BP, Henderson M, Welch CA. (1988) Executive functions in unipolar depression before and after electroconvulsive therapy. *Int J Neurosci* 38:287–97.

Jones G, Callender K. (1981) Northwick Park ECT trial [letter]. *Lancet 1*: 500–1.

Jones RM, Knight PR. (1981) Cardiovascular and hormonal responses to electroconvulsive therapy. Modification of an exaggerated response in an hypertensive patient by beta-receptor blockade. *Anaesthesia 36*: 795–9.

Kahn RL, Fink M. (1959) Personality factors in behavioral response to electroshock therapy. *Neuropsychiatry 1*:45–49.

Kahn RL, Fink M. (1960) Prognostic value of Rorschach criteria in clinical reponse to convulsive therapy. *Journal of Neuropsychiatry 1*:242–5.

Kahn RL, Pollack M, Fink M. (1959) Sociopsychologic aspects of psychiatric treatment in a voluntary mental hospital: Duration of hospitalization, discharge ratings and diagnosis. *Arch Gen Psychiatry 1*:565–74.

Kalayam B, Alexopoulos GS. (1989) Nifedipine in the treatment of blood pressure rise after ECT. *Convuls Ther 5*:110–3.

Kalayam B, Steinhart MJ. (1981) A survey of attitudes on the use of electroconvulsive therapy. *Hosp Community Psychiatry 32*:185–8.

Kalinowsky LB. (1939) Electric-convulsion therapy in schizophrenia. *Lancet* 2:1232–3.

Kalinowsky L. (1945) Organic psychotic syndromes occurring during electric convulsive therapy. *Archives of Neurology and Psychiatry 53*: 269–73.

Kalinowsky LB. (1947) Epilepsy and convulsive therapy. *Res Publ Assoc Res Nerv Ment Dis 26*:175–83.

Kalinowsky LB. (1956a) The danger of various types of medication during electric convulsive therapy. *Am J Psychiatry 112*:745–6.

Kalinowsky LB. (1956b) Additional remarks on the danger of premedication in electric convulsive therapy. *Am J Psychiatry 113*:79–80.

Kalinowsky LB. (1982) The history of electroconvulsive therapy. In: R Abrams, WB Essman, eds. *Electroconvulsive Therapy: Biological Foundations and Clinical Applications.* New York: Spectrum Publications. pp. 1–6.

Kalinowsky LB. (1986) History of convulsive therapy. *Ann N Y Acad Sci 462*: 1–4.

Kalinowsky L, Hoch PH. (1952) *Shock Treatment, Psychosurgery and Other Somatic Treatments in Psychiatry* New York: Grune and Stratton.

Kalinowsky LB, Kennedy F. (1943) Observations in electric shock therapy applied to problems of epilepsy. *J Nerv Ment Dis 98*:56–67.

Kalinowsky LB, Hippius H, Klein HE. (1982) *Biological Treatments in Psychiatry.* New York: Grune and Stratton.

Kane FJ. (1963) Transient neurological symptoms accompanying ECT. *Am J Psychiatry 119*:786–7.

Kantor SJ, Glassman AH. (1977) Delusional depressions: natural history and response to treatment. *Br J Psychiatry 131*:351–60.

Kapur S, Mann JJ. (1993) Antidepressant action and the neurobiologic effects of ECT: human studies. In: CE Coffey, ed. *The Clinical Science of Electroconvulsive Therapy*. Washington DC: American Psychiatric Press. pp. 235–50.

Karel R. (1991) California to consider bill restricting ECT. *Psychiatric News*, May 17.

Karliner W. (1978) ECT for patients with CNS disease. *Psychosomatics 19*: 781–3.

Katona CLE, Aldridge CR. (1984) Prediction of ECT response. *Neuropharmacology 23*:281–3.

Katona CL, Aldridge CR, Roth M, Hyde J. (1987) The dexamethasone suppression test and prediction of outcome in patients receiving ECT. *Br J Psychiatry 150*:315–8.

Kaufman KR. (1994) Asystole with electroconvulsive therapy. *J Intern Med 235*:275–77.

Kaufman KR, Finstead BA, Kaufman ER. (1986) Status epilepticus following electroconvulsive therapy. *Mt Sinai J Med 53*:119–22.

Kay DW, Fahy T, Garside RF. (1970) A seven-month double-blind trial of amitriptyline and diazepam in ECT-treated depressed patients. *Br J Psychiatry 17*:667–71.

Kearns A. (1987) Cotard's syndrome in a mentally handicapped man. *Br J Psychiatry 150*:112–4.

Kellner CH, Bachman DL. (1992) Hallucination after intravenous caffeine. *Am J Psychiatry 149*:422.

Kellner CH, Batterson R. (1989) Low-dose caffeine in ECT. *Convuls Ther 5*: 189–90.

Kellner CH, Burns CM, Bernstein HJ, Monroe RR. (1991) Electrode placement in maintenance ECT. *Convuls Ther 7*:61–2.

Kelway B, Simpson KH, Smith RJ, Halsall P. (1986) Effects of atropine and glycopyrrolate on cognitive function following anesthesia and electroconvulsive therapy (ECT). *Int J Clin Pharmacology 1*:296–302.

Kendell B, Pratt RTC. (1983) Brain damage and ECT. *Br J Psychiatry 143*: 99–100.

Kendell RE, Cooper JE, Gourlay AJ, Copeland JR. (1971) Diagnostic criteria of American and British psychiatrists. *Arch Gen Psychiatry 25*: 123–30.

Kerr RA, McGrath JJ, O'Kearney RT, Price J. (1982) ECT: misconceptions and attitudes. *Aust N Z J Psychiatry 16*:43–49.

Kety S. (1974) Biochemical and neurochemical effects of electroconvulsive shock. In: M Fink, S Kety, J McGaugh, TA Williams, eds. *Psychobiology of Convulsive Therapy*. J. Wiley & Sons: New York. pp. 285–294.

Kety SS, Woodford RB, Harmel MH, Freyhand FA, Appel KE, Schmidt CF. (1948) Cerebral blood flow and metabolism in schizophrenia: The effects of barbiturate semi-narcosis, insulin coma and electroshock. *Am J Psychiatry 104*:765–70.

Kety S, Javoy F, Thierry AM, Julou L, Glowinski J. (1967) A sustained effect of electroconvulsive shock on the turnover of norepinephrine in the central nervous system of the rat. *Proc Natl Acad Sci 58*: 1249–54.

Khan A, Nies A, Johnson G, Becker J. (1985) Plasma catecholamines and ECT. *Biol Psychiatry 20*:799–804.

Khoury GF, Benedetti C. (1989) T-wave changes associated with electroconvulsive therapy. *Anesth Analg 69:*677–9.

King BH, Liston EH. (1990) Proposals for the mechanism of action of convulsive therapy: a synthesis. *Biol Psychiatry 27*:76–94.

King PD. (1960) Chlorpromazine and electroconvulsive therapy in the treatment of newly hospitalized schizophrenics. *Journal of Clinical and Experimental Psychopathology 21*:101–5.

Kirkegaard C. (1987) Effects of ECT on the TRH stimulation test. *Psychoneuroendocrinology 12*:491–3.

Kirkegaard C, Carroll BJ. (1980) Dissociation of TSH adrenocortical disturbances in endogenous depression. *Psychiatry Res 3*:253–64.

Kirkegaard C, Norlem N, Lauridsen UB, Bjorum N. (1977) Prognostic value of thyrotropin-releasing hormone stimulation test in endogenous depression. *Acta Psychiatr Scand 52*:170–7.

Kirstein L, Ottosson JO. (1960) Experimental studies of electroencephalographic changes following electroconvulsive therapy. *Acta Psychiatrica et Neurologica Scandinavica Supplement 145*:60–102.

Kitamura T, Page AJ. (1984) Electrocardiographic changes following electroconvulsive therapy. *Eur Arch Psychiatry Neurol Sci 234*:147–8.

Klimes I, Vigas M, Jurcovicova J, Wiedermann V. (1978) Serum prolactin after electroconvulsive therapy. *Endokrinologie 72*:371–3.

Klotz M. (1955) Serial electroencephalographic changes due to electrotherapy. *Diseases of the Nervous System 16*:120–1.

Kolb LC, Vogel VH. (1942) The use of shock therapy in 305 mental hospitals. *Am J Psychiatry 99*:90–100.

Kolbeinsson H, Arnaldsson OS, Petursson H, Skulason S. (1986) Computed tomographic scans in ECT-patients. *Acta Psychiatr Scand 73*: 28–32.

Kolbeinsson H, Petursson H. (1988) Electroencephalographic correlates of electroconvulsive therapy. *Acta Psychiatr Scand 78*:162–8.

Koo JY, Chien CP. (1986) Coma following ECT and intravenous droperidol: case report. *J Clin Psychiatry 47*:94–95.

Korin H, Fink M, Kwalwasser S. (1956) Relation of changes in memory and learning to improvement in electroshock. *Confinia Neurologica 16*: 88–96.

Kovac AL, Goto H, Arakawa K, Pardo MP. (1990) Esmolol bolus and infusion attenuates increases in blood pressure and heart rate during electro-convulsive therapy. *Can J Anesth 37*:58–62.

Kramer BA. (1985) Use of ECT in California, 1977–1983. *Am J Psychiatry 142*:1190–2.

Kramer BA. (1986) Severe confusion in a patient receiving electroconvulsive therapy and atenolol. *J Nerv Ment Dis 174*:562–563.

Kramer BA. (1990) Maintenance electroconvulsive therapy in clinical practice. *Convuls Ther 6*:279–86.

Kramer BA. (1996) Use of ECT in California, revisited: 1984–1990 [abstract]. *Convuls Ther 12*:76.

Kramer BA, Afrasiabi A. (1991) Atypical cholinesterase and prolonged apnea during electroconvulsive therapy. *Convuls Ther 7*:129–32.

Kramer BA, Allen RE, Friedman B. (1986) Atropine and glycopyrrolate as ECT preanesthesia. *J Clin Psychiatry 47*:199–200.

Kramer BA, Pollock VE, Schneider LS, Gray GE. (1989) Interrater reliability of MECTA SR-1 seizure duration. *Biol Psychiatry 25*:642–4.

Kraus RP, Remick RA. (1982) Diazoxide in the management of severe hypertension after electroconvulsive therapy. *Am J Psychiatry 139*: 504–5.

Kriss A, Blumhardt LD, Halliday AM, Pratt RT (1978) Neurological asymmetries immediately after unilateral ECT. *J Neurol Neurosurg Psychiatry 41*:1135–44.

Kriss A, Halliday AM, Halliday E, Pratt RT. (1980) Evoked potentials following unilateral ECT. II. The flash evoked potential. *Electroencephalogr Clin Neurophysiol 48*:490–501.

Kronfol Z, Hamsher KD, Digre K, Waziri R. (1978) Depression and hemispheric functions: changes associated with unilateral ECT. *Br J Psychiatry 132*:560–7.

Krueger RB, Fama JM, Devanand DP, Prudic J, Sackeim HA. (1993) Does ECT permanently alter seizure threshold? *Biol Psychiatry 33*:272–6.

Krystal AD, Weiner RD, Coffey CE, et al. (1992) EEG evidence of more "intense" seizure activity with bilateral ECT. *Biol Psychiatry 31*: 617–21.

Krystal AD, Weiner RD, Coffey CE. (1995) The ictal EEG as a marker of adequate stimulus intensity with unilateral ECT. *J Neuropsychiatry 7*: 295–303.

Krystal AD, Weiner RD, Gasseert D, et al. (1996) The relative ability of three ictal EEG frequency bands to differentiate ECT seizures on the basis of electrode placement, stimulus intensity, and therapeutic response. *Convuls Ther 12*:13–24.

Krystal AD, Weiner RD, McCall WV, et al. (1993) The effects of ECT stimulus dose and electrode placement on the ictal electroencephalogram: an intra-individual cross-over study. *Biol Psychiatry 34*:759–67.

Krystal AD, Weiner RD. (1994) ECT seizure therapeutic adequacy. *Convuls Ther 10*:153–64.

Krystal AD, Weiner RS. (1995) ECT seizure duration: reliability of manual and computer-automated determinations. *Convuls Ther 11*:158–69.

Kupfer D. (1986) The sleep EEG in diagnosis and treatment of depression. In: AJ Rush, KZ Altshuler, eds. *Depression: Basic Mechanisms, Diagnosis, and Treatment.* Guilford Press: New York. pp. 102–25.

Kurland AA, Turek IS, Brown CC, Wagman AM. (1976) Electroconvulsive therapy and EEG correlates in depressive disorders. *Compr Psychiatry 17*:581–9.

Kurokawa Y, Ueno T, Obara T, Gotohda T, Fukatsu R, Yamashita I. (1989) Hyperkinetic mutism within the scope of consciousness disorder in a case of systemic lupus erythematosus. *Jpn J Psychiatry Neurol 43*: 89–96.

Kwentus JA, Hart RP, Calabrese V, Hekmati A. (1986) Mania as a symptom of multiple sclerosis. *Psychosomatics 27*:729–31.

Kwentus JA, Schulz SC, Hart RP. (1984) Tardive dystonia, catatonia, and electroconvulsive therapy. *J Nerv Ment Dis 172*:171–3.

Laird DM. (1955) Convulsive therapy in psychoses accompanying pregnancy. *N Engl J Med 252*:934–6.

Lam RW. (1990) Treatment of depression in patients with dementia. *Am J Psychiatry 147*:130–1.

Lambourn J, Gill D. (1978) A controlled comparison of simulated and real ECT. *Br J Psychiatry 133*:514–9.

Lamy S, Bergsholm P, d'Elia G. (1994) The antidepressant efficacy of high-dose nondominant long-distance parietotemporal and bitemporal electroconvulsive therapy. *Convuls Ther 10*:43–52.

Lancaster NP, Steinert RR, Frost I. (1958) Unilateral electro-convulsive therapy. *Journal of Mental Science 104*:221–7.

Lane RD, Zeitlin SB, Abrams R, Swartz CM. (1989) Differential effects of right unilateral and bilateral ECT on heart rate. *Am J Psychiatry 146*: 1041–3.

Lane R, Novelly R, Cornell C, Zeitlin S, Schwartz G. (1988) Asymmetric hemispheric control of heart rate [abstract]. *Psychophysiology 25*:464.

Langer G, Neumark J, Koining G, Graf M, Schonbeck G. (1985) Rapid psychotherapeutic effects of anesthesia with isoflurane (ES narcotherapy) in treatment-refractory depressed patients. *Neuropsychobiology 14*: 118–20.

Langer G, Karazman R, Neumark J, Saletu B, Schonbeck G, Grunberger J, Dittrich R, Petriceck W, Hoffman P, Linzmayer L, Anderer P, Steinberger K. (1995) Isoflurane narcotherapy in depressive patients refractory to conventional antidepressant drug treatment. *Neuropsychobiology 31*:182–94.

Langsley DG, Enterline JD, Hickerson GX. (1959) Comparison of chlorpromazine and EST in treatment of acute schizophrenic and manic reactions. *Archives of Neurology Psychiatry 81*:384–91.

Larson G, Swartz CM. (1986) Differences between first and second electroconvulsive treatments given in the same session. *Convuls Ther 2*:191–6.

Larson G, Swartz C, Abrams R. (1984) Duration of ECT-induced tachycardia as a measure of seizure length. *Am J Psychiatry 141*:1269–71.

Latey RH, Fahy TJ. (1985) Electroconvulsive therapy in the Republic of Ireland 1982: a summary of findings. *Br J Psychiatry 147*:438–9.

Lauterbach EC, Moore NC. (1990) Parkinsonism-dystonia syndrome and ECT [letter]. *Am J Psychiatry 147*:1249–50.

Lawson JS, Inglis J, Delva NJ, Rodenburg M, Waldron JJ, Letemendia FJ. (1990) Electrode placement in ECT: cognitive effects. *Psychol Med 20*:335–44.

Lazarus A. (1986) Treatment of neuroleptic malignant syndrome with electroconvulsive therapy. *J Nerv Ment Dis 174*:47–9.

Lebensohn ZM, Jenkins RB. (1975) Improvement of Parkinsonism in depressed patients treated with ECT. *Am J Psychiatry 132*:283–5.

Lebrun-Grandie P, Baron JC, Soussaline R, Loch'h C, Sastre J, Bousser MG. (1983) Coupling between regional blood flow and oxygen utilization in the normal human brain. *Arch Neurol 40*:230–6.

Lee JT, Erbguth PH, Stevens WC, Sack RL. (1985) Modification of electroconvulsive therapy induced hypertension with nitroglycerine ointment. *Anesthesiology 62*:793–6.

Leechuy I, Abrams R. (1987) Postictal delirium (and recovery from melancholia) after left-unilateral ECT. *Convuls Ther 3*:65–8.

Leechuy I, Abrams R, Kohlhaas J. (1988) ECT-induced postictal delirium and electrode placement. *Am J Psychiatry 145*:880–1.

Lehmann L, Liddell J. (1969) Human cholinesterase (pseudocholinesterase): genetic variants and their recognition. *Br J Anaesth 41*:235–44.

Lerer B. (1984) Electroconvulsive shock and neurotransmitter receptors: implications for mechanism of action and adverse effects of electroconvulsive therapy. *Biol Psychiatry 19*:361–83.

Lerer B. (1987) Neurochemical and other neurobiological consequences of ECT: implications for the pathogenesis and treatment of affective disorders. In: HY Meltzer, ed. *Psychopharmacology: The Third Generation of Progress.* Raven Press: New York.

Lerer B, Belmaker RH. (1982) Receptors and the mechanism of action of ECT. *Biol Psychiatry 17*:497–511.

Lerer B, Shapira B. (1986) Optimum frequency of electroconvulsive therapy: implications for practice and research. *Convuls Ther 2*:141–4.

Lerer B, Shapira B. (1989) In reply [letter]. *Convuls Ther 5*:364–5.

Lerer B, Sitaram N. (1983) Clinical strategies for evaluating ECT mechanisms—pharmacological, biochemical and psychophysiological approaches. *Prog Neuropsychopharmacol Biol Psychiatr 7*:309–33.

Lerer B, Shapira B, Calev A, Tubi N, Drexler H, Kindler S, Lidsky D, Schwartz JE. (1995) Antidepressant and cognitive effects of twice-versus three-times-weekly ECT. *Am J Psychiatry 152*:564–70.

Letemendia JF, Delva NJ, Rodenberg M, Lawson JS, Inglis J, Waldron JJ,

Lywood DW. (1993) Therapeutic advantage of bifrontal electrode placement in ECT. *Psychol Med 23*:349–60.

Levy LA, Savit JM, Hodes M. (1983) Parkinsonism: improvement by electro-convulsive therapy. *Arch Phys Med Rehabil 64*:432–3.

Levy R. (1968) The clinical evaluation of unilateral electroconvulsive therapy. *Br J Psychiatry 114*:459–63.

Levy SD, Levy SB. (1987) Electroconvulsive therapy in two former neuro-surgical patients: Skull prosthesis and ventricular shunt. *Convuls Ther 3*:46–8.

Levy SD. (1988) 'Cuff' monitoring, osteoporosis, and fracture. *Convuls Ther 4*:248–9.

Lewis WH, Jr, Richardson DJ, Gahagan LH. (1955) Cardiovascular distur-bances and their management in modified electrotherapy for psychiatric illness. *N Engl J Med 252*:1016–20.

Liang RA, Lam RW, Aneill RJ. (1988) ECT in the treatment of mixed de-pression and dementia. *Br J Psychiatry 152*:281–4.

Liberson WT. (1944) New possibilities in electric convulsive therapy: brief stimulus technique. *Digest of Neurology and Psychiatry 12*:368.

Liberson WT. (1948) Brief stimulus therapy. Physiological and clinical obser-vations. *Am J Psychiatry 105*:28–9.

Liberson WT. (1953) Current evaluation of electric convulsive therapy—cor-relation of the parameters of electric current with physiologic and psy-chologic changes. *Res Publ Assoc Res Nerv Ment Dis 31*:199–231.

Liberson WT, Wilcox P. (1945) Electric convulsive therapy: Comparison of "brief stimulus technique" with Friedman-Wilcox-Reiter technique. *Digest of Neurology and Psychiatry 8*:292–302.

Liberson WT, Kaplan JA, Sherer IW, Trehub A. (1956) Correlations of EEG and psychological findings during intensive brief stimulus therapy. *Confinia Neurologica 16*:116–25.

Liberzon I, DeQuardo JR, Sidell G, Mazzara C, Tandon R. (1947) Post-ECT dyskinesia. *Convuls Ther 7*:40–4.

Lidbeck WL. (1944) Pathologic changes in the brain after electric shock: an experimental study on dogs. *J Neuropathol Exp Neurol 3*:81–6.

Liebowitz NR, El-Mallakh RS. (1993) Cardiac arrest during ECT: a cholin-ergic phenomenon? *J Clin Psychiatry 54*:279–80.

Lingley JR, Robbins LL. (1947) Fractures following electroshock therapy. *Radiology 48*:124–8.

Linkowski P, Mendlewicz J, Kerkhofs M, Leclercq R, Golstein J, Brasseur M, et al. (1987) 24-hour profiles of adrenocorticotropin, cortisol, and growth hormone in major depressive illness: effect of antidepressant treatment. *J Clin Endocrinol Metab 65*:141–52.

Linnoila M, Karoum F, Potter WZ. (1983) Effects of antidepressant treatments on dopamine turnover in depressed patients. *Arch Gen Psychiatry 40*:1015–7.

Linnoila M, Miller TL, Bartko J, Potter WZ. (1984) Five antidepressant treatments in depressed patients. Effects on urinary serotonin and 5-hydroxyindoleacetic acid output. *Arch Gen Psychiatry 41*:688–92.

Lipkin KM, Dyrud J, Meyer GG. (1970) The many faces of mania. *Arch Gen Psychiatry 22*:262–7.

Lipman RS, Backup C, Bobrin Y, Delaplane JM, Doeff J, Gittleman S, Joseph R, Kanefield, M. (1986a) Dexamethasone suppression test as a predictor of response to electroconvulsive therapy. I. Inpatient treatment. *Convuls Ther 2*:151–60.

Lipman RS, Uffner W, Schwalb N, Ravetz R, Lief B, Levy S. (1986b) Dexamethasone suppression test as a predictor of response to electroconvulsive therapy. II. Six-month follow-up. *Convuls Ther 2*:161–7.

Lippmann S, Manshadi M, Wehry M, Byrd R, Past W, Keller W, Schuster J, Elams, Meyer D, O'Daniel R. (1985) 1,250 electroconvulsive treatments without evidence of brain injury. *Br J Psychiatry 147*: 203–4.

Lisanby SH, Devanand DP, Prudic J, Pierson D, Nobler M, Fitzsimons L, Sackeim HA. (1997) Prolactin response to ECT: effects of electrode placement and stimulus dosage. *Biol Psychiatry* in press.

Lisanby SH, Devanand DP, Nobler MS, Prudic J, Mullen L, Sackeim HA. (1996) Exceptionally high seizure thresholds: ECT device limitations. *Convuls Ther 12*:156–64.

Liskow BI. (1985) Relationship between neuroleptic malignant syndrome and malignant hyperthermia [letter]. *Am J Psychiatry 142*:390.

Liston EH, Salk JD. (1990) Hemodynamic responses to ECT after bilateral adrenalectomy. *Convuls Ther 6*:160–4.

Liston EH, Sones DE. (1990) Postictal hyperactive delirium in ECT: management with midazolam. *Convuls Ther 6*:19–25.

Liston EH, Guze BH, Baxter LR, Jr, Richeimer SH, Gold ME. (1988) Motor versus EEG seizure duration in ECT. *Biol Psychiatry 24*:94–6.

Liu JC. (1949) Nerve cell changes resulting from starvation. *Anat Rec 103*: 68.

London SW, Glass DD. (1985) Prevention of electroconvulsive therapy-induced dysrhythmias with atropine and propranolol. *Anesthesiology 62*:819–22.

Loo H, Kuche H, Benkelfat C. (1985) Electroconvulsive therapy during anticoagulant therapy. *Convuls Ther 1*:258–62.

Loo H, Galinowski A, Boccara I, Richard A. (1988) Interet de la sismotherapie d'entretien dans les depressions recurrentes: a propos de 4 observations. *Encephale 14*:39–41.

Loo H, Galinowski A, De Carvalho W, Bourdel MC, Poirier MF. (1991) Use of maintenance ECT for elderly depressed patients. *Am J Psychiatry 148*:810.

Lotstra F, Linkowski P, Mendlewicz J. (1983) General anesthesia after neuroleptic malignant syndrome. *Biol Psychiatry 18*:243–7.

Lovett-Doust JW, Raschka LB. (1975) Enduring effects of modified ECT on the cerebral circulation in man. A computerized study by cerebral impedance plethysmography. *Psychiatr Clin 8*:293–303.

Lowinger P, Huston PE. (1953) Electric shock in psychosis with cerebral spastic paralysis. *Diseases of the Nervous System 14*:2–4.

Lown B. (1979) Sudden cardiac death: The major challenge confronting contemporary cardiology. *Am J Cardiol 43*:313.

Lunn RJ, Savageau MM, Beatty WW, Gerst JW, Staton RD, Brumback RA. (1981) Anesthetics and electroconvulsive therapy seizure duration: implications for therapy from a rat model. *Biol Psychiatry 16*: 1163–75.

Lunn V, Trolle E. (1949) On the initial impairment of consciousness following electric convulsive therapy. *Acta Psychiatr Scand 24*:33–58.

Lurie SN, Coffey CE. (1990) Caffeine-modified electroconvulsive therapy in depressed patients with medical illness. *Clin Psychiatry 51*:154–7.

Lykouras E, Malliaras D, Christodoulou GN, Papakostas Y, Voulgari A, Tzonou A, et al. (1986) Delusional depression: phenomenology and response to treatment. A prospective study. *Acta Psychiatr Scand 73*: 324–9.

Lykouras L, Markianos M, Hatzimanolis J, Malliaras D, Stefanis C. (1990) Biogenic amine metabolites during electroconvulsive therapy of melancholic patients. *Convuls Ther 6*:266–72.

Lykouras L, Markianos M, Augoustides A, Papakostas Y, Stefanis C. (1993) Evaluation of TSH and prolactin responses to TRH as predictors of the therapeutic effect of ECT in depression. *Eur Neuropsychopharmacol 3*:81–3.

Mac DS, Pardo MP. (1983) Systemic lupus erythematosus and catatonia: a case report. *J Clin Psychiatry 44*:155–6.

Mackenzie TB, Price TR, Tucker GJ, Culver, CM. (1985) Early change in cognitive performance accompanying bilateral ECT. *Convuls Ther 1*: 183–9.

Malek-Ahmadi P, Weddige RL. (1988) Tardive dyskinesia and electroconvulsive therapy. *Convuls Ther 4*:328–31.

Malek-Ahmadi P, Sedler RR. (1989) Electroconvulsive therapy and asymptomatic meningioma. *Convuls Ther 5*:168–70.

Malek-Ahmadi P, Beceiro JB, McNeil BW, Weddige RL. (1990) Electroconvulsive therapy and chronic subdural hematoma. *Convuls Ther 6*: 38–41.

Maletzky BM. (1978) Seizure duration and clinical effect in electroconvulsive therapy. *Compr Psychiatry 19*:541–50.

Maletzky BM. *Multiple-Monitored Electroconvulsive Therapy*. (1981) Boca Raton, FL: CRC Press.

Maletzky BM. (1986) Conventional and multiple-monitored electroconvulsive therapy: a comparison in major depressive episodes. *J Nerv Ment Dis 174*:257–64.

Malitz S, Sackeim HA, Decina P, Kanzler M, Kerr B. (1986) The efficacy of electroconvulsive therapy: dose-response interactions with modality. *Ann N Y Acad Sci 462*:56–64.

Malmivuo, Plonsey. (1995) *Bioelectromagnetism*. New York: Oxford University Press. p. 64.

Malsch E, Gratz I, Mani S, Backup C, Levy S, Allen E. (1994) Efficacy of electroconvulsive therapy after propofol and methohexital anesthesia. *Convuls Ther 10*:212–19.

Maltbie AA, Wingfield MS, Volow MR, Weiner RD, Sullivan JL, Cavenar JO, Jr. (1980) Electroconvulsive therapy in the presence of brain tumor. Case reports and an evaluation of risk. *J Nerv Ment Dis 168*:400–5.

Mandel M. (1975) Electroconvulsive therapy for chronic pain associated with depression. *Am J Psychiatry 132*:632–6.

Mandel MR, Miller AL, Baldessarini RJ. (1980) Intoxication associated with lithium and ECT. *Am J Psychiatry 137*:1107–9.

Mandel M. (1980) Review of Breggin P. *Electroshock: Its Brain Disabling Effects. N Engl J Med 303*:402.

Mander AJ, Whitfield A, Kean D, Smith MA, Douglas RH, Kendell RE. (1987) Cerebral and brain stem changes after ECT revealed by nuclear magnetic resonance imaging. *Br J Psychiatry 151*:69–71.

Maneksha FR. (1991) Hypertension and tachycardia during electroconvulsive therapy: to treat or not to treat? *Convuls Ther 7*:28–35.

Manly DT, Swartz CM. (1994) Asymmetric bilateral right frontotemporal left frontal stimulus electrode placement: comparisons with bifrontotemporal and unilateral placements. *Convuls Ther 10*:267–70.

Mann JJ, Brown RD, Mason BJ, Halper JP, Sweeney JP, Kocsis JH, Manevitz A. (1985) Alteration of adrenergic receptor responsivity by electroconvulsive therapy. In: C Shagass, ed. *Biological Psychiatry*: Proceedings of the Fourth World Congress of Biological Psychiatry (1985). New York: Elsevier. pp. 867–70.

Mann JJ, Mahler JC, Wilner PJ, Halper JP, Brown RP, Johnson KS, et al. (1990) Normalization of blunted lymphocyte β-adrenergic responsivity in melancholic inpatients by a course of electroconvulsive therapy. *Arch Gen Psychiatry 47*:461–4.

Mann SC, Caroff SN, Bleier HR, Welz WK, Kling MA, Hayashida M. (1986) Lethal catatonia. *Am J Psychiatry 143*:1374–81.

Manning EL, Hollander WM. (1954) Glaucoma and electroshock therapy. *Am J Ophthalmol 37*:857–9.

Mansheim P. (1983) ECT in the treatment of a depressed adolescent with meningomyelocele, hydrocephalus, and seizures. *J Clin Psychiatry 44*: 385–6.

Marco LA, Randels PM. (1979) Succinylcholine drug interactions during electroconvulsive therapy. *Biol Psychiatry 14*:433–45.

Marjerrison G, James J, Reichert H. (1975) Unilateral and bilateral ECT: EEG findings. *Canadian Psychiatric Association Journal 20*:257–66.

Markianos M, Papakostas Y, Stefanis C. (1987) The patterns of prolactin release by ECT and TRH compared. *Life Sci 41*:1273–6.

Martensson B, Bartfai A, Hallen B, Hellstrom C, Junthe T, Olander M. (1994) A comparison of propofol and methohexital as anesthetic agents for ECT: effects on seizure duration, therapeutic outcome, and memory. *Biol Psychiatry 35*:179–89.

Martin BA, Kramer PM. (1982) Clinical significance of the interaction between lithium and a neuromuscular blocker. *Am J Psychiatry 139*: 1326–28.

Martin RD, Flegenheimer WV. (1971) Psychiatric aspects of the management of the myasthenic patients. *Mt Sinai J Med 38*:594–601.

Mathe AA, Bergman P, Aperia B, Wetterberg L. (1987) Electroconvulsive therapy and plasma prostaglandin E2 metabolite in major depressive disorder. *Prog Neuropsychopharmacol Biol Psychiatry 11*:701–7.

Mathisen KS, Pettinati HM. (1987) Meta-analysis of effects of electrode placements. *Convuls Ther 3*:69–70.

Mattes JA, Pettinati HM, Stephens S, Robin SE, Willis KW. (1990) A placebo-controlled evaluation of vasopressin for ECT-induced memory impairment. *Biol Psychiatry 27*:289–303.

Matthew JR, Constan E. (1964) Complications following ECT over a three-year period in a state institution. *Am J Psychiatry 120*:1119–20.

Maxwell RD. (1968) Electrical factors in electroconvulsive therapy. *Acta Psychiatr Scand 44*:436–48.

McAllister DA, Perri MG, Jordan MC, Rauscher FP, Sattin A. (1987) Effects of ECT given two vs three times weekly. *Psychiatry Res 21*:63–9.

McAllister TW, Price TR. (1982) Severe depressive pseudodementia with and without dementia. *Am J Psychiatry 139*:626–9.

McAndrew J, Berkey B, Matthews C. (1967) The effects of dominant and nondominant unilateral ECT as compared to bilateral ECT. *Am J Psychiatry 124*:483–90.

McCabe MS. (1976) ECT in the treatment of mania: a controlled study. *Am J Psychiatry 133*:688–91.

McCabe MS, Norris B. (1977) ECT versus chlorpromazine in mania. *Biol Psychiatry 12*:245–54.

McCall WV. (1996) Asystole in electroconvulsive therapy: report of four cases. *J Clin Psychiatry 57*:199–203.

McCall WV, Farah A. (1995) Greater ictal EEG regularity during RUL ECT is associated with greater treatment efficacy [abstract]. *Convuls Ther 11*:69.

McCall WV, Shelp FE, Weiner RD, Austin S, Norris J. (1993a) Convulsive threshold differences in right unilateral and bilateral ECT. *Biol Psychiatry 34*:606–11.

McCall WV, Reid S, Rosenquist P, Foreman A, Kiesow-Webb N. (1993b) A reappraisal of the role of caffeine in ECT. *Am J Psychiatry 150*: 1543–45.

McCall WV, Farah BA, Reboussin D, Colenda CC. (1995) Comparison of the efficacy of titrated, moderate-dose and fixed, high-dose right unilateral ECT in elderly patients. *Am J Geriatr Psychiatry 3*:317–24.

McCall WV, Reid S, Ford M. (1994) Electrocardiographic and cardiovascular effects of subconvulsive stimulation during titrated right unilateral ECT. *Convuls Ther 10*:25–33.

McCall WV, Weiner RD, Carroll BJ, Shelp FE, Ritchie JC, Austin S, Norris RN. (1996) Serum prolactin, electrode placement, and the convulsive threshold during ECT. *Convuls Ther 12*:81–5.

McCall WV, Shelp FE, Weiner RD, Austin S, Harrill A. (1991) Effects of labetalol on hemodynamics and seizure duration during ECT. *Convuls Ther 7*:5–14.

McClelland R, McAllister G. (1988) Comparison of electrical measurements on constant voltage and constant current ECT machines. *Br J Psychiatry 153*:126–7.

McCreadie RG, Phillips K, Robinson AD, Gilhooly G, Crombie W. (1989) Is electroencephalographic monitoring of electroconvulsive therapy useful? *Br J Psychiatry 154*:229–31.

McDonald IM, Perkins M, Marjerrison G, Podilsky M. (1966) A controlled comparison of amitriptyline and electroconvulsive therapy in the treatment of depression. *Am J Psychiatry 122*:1427–31.

McKenna G, Engle RP, Jr, Brooks H, Dalen J. (1970) Cardiac arrhythmias during electroshock therapy: significance, prevention, and treatment. *Am J Psychiatry 127*:530–3.

Meco G, Casacchia M, Carchedi F, Falaschi P, Rocco A, Frajese G. (1978) Prolactin response to repeated electroconvulsive therapy in acute schizophrenia. *Lancet 2*:999.

Medical Research Council. Clinical trial of the treatment of depressive illness. *Br Med J 5439*:881–6.

Medlicott RW. (1948) Brief stimuli electroconvulsive therapy. *N Z Med J 47*: 29–37.

Meduna LJ. (1932) Klinische und anatomische Beitrag zür Frage der genuinen Epilepsie. *Deutsche Zeitung der Nervenkrankheiten 129*:17–42.

Meduna LJ. (1934) Über experimentelle Campherepilepsie. *Arch Psychiatr Nervenkr 102*:333–9.

Meduna L. (1985) Autobiography. Part 1. *Convuls Ther 1*:43–57.

Meisel A, Roth LH, Lidz CW. (1977) Toward a model of the legal doctrine of informed consent. *Am J Psychiatry 134*:285–9.

Meldrum BS. (1986) Neuropathological consequences of chemically and electrically induced seizures. *Ann N Y Acad Sci 462*:186–93.

Mendels J. (1965a) Electroconvulsive therapy and depression: I. The prognostic significance of clinical factors. *Br J Psychiatry 111*:675–81.

Mendels J. (1965b) Electroconvulsive therapy and depression: II. Significance of endogenous and reactive syndromes. *Br J Psychiatry 111*: 682–6.

Mendels J. (1965c) Electroconvulsive therapy and depression: III. A method for prognosis. *Br J Psychiatry 111*:687–90.

Mendels J. (1967) The prediction of response to electroconvulsive therapy. *Am J Psychiatry 124*:153–9.

Menken M, Safer J, Goldfarb C, Varga E. (1979) Multiple ECT: morphologic effects. *Am J Psychiatry 36*:453.

Mensah GA, Schoen RE, Devereux RB. (1990) Intracardiac thrombi in patients undergoing electroconvulsive therapy. *Am Heart J 119*:684–5.

Merrill RD. (1990) ECT for a patient with profound mental retardation. *Am J Psychiatry 147*:256–7.

Merritt HH, Putnam TJ. (1938) New series of anticonvulsant drugs tested by experiments on animals. *Archives of Neurology and Psychiatry 39*: 1003–15.

Messina AG, Paranicas M, Katz B, Markowitz J, Yao F-S, Devereux RB. (1992) Effect of electroconvulsive therapy on the electrocardiogram and echocardiogram. *Anesth Analg 75*:511–14.

Mielke DH, Winstead DK, Goethe JW, Schwartz BD. (1984) Multiple-monitored electroconvulsive therapy: safety and efficacy in elderly depressed patients. *J Am Geriatr Soc 32*:180–2.

Miller AL, Faber RA, Hatch JP, Alexander HE. (1985) Factors affecting amnesia, seizure duration, and efficacy in ECT. *Am J Psychiatry 142*: 692–6.

Miller DH, Clancy J, Cummings E. (1953) A comparison between unidirectional current nonconvulsive electrical stimulation given with Reiter's machine, standard alternating current electroshock and pentothal in chronic schizophrenia. *Am J Psychiatry 109*:617–20.

Miller E. (1970) The effect of ECT on memory and learning. *Br J Med Psychol 43*:57–62.

Miller ME, Gabriel A, Herman G, Stern A, Shagong U, Klupersmith J. (1987) Atropine sulfate premedication and cardiac arrhythmia in electroconvulsive therapy (ECT). *Convuls Ther 3*:10–17.

Milstein V, Small JG, Klapper MH, Small IF, Miller MJ, Kellams JJ. (1987) Uni- versus bilateral ECT in the treatment of mania. *Convuls Ther 3*: 1–9.

Mindham RH, Howland C, Shepherd M. (1973) An evaluation of continuation therapy with tricyclic antidepressants in depressive illness. *Psychol Med 3*:5–17.

Misiaszek J, Cork RC, Hameroff SR, Finley J, Weiss IL. (1984) The effect of electroconvulsive therapy on plasma β-endorphin. *Biol Psychiatry 19*: 450–5.

Mitchell P, Smythe G, Torda T. (1990) Effect of the anesthetic agent propofol on hormonal responses to ECT. *Biol Psychiatry 28*:315–24.

Mitchell P, Torda T, Hickie I, Burke C. (1991) Propofol as an anaesthetic agent for ECT: effect on outcome and length of course. *Aust N Z J Psychiatry 25*:255–61.

Modigh K, Balldin J, Eriksson E, Granerus AK, Walinder J. (1984) Increased responsiveness of dopamine receptors after ECT: a review of experimental and clinical evidence. In: B Lerer, RD Weiner, RH Belmaker, eds. *ECT: Basic Mechanisms*. London: John Libbey. pp. 18–27.

Moir DC, Crooks J, Cornwell WB, O'Malley K, Dingwall-Fordyce I, Turnbull MJ, et al. (1972) Cardiotoxicity of amitriptyline. *Lancet 2*: 561–4.

Monke JV. (1952) Electroconvulsive therapy following surgical correction of aortic coarctation by implantation of an aortic isograft. *Am J Psychiatry 109*:378–9.

Moore MB. (1960) Electroconvulsive therapy and the aorta. *Can Med Assoc J 83*:1258–9.

Moore NP. (1943) The maintenance treatment of chronic psychotics by electrically induced convulsions. *J Ment Sci 89*:257–69.

Moore RA. (1977) The electroconvulsive therapy fight in California. *J Forensic Sci 22*:845–50.

Moriarty JD, Siemens JC. (1947) Electroencephalographic study of electric shock therapy. *Arch Neurol Psychiatry 57*:693–711.

Mosovich A, Katzenelbogen S. (1948) Electroshock therapy, clinical and electroencephalographic studies. *J Nerv Ment Dis 107*:517–30.

Mowbray RM. (1959) Historical aspects of electric convulsant therapy. *Scott Med J 4*:373–8.

Mulgaokar GD, Dauchot PJ, Duffy JP, Anton AH. (1985) Noninvasive assessment of electroconvulsive-induced changes in cardiac function. *J Clin Psychiatry 46*:479–82.

Muller DJ. (1971) Unilateral ECT. (One year's experience at a city hospital). *Diseases of the Nervous System 32*:422–4.

Murray GB, Shea V, Conn DK. (1986) Electroconvulsive therapy for post-stroke depression. *J Clin Psychiatry 47*:258–60.

Nakajima T, Daval JL, Gleiter CH, Deckert J, Post RM, Marangos PJ. (1989) C-fos mRNA expression following electrical-induced seizure and acute nociceptive stress in mouse brain. *Epilepsy Res 4*:156–9.

National Institutes of Health. (1985) Consensus Conference: Electroconvulsive therapy. *JAMA 254*:2103–8.

Nelson JP, Rosenberg DR. (1991) ECT treatment of demented elderly patients with major depression: a retrospective study of efficacy and safety. *Convuls Ther 7*:157–65.

Nemeroff CB, Bissette G, Akil H, Fink M. (1991) Neuropeptide concentrations in the cerebrospinal fluid of depressed patients treated with electroconvulsive therapy: corticotrophin-releasing factor, β-endorphin and somatostatin. *Br J Psychiatry 158*:59–63.

Nerozzi D, Graziosi S, Melia E, Aceti F, Magnani A, Fiume S, Fraioli F, Frajese G. (1987) Mechanism of action of ECT in major depressive disorders: a neuroendocrine interpretation. *Psychiatry Res 20*: 207–13.

Neuberger K, Whitehead RH, Rutledge EK, Ebaugh FG (1942) Pathologic changes in the brains of dogs given repeated electric shocks. *Am J Ment Sci 204*:381–7.

Newman ME, Lerer B. (1988) Chronic electroconvulsive shock and desipramine reduce the degree of inhibition by 5-HT and carbachol of forskolin-stimulated adenylate cyclase in rat hippocampal membranes. *Eur J Pharmacol 148*:257–60.

News and Notes. (1992) Dick Cavett and ECT. *Convuls Ther 8*:300–1.

Nilsen SM, Willis KW, Pettinati HM. (1986) Instrument review: initial impression of two new brief-pulse electroconvulsive therapy machines. *Convuls Ther 2*:43–54.

Nilsen-Stevens SM, Pettinati HM, Willis KW, Bedient L, Greenberg RM, Zomorodi A. (1990) Clinical review of Medcraft Corporation's new brief-pulse ECT device. *Convuls Ther 6*:42–53.

Nobler MS, Sackeim HA, Solomou M, et al. (1993) EEG manifestations during ECT: effects of electrode placement and stimulus intensity. *Biol Psychiatry 34*:321–30.

Nobler MS, Sackeim HA, Prohovnik I, et al. (1994) Regional cerebral blood flow in mood disorders, III: Treatment and clinical response. *Arch Gen Psychiatry 51*:884–97.

Nolen WA, Zwaan WA. (1990) Treatment of lethal catatonia with electroconvulsive therapy and dantrolene sodium: a case report. *Acta Psychiatr Scand 82*:90–2.

Nutt DJ, Gleiter CH, Glue P. (1989) Neuropharmacological aspects of ECT: in search of the primary mechanism of action. *Convuls Ther 5*: 250–60.

Nyirö J, Jablonsky A. (1929) Einige daten zur prognose der Epilepsie, mit besonderer rucksicht auf die konstitution. *Psychiatr Neurol Wochenschr 31*:547–9.

Nyström S. (1964) On relation between clinical factors and efficacy of E.C.T. in depression. *Acta Psychiatr Scand Suppl 181*:115–8.

O'Brien PD, Morgan DH. (1991) Bladder rupture during ECT. *Convuls Ther 7*:56–9.

O'Connell BK, et al. (1988) Neuronal lesions in mercaptopropionic acid-induced status epilepticus. *Acta Neuropathol (Berl) 77*:47–54

O'Dea JPK, Gould D, Hallberg M, Wieland RG. (1978) Prolactin changes during electroconvulsive therapy. *Am J Psychiatry 135*:609–11.

O'Dea JPK, Llerna LA, Hallberg M, Wieland RG. (1979) Specificity of pituitary responses to electroconvulsive therapy. *J Irish Med Assoc 72*: 490–2.

O'Donnell MP, Webb MGT. (1986) Post-ECT blood pressure rise and its relationships to cognitive and affective change. *Br J Psychiatry 149*: 494–7.

O'Flaherty D, Husain MM, Moore M, Wolff TR, Sills S, Giesecke AH. (1992) Circulatory responses during electroconvulsive therapy: the comparative effects of placebo, esmolol and nitroglycerin. *Anesthesia 47*: 563–67.

Ohman R, Walinder J, Balldin J, Wallin L, Abrahamsson L. (1976) Prolactin response to electroconvulsive therapy. *Lancet 2*:936–8.

Olesen AC, Lolk A, Christensen P. (1989) Effect of a single nighttime dose of oxazepam on seizure duration in electroconvulsive therapy. *Convuls Ther 5*:3–7.

Osborne RG, Tunakan B, Barmore J. (1963) Anaesthetic agent in electroconvulsive therapy: A controlled comparison. *J Nerv Ment Dis 137*: 297–300.

Ottosson J-O. (1960) Experimental studies of the mode of action of electroconvulsive therapy. *Acta Psychiatrica et Neurologica Scandinavica Suppl 145*:1–141.

Ottosson J-O. (1962a) Electroconvulsive therapy of endogenous depression: An analysis of the influence of various factors on the efficacy of therapy. *Journal of Mental Science 108*:694–703.

Ottosson J-O. (1962b) Electroconvulsive therapy—Electrostimulatory or convulsive therapy? *Journal of Neuropsychiatry 3*:216–20.

Ottosson J-O. (1962c) Seizure characteristics and therapeutic efficiency in electroconvulsive therapy: An analysis of the antidepressive efficiency of grand mal and lidocaine-modified seizures. *J Nerv Ment Dis 135*: 239–51.

Ottosson J-O. (1968) Psychological theories of ECT: a review. Psychological or physiological theories of ECT. *International Journal of Psychiatry 5*:170–4.

Ottosson J-O. (1992) Ethics of electroconvulsive therapy. *Convuls Ther 8*: 233–36.

Ottosson J-O. (1995) Ethical aspects of research and practice of ECT [lecture]. *Convuls Ther 11*:288–99.

Overall JE, Rhoades HM. (1987) A comment on the efficacy of unilateral versus bilateral ECT. *Convuls Ther 2*:245–52.

Overall JE, Rhoades HM. (1987) A reply to Mathisen and Pettinati [letter]. *Convuls Ther 3*:70.

Owens DG, Johnstone EC, Crow TJ, Frith CD, Jagoe JR, Kreel L. (1985) Lateral ventricular size in schizophrenia: relationship to the disease process and its clinical manifestations. *Psychol Med 15*:27–41.

Pacella BL, Barrera ES, Kalinowsky L. (1942) Variations in the electroencephalogram associated with electric shock therapy in patients with mental disorders. *Arch Neurol Psychiatry 47*:367–84.

Packman PM, Meyer DA, Verdun RM. (1978) Hazards of succinylcholine administration during electrotherapy. *Arch Gen Psychiatry 35*: 1137–41.

Paivio A. (1969) Mental imagery in associative learning and memory. *Psychol Rev 76*:241–63.

Paivio A. (1971) *Imagery and Verbal Processes*. New York: Holt, Rinehart and Winston.

Palmer RL, Mani C, Abdel-Kariem MAA, Brandon S. (1990) Dexamethasone suppression tests in the context of a double-blind trial of electroconvulsive therapy and simulated ECT. *Convuls Ther* 6:13–8.

Pande AC, Krugler T, Haskett RF, Greden JF, Grunhaus LJ. (1988) Predictors of response to electroconvulsive therapy in major depressive disorder. *Biol Psychiatry* 24:91–3.

Pande AC, Grunhaus LJ, Aisen AM, Haskett RF. (1990) A preliminary magnetic resonance imaging study of ECT-treated depressed patients. *Biol Psychiatry* 27:102–4.

Papakostas Y, Fink M, Lee J, Irwin P, Johnson L. (1981) Neuroendocrine measures in psychiatric patients: course and outcome with ECT. *Psychiatr Res* 4:55–64.

Papakostas Y, Stefanis C, Sinouri A, Trikkas G, Papadimitriou G, Pittoulis S. (1984) Increases in prolactin levels following bilateral and unilateral ECT. *Am J Psychiatry* 141:1623–4.

Papakostas YG, Stefanis CS, Markianos M, Papadimitrious GN. (1985) Naloxone fails to block ECT-induced prolactin increase. *Biol Psychiatry* 20:1326–7.

Papakostas Y, Markianos M, Papadimitriou G, Stefanis C. (1986a) Prolactin response induced by ECT and TRH. *Br J Psychiatry* 148:721–3.

Papakostas Y, Stefanis C, Markianos M, Papadimitriou G. (1986b) Electrode placement and prolactin response to electroconvulsive therapy. *Convuls Ther* 2:99–107.

Papakostas Y, Markianos M, Stefanis C. (1988) Methysergide reduces the prolactin response to ECT. *Biol Psychiatry* 24:465–8.

Papakostas Y, Markianos M, Papadimitriou G, Stefanis C. (1990) Thyrotropin and prolactin secretion during ECT: implications for the mechanism of ECT action. *Convuls Ther* 6:214–20.

Parab AL, Chaudhari LS, Apte J. (1992) Use of nitroglycerine ointment to prevent hypertensive response during electroconvulsive therapy—a study of 50 cases. *J Postgrad Med* 38:55–7.

Partap M, Jos CJ, Dye CJ. (1983) Vasopressin-8-lysine in prevention of ECT-induced amnesia. *Am J Psychiatry* 140:946–7.

Paulson GW. (1967) Exacerbation of organic brain disease by electroconvulsive treatment. *North Carolina Medical Journal* 28:328–31.

Pearlman C. (1990) Neuroleptic malignant syndrome and electroconvulsive therapy. *Convuls Ther* 6:251–4.

Pearlman C, Richmond J. (1990) New data on the methohexital-thiopental-arrhythmia issue. *Convuls Ther* 6:221–3.

Pearlman T, Loper M, Tillery L. (1990) Should psychiatrists administer anesthesia for ECT? *Am J Psychiatry* 147:1553–6.

Penfield W, Jasper H. (1954) *Epilepsy and Functional Anatomy of the Human Brain*. Boston: Little Brown.

Penfield W, von Kalman S, Cipriani A. (1939) Cerebral blood flow during induced epileptiform seizures in animals and man. *J Neurophysiol 2*: 257–67,

Penney JF, Dinwiddie SH, Zorumski CF, Wetzel RD. (1990) Concurrent and close temporal administration of lithium and ECT. *Convuls Ther 6*: 139–45.

Perrin GM. (1961) Cardiovascular aspects of electric shock therapy. *Acta Psychiatr Neurol Scand 36*:1–45.

Perris C, d'Elia G. (1966) A study of bipolar (manic-depressive) and unipolar recurrent depressive psychoses. IX. Therapy and prognosis. *Acta Psychiatr Scand 42*:153–71.

Perry GF. (1983) ECT for dementia and catatonia [letter]. *J Clin Psychiatry 44*:117.

Perry P, Tsuang MT. (1979) Treatment of unipolar depression following electroconvulsive therapy. Relapse rate comparisons between lithium and tricyclic therapies following ECT. *J Affect Disord 1*:123–9.

Peters SG, Wochos DN, Peterson GC. (1984) Status epilepticus as a complication of concurrent electroconvulsive and theophylline therapy. *Mayo Clin Proc 59*:568–70.

Peterson G. (1991) San Francisco official attacks ECT. *The Psychiatric Times*, May.

Pettinati HM. (1994) Speed of ECT? [letter]. *Convuls Ther* 69–71.

Pettinati HM, Rosenberg J. (1984) Memory self-ratings before and after electroconvulsive therapy: depressive- vs ECT-induced. *Biol Psychiatry 10*: 539–48.

Pettinati HM, Nilsen S. (1985) Missed and brief seizures during ECT: differential response between unilateral and bilateral electrode placement. *Biol Psychiatry 20*:506–14.

Pettinati HM, Mathisen KS, Rosenberg J, Lynch JF. (1986) Meta-analytical approach to reconciling discrepancies in efficacy between bilateral and unilateral electroconvulsive therapy. *Convuls Ther 2*:7–17.

Pettinati HM, Milner B, Ergin AB. (1989) Memory deficits and electrical stimulation intensity with unilateral ECT. Presented at the 44th Annual Meeting of the Society of Biological Psychiatry, San Francisco.

Pettinati HM, Stephens RN, Willis KM, Robin S. (1990) Evidence for less improvement in depression in patients taking benzodiazepines during unilateral ECT. *Am J Psychiatry 147*:1029–35.

Pettinati HM, Tamburello BA, Ruetsch CR, Kaplan FN. (1994) Patient attitudes toward electroconvulsive therapy. *Psychopharmacol Bull 30*: 471–75.

Philibert RA, Richards L, Lynch CF, Winokur G. (1995) Effect of ECT on mortality and clinical outcome in geriatric unipolar depression. *J Clin Psychiatry 56*:390–94.

Pinel JP, Van Oot PH. (1975) Generality of the kindling phenomenon: some clinical implications. *Can J Neurol Sci 2*:467–75.

Pinel JP, Van Oot PH. (1977) Intensification of the alcohol withdrawal syndrome following periodic electroconvulsive shocks. *Biol Psychiatry 12*: 479–86.

Pippard J, Ellam L. (1981) *Electroconvulsive Treatment in Great Britain, 1980.* London: Gaskell.

Pitts FM, Jr, Desmarias GM, Stewart W, Schaberg K. (1965) Induction of anesthesia with methohexital and thiopental in electroconvulsive therapy. *N Engl J Med 273*:353–60.

Pitts FN, Jr. (1982) Medical physiology of ECT. In: R Abrams, WB Essman, eds. *Electroconvulsive Therapy: Biological Foundations and Clinical Applications.* New York: Spectrum Publications. pp. 57–90.

Pollard BJ, O'Leary J. (1981) Guedel airway and tooth damage. *Anaesthesia and Intensive Care 9*:395.

Pollitt JD. (1965) Suggestions for a physiological classification of depression. *Br J Psychiatry 111*:489–95.

Pomeranze J, Karliner W, Triebel WA, King EJ. (1968) Electroshock therapy in presence of serious organic disease. Depression and aortic aneurysm. *Geriatrics 23*:122–4.

Pope HG, Lipinski JF. (1978) Diagnosis in schizophrenia and manic-depressive illness: a reassessment of the specificity of "schizophrenic" symptoms in the light of current research. *Arch Gen Psychiatry 35*: 811–28.

Pope H, Lipinski JF, Cohen BM, Axelrod DT. (1980) "Schizoaffective disorder": An invalid diagnosis? A comparison of schizoaffective disorder, schizophrenia, and affective disorder. *Am J Psychiatry 137*:921–7.

Position Paper on Electro-Convulsive Therapy of the Ontario Medical Association and the Ontario Psychiatric Association [excerpt]. (1985) *Schedule "H" of Report of the Electroconvulsive Therapy Review Committee.* Ontario: Ontario Government Bookstore. p. 87. December.

Posner JB, Plum F, Van Poznak A. (1969) Cerebral metabolism during electrically induced seizures in man. *Arch Neurol 20*:388–95.

Post RM. (1990) ECT: the anticonvulsant connection [comment]. *Neuropsychopharmacology 3*:73–82.

Post RM, Putnam F, Contel NR, Goldman B. (1984) Electroconvulsive seizures inhibit amygdala kindling: implications for mechanisms of action in affective illness. *Epilepsia 25*:234–9.

Post RM, Putnam F, Uhde TW, Weiss SRB. (1986) Electroconvulsive therapy as an anticonvulsant: Implications for its mechanism of action in affective illness. *Ann N Y Acad. Sci 462*:376–88.

Powell JC, Silveira WR, Lindsay R. (1988) Pre-pubertal depressive stupor: a case report. *Br J Psychiatry 153*:689–92.

Powers P, Douglass TS, Waziri R. (1976) Hyperpyrexia in catatonic states. *Diseases of the Nervous System 37*:359–61.

Prakash R, Leavell SR. (1984) Status epilepticus with unilateral ECT: case report. *J Clin Psychiatry 45*:403–4.

Pratt RT, Warrington EK, Halliday AM. (1971) Unilateral ECT as a test for cerebral dominance, with a strategy for treating left-handers. *Br J Psychiatry 119*:79–83.

Price TR. (1981) Unilateral electroconvulsive therapy for depression [letter]. *N Engl J Med 304*:53.

Price TR. (1982a) Short- and long-term cognitive effects of ECT: Part I— Effects on memory. *Psychopharmacol Bull 18*:81–91.

Price TR. (1982b) Short- and long-term cognitive effects of ECT: Part II— Effects on nonmemory associated cognitive functions. *Psychopharmacol Bull 18*:91–101.

Price TR, Levin R. (1978) The effects of electroconvulsive therapy on tardive dyskinesia. *Am J Psychiatry 135*:991–3.

Price TR, Tucker GJ. (1977) Psychiatric and behavioral manifestations of normal pressure hydrocephalus. *J Nerv Ment Dis 164*:51–5.

Price TR, Mackenzie TB, Tucker GJ, Culver C. (1978) The dose-response ratio in electroconvulsive therapy: a preliminary study. *Arch Gen Psychiatry 35*:1131–6.

Price TR, McAllister TW. (1989) Safety and efficacy of ECT in depressed patients with dementia: a review of clinical experience. *Convuls Ther 5*:1–74.

Proctor LD, Goodwin JE. (1943) Comparative electroencephalographic observations following electroshock therapy using raw 60 cycle alternating and unidirectional fluctuating current. *Am J Psychiatry 99*: 525–30.

Prohovnik I, Sackeim HA, Decina P, Malitz S. (1986) Acute reductions of regional cerebral blood flow following electroconvulsive therapy: interactions with modality and time. *Ann N Y Acad Sci 462*: 249–62.

Prudic J, Sackeim HA, Decina P, Hopkins N, Ross FR, Malitz S. (1987) Acute effects of ECT on cardiovascular functioning: relations to patient and treatment variables. *Acta Psychiatr Scand 75*:344–51.

Prudic J, Devanand DP, Sackeim HA, Decina P, Kerr B. (1989) Relative response of endogenous and non-endogenous symptoms to electroconvulsive therapy. *J Affect Disord 16*:59–64.

Prudic J, Sackeim HA, Devanand DP, Krueger RB, Settembrino JM. (1994) Acute cognitive effects of subconvulsive stimulation. *Convuls Ther 10*: 4–24.

Public Health Service. (1994) New directions for ECT research. *Psychopharmacol Bull*, Public Health Service publication #94–3707.

Raichel ME, Eichling JO, Grubb RL, Hartman BK. (1976) Central noradrenergic regulation of brain microcirculation. In: M Hanna, H Papius, W Feindel, eds. *Dynamics of Brain Edema*. New York: Springer-Verlag. pp. 11–7.

Railton R, Fisher J, Sinclair A, Shrigmankar JM. (1987) Comparison of electrical measurements on constant voltage and constant current ECT machines. *Br J Psychiatry 151*:244–7.

Railton R. (1987) Comparison of electrical measurements on constant voltage and constant current ECT machines [letter]. *Br J Psychiatry 151*: 701.

Rampton AJ, Griffin RM, Stuart CS, Durcan JJ, Huddy NC, Abbott MA. (1989) Comparison of methohexital and propofol for electroconvulsive therapy: effects on hemodynamic responses and seizure duration. *Anesthesiology 70*:412–7.

Rao KM, Gangadhar BN, Janakiramaiah N. (1993) Nonconvulsive status epilepticus after the ninth electroconvulsive therapy. *Convuls Ther 9*: 128–34.

Raskind M, Orenstein H, Weitzman RE. (1979) Vasopressin in depression. *Lancet 1*:164.

Rasmussen KG, Abrams R. Treatment of Parkinson's disease with electroconvulsive therapy. *Psychiatr Clin North Am 14*:925–933, 1991.

Rasmussen KG, Abrams R: The role of electroconvulsive therapy in Parkinson's disease. In: Huber S, Cummings J, eds. *Neurobehavioral Aspects of Parkinson's Disease.* New York: Oxford University Press, 1992. pp. 252–270.

Rasmussen KG, Zorumski CF. (1993) Electroconvulsive therapy in patients taking theophylline. *J Clin Psychiatry 54*:427–31.

Rasmussen KG, Zorumski CF, Jarvis MR. (1994) Possible impact of stimulus duration on seizure threshold in ECT. *Convuls Ther 10*:177–80.

Rausch JL, Rich CL, Risch SC. (1988) Platelet serotonin transport after a single ECT. *Psychopharmacology 95*:139–41

Ray I. (1975) Side effects from lithium. *Can Med Assoc J 112*:417–9.

Räsänen J, Martin DJ, Downs JB, Hodges MR. (1988) Oxygen supplementation during electroconvulsive therapy. *Br J Anaesth 61*:593–7.

Reed RR, Ciesel C, Owens G. (1971) Induced seizures as therapy of experimental strokes in dogs. *J Neurosurgery 34*:178–84.

Regestein QR, Reich P. (1985) Electroconvulsive therapy in patients at high risk for physical complications. *Convuls Ther 1*:101–14.

Regestein QR, Kahn CB, Siegel AJ, Blacklow RS, Genack A. (1971) A case of catatonia occurring simultaneously with severe urinary retention. *J Nerv Ment Dis 152*:432–5.

Regestein QR, Murawski BJ, Engle RP. (1975) A case of prolonged, reversible dementia associated with abuse of electroconvulsive therapy. *J Nerv Ment Dis 161*:200–3.

Reichert H, Benjamin J, Keegan D, Marjerrison G. (1976a) Bilateral and non-dominant unilateral ECT. Part I—Therapeutic efficacy. *Canadian Psychiatric Association Journal 21*:69–78.

Reichert H, Benjamin J, Neufeldt AH, Marjerrison G. (1976b) Bilateral and non-dominant unilateral ECT. Part II—Development of prograde effects. *Canadian Psychiatric Association Journal 21*:79–86.

Reid AH. (1972) Psychoses in adult mental defectives. I. Manic depressive psychosis. *Br J Psychiatry 120*:205–12.

Reitan RM. (1955) An investigation of the validity of Halstead's measures of biological intelligence. *Arch Neurol Psychiatry 73*:28–35.

Reiter-Theil S. (1992) Autonomy and beneficence: ethical issues in electroconvulsive therapy. *Convuls Ther 8*:237–44.

Remick RA, Maurice WL. (1978) ECT in pregnancy [letter]. *Am J Psychiatry* *135*:761–2.

Repke JT, Berger NG. (1984) Electroconvulsive therapy in pregnancy. *Obstet Gynecol 63*:39S–41S.

Ribot T. (1882) *Diseases of Memory: An Essay in Positive Psychology.* New York: D. Appleton & Co.

Rice EH, Sombrotto LB, Markowitz JC, Leon AC. (1994) Cardiovascular morbidity in high-risk patients. *Am J Psychiatry 151*:1637–41.

Rich CL, Black NA. (1985) The efficiency of ECT: II. Correlation of specific treatment variables to response rate in unilateral ECT. *Psychiatry Res 16*:147–54.

Rich CL, Woodruff RA, Jr, Cadoret R, Craig A, Pitts FN, Jr. (1969) Electrotherapy: the effects of atropine on EKG. *Diseases of the Nervous System 30*:622–6.

Rich CL, Cunningham LA, Maher CC, Woodruff RA. (1975a) The effect of modified ECT on serum creatine phophokinase, I. With intravenous atropine. *Diseases of the Nervous System 36*:653–5.

Rich CL, Cunningham LA, Maher CC, Woodruff RA. (1975b) The effect of modified ECT on serum creatine phosphokinase. II. With subcutaneous atropine. *Diseases of the Nervous System 36*:655–6.

Rich CL, Spiker DG, Jewell SW, Neil JF. (1984) DSM-III, RDC, and ECT: depressive subtypes and immediate response. *J Clin Psychiatry 45*: 14–8.

Rich CL, Spiker DG, Jewell SW, Neil JF, Phillipson M. (1986) ECT response in psychotic versus nonpsychotic unipolar depressives. *J Clin Psychiatry 47*:123–5.

Ries RK. (1985) Poor interrater reliability of MECTA EEG seizure duration measurement during ECT. *Biol Psychiatry 20*:94–8.

Ries RK. (1987) *Informed ECT for Patients and Families: Informed ECT for Health Professionals; Shock Therapy* [videotape reviews]. *Hosp Community Psychiatry 38*:137–8.

Ries R, Bokan J. (1979) Electroconvulsive therapy following pituitary surgery. *J Nerv Ment Dis 167*:767–8.

Rifkin A. (1988) ECT versus tricyclic antidepressants in depression: a review of the evidence. *J Clin Psychiatry 49*:3–7.

Roberts JM. (1959a) Prognostic factors in the electroshock treatment of depressive states: I. Clinical features from history and examination. *J Ment Sci 105*:693–702.

Roberts JM. (1959b) Prognostic factors in the electroshock treatment of depressive states: II. The application of specific tests. *J Ment Sci 105*: 703–13.

Roberts MA, Attah JR. (1988) Carbamazepine and ECT. *Br J Psychiatry 53*:418.

Roberts R, Owens G, Vilisenkas J, Thomas DD. (1972) Induced seizures as therapy for experimental stroke in monkeys. *J Neurosurgery 37*: 711–4.

Robertson AD, Inglis J. (1978) Memory deficits after electroconvulsive therapy: cerebral asymmetry and dual-encoding. *Neuropsychologia 16*: 179–87.

Robin AA, Harris JA. (1962) A controlled trial of imipramine and electroplexy. *J Ment Sci 106*:217–9.

Robin A, DeTissera S. (1982) A double-blind controlled comparison of the therapeutic effects of low and high energy electroconvulsive therapies. *Br J Psychiatry 141*:357–66.

Robin A, Binnie CD, Copas JB. (1985) Electrophysiological and hormonal responses to three types of electroconvulsive therapy. *Br J Psychiatry 147*:707–12.

Robins MA, Attah JR. (1988) Carbamazepine and ECT. *Br J Psychiatry 153*: 418.

Roccaforte WH, Burke WJ. (1989) ECT following craniotomy. *Psychosomatics 30*:99–101.

Rochford G, Williams M. (1962) Development and breakdown of the use of names. *J Neurol Neurosurg Psychiatry 25*:222.

Rogers MC, Battit G, McPeek B, Todd D. (1978) Lateralization of sympathetic control of the human sinus node: ECG changes of stellate ganglion block. *Anesthesiology 48*:139–41.

Roith AI. (1959) Status epilepticus as a complication of E.C.T. *Br J Clin Pract 13*:711–2.

Rollason WN, Sutherland MS, Hall DJ. (1971) An evaluation of the effect of methohexitone and propanidid on blood pressure, pulse rate and cardiac arrhythmia during electroconvulsive therapy. *Br J Anaesth 43*: 160–6.

Rosen AD, Gur RC, Sussman N, Gur RE, Hartig H. (1982) Hemispheric asymmetry in the control of heart rate. *Abstracta Soc Neurosci 8*: 917.

Rosenberg R, Vorstrup S, Andersen A, Bolwig TG. (1988) Effect of ECT on cerebral blood flow in melancholia assessed with SPECT. *Convuls Ther 4*:62–73.

Rosenfeld JE, Glassberg S, Sherrid M. (1988) Administration of ECT 4 years after aortic aneurysm dissection. *Am J Psychiatry 145*:128–9.

Rosenquist PB, McCall WV, Farah A, Reboussin DM. (1994) Effects of caffeine pretreatment on measures of seizure impact. *Convuls Ther 10*: 181–85.

Rossi A, Stratta P, Nistico R, Sabatini MD, DiMichele V, Casacchia M. (1990) Visuospatial impairment in depression: a controlled ECT study. *Acta Psychiatr Scand 81*:245–9.

Roth LH, Meisel A, Lidz CW. (1977) Tests of competency to consent to treatment. *Am J Psychiatry 134*:279–84.

Roth M. (1951) Changes in the EEG under barbiturate anesthesia produced by electro-convulsive treatment and their significance for the theory of ECT action. *Electroencephalogr Clin Neurophysiol 3*:261–80.

Roth SD, Mukherjee S, Sackeim HA. (1988) Electroconvulsive therapy in a patient with mania, parkinsonism, and tardive dyskinesia. *Convuls Ther* 4:92–7.

Roueche B. (1974) As empty as Eve. *The New Yorker*, Sept. 9. pp. 34–48.

Rouse EC. (1988) Propofol for electroconvulsive therapy. A comparison with methohexitone. Preliminary report. *Anaesthesia 43:Suppl*, 61–4.

Royal College of Psychiatrists. (1989) *The Practical Administration of Electroconvulsive Therapy (ECT)*. ECT Sub-committee of the Research Committee. London: Gaskell.

Royal College of Psychiatrists. (1995) *The ECT Handbook: The Second Report of the Royal College of Psychiatrists' Special Committee on ECT*. London: Royal College of Psychiatrists.

Rudorfer MV, Hsiao JK, Risby ED, Linnoila M, Potter WZ. (1986) Biochemical effects of ECT versus antidepressant drugs. *New Research Abstracts*. Washington DC: American Psychiatric Association. p. 110.

Rudorfer MV, Linnoila M, Potter WZ. (1987) Combined lithium and electroconvulsive therapy: pharmacokinetic and pharmacodynamic interactions. *Convuls Ther 3*:40–5.

Ruedrich SL, Chu CC, Moore SL. (1983) ECT for major depression in a patient with acute brain trauma. *Am J Psychiatry 140*:928–9.

Rummans TA, Bassingthwaigte ME. (1991) Severe medical and neurologic complications associated with near-lethal catatonia treated with electroconvulsive therapy. *Convuls Ther 7*:121–4.

Ryan RJ, Swanson DW, Faiman C, Mayberry WE. Spadoni AJ. (1970) Effects of convulsive electroshock on serum concentrations of follicle stimulating hormone, luteinizing hormone, thyroid stimulating hormone and growth hormone in man. *J Clin Endocrinol Metab 30*:51.

Sackeim HA. (1989) ECT: twice or thrice a week? *Convuls Ther 5*:362–4.

Sackeim HA. (1991a) Optimizing unilateral electroconvulsive therapy. *Convuls Ther 7*:201–212.

Sackeim HA. (1991b) Are ECT devices underpowered? *Convuls Ther 7*: 233–6.

Sackeim HA. (1994a) Physical properties of the ECT stimulus [Response to commentaries]. *Convuls Ther 10*:140–52.

Sackeim HA. (1994b) Central issues regarding the mechanisms of action of electroconvulsive therapy: directions for future research. *Psychopharmacol Bull 30*:281–308.

Sackeim HA. (1994c) Magnetic stimulation therapy and ECT [commentary]. *Convuls Ther 10*:255–58.

Sackeim HA, Decina P, Prohovnik I, Malitz S, Resor SR. (1983a) Anticonvulsant and antidepressant properties of electroconvulsive therapy: a proposed mechanism of action. *Biol Psychiatry 18*:1301–10.

Sackeim HA, Decina P, Malitz S, Hopkins N, Yudofsky SC, Prohovnik I. (1983b) Postictal excitement following bilateral and right-unilateral ECT. *Am J Psychiatry 140*:1367–8.

Sackeim HA, Decina P, Kanzler M, Kerr B, Malitz S. (1987a) Effects of electrode placement on the efficacy of titrated, low dosage ECT. *Am J Psychiatry 144*:1449–55.

Sackeim HA, Decina P, Prohovnik I, Portnoy S, Kanzler M, Malitz S. (1986a) Dosage, seizure threshold, and the antidepressant efficacy of electroconvulsive therapy. *Ann N Y Acad Sci 462*:398–410.

Sackeim HA, Devanand DP, Prudic J. (1991) Stimulus intensity, seizure threshold, and seizure duration: impact on efficacy and safety of electroconvulsive therapy. In: CH Kellner, ed. *Electroconvulsive Therapy: The Psychiatric Clinics of North America*, Vol. 14, Philadelphia: WB Saunders. pp. 803–43.

Sackeim HA, Greenberg MS, Weiman MA, Gur RC, Hungerbuhler JP, Geshwind N. (1982) Hemispheric asymmetry in the expression of positive and negative emotions: Neurologic evidence. *Arch Neurol 39*:210–8.

Sackeim HA, Long J, Luber B, et al. (1994) Physical properties and quantification of the ECT stimulus: I. Basic principles. *Convuls Ther 10*:93–123.

Sackeim HA, Luber BL, Katzman GP, Moeller JR, Prudic J, Devanand DP, Nobler MS. (1996) The effects of electroconvulsive therapy on quantitative EEG: relationship to clinical outcome. *Arch Gen Psychiatry 53*: 814–24.

Sackeim HA, Portnoy S, Neeley P, Steif BL, Decina P, Malitz S. (1986b) Cognitive consequences of low-dosage electroconvulsive therapy. *Ann N Y Acad Sci 462*:326–40.

Sackeim HA, Prudic J, Devanand DP, et al. (1992) In reply: Stimulus dosing strategies and the efficacy of unilateral ECT. *Convuls Ther 8*:46–52.

Sackeim HA, Prudic J, Devanand DP, Kiersky JE, Fitzimons L, Moody BJ, McElhiney MC, Coleman EZ, Settembrino JM. (1993) Effects of stimulus intensity and electrode placement on the efficacy and cognitive effects of electroconvulsive therapy. *N Engl J Med 328*:839–46.

Sackeim HA, Decina P, Prohovnik I, Malitz S. (1987b) Seizure threshold in electroconvulsive therapy: effects of sex, age, electrode placement, and number of treatments. *Arch Gen Psychiatry 44*:355–60.

Sackeim HA, Decina P, Portnoy S, Neeley P, Malitz S. (1987c) Studies of dosage, seizure threshold, and seizure duration in ECT. *Biol Psychiatry 22*:249–68.

Sackeim HA, Devanand DP, Prudic J. (1991) Stimulus intensity, seizure threshold, and seizure duration: Impact on the efficacy and safety of electroconvulsive therapy. *Psychiatr Clin North Am 14*:803–843.

Sackeim HA, Prudic J, Devanand DP, Krueger RB (1992) Stimulus dosing strategies and the efficacy of unilateral ECT. *Convuls Ther 8*: 46–52.

Salmon JB, Hanna MH, Williams TB, Wheeler M. (1988) Thalamic pain— the effect of electroconvulsive therapy (ECT). *Pain 33*:67–71.

Salzman C. (1970) *Resident Guide to the Use of Electroconvulsive Therapy*. Boston: Massachusetts Mental Health Center Monograph.

Salzman C. (1977) ECT and ethical psychiatry. *Am J Psychiatry 134*: 1006–9.

Sandford JL. (1966) Electric and convulsive treatments in psychiatry. *Diseases of the Nervous System 27*:333–8.

Savitsky N, Karliner W. (1951) Electroshock therapy and multiple sclerosis. *N Y J Med 51*:788.

Savitsky N, Karliner W. (1953) Electroshock in the presence of organic disease of the nervous system. *Journal of Hillside Hospital 2*:3–22.

Schillinger D. (1987) Nifedipine in hypertensive emergencies—a prospective study. *J Emerg Med 5*:463–73.

Schultz H, Muller J, Roth B, Stein J. (1968) Das bioelektrische Bild wahrend der Krampfbehandlung in narkose und relaxation bei endogenen psychosen. *Archiv für Psychiatrie und Nervenkrankheiten 211*: 414–32.

Schwartz M. (1985) Computed tomography and ECT. *Convuls Ther 1*:70–1.

Scott AIF. Commentary in Cooper SJ, Scott AIF, Whalley LJ. (1990) A neuroendocrine view of ECT. *Br J Psychiatry 157*:740–3.

Scott AIF. (1995) Does ECT alter brain structure? [letter] *Am J Psychiatry 152*:1403.

Scott AI, Riddle W. (1989) Status epilepticus after electroconvulsive therapy. *Br J Psychiatry 155*:119–121.

Scott AIF, Turnbull LW, Blane A, Douglas RHB. (1991) Electroconvulsive therapy and brain damage [letter]. *Lancet 338*:264.

Scott A, Whalley L. (1986) Hormone release by electroconvulsive therapy. *Lancet 2*:581–2.

Scott AI, Whalley LJ, Bennie J, Bowler G. (1986) Oestrogen-stimulated neurophysin and outcome after electroconvulsive therapy. *Lancet 1*:1411–4.

Scott AI. (1989) Which depressed patients will respond to electroconvulsive therapy? the search for biological predictors of recovery. *Br J Psychiatry 154*:8–17.

Scott AI, Shering P, Dykes S. (1989a) Would monitoring by electroencephalogram improve the practice of electroconvulsive therapy? *Br J Psychiatry 154*:853–7.

Scott AIF, Milner JB, Shering PA. (1989b) Diminished TSH release after a course of ECT: altered monoamine function or seizure activity? *Psychoneuroendocrinology 14*:425–31.

Scott AI, Douglas RH, Whitfield A, Kendell RE. (1990) Time course of cerebral magnetic resonance changes after electroconvulsive therapy. *Br J Psychiatry 156*:551–3.

Scott AI, Turnbull LW. (1990) Do repeated courses of ECT cause brain damage detectable by MRI? *Am J Psychiatry 147*:371–2.

Seager CP, Bird RL. (1962) Imipramine with electrical treatment in depression—a controlled trial. *J Ment Sci 108*:704–7.

Selvin BL. (1987) Electroconvulsive therapy—1987. *Anesthesiology 67*: 367–385.

Senter NW, Winslade WJ, Liston EH, Mills MJ. (1984) Electroconvulsive therapy: the evolution of legal regulation. *American Journal of Social Psychiatry* 4:11–5.

Serra G, Argiolas A, Fadda F, Melis MR, Gessa GL. (1981) Repeated electroconvulsive shock prevents the sedative effect of small doses of apomorphine. *Psychopharmacology* 73:194–6.

Shagass C, Jones AL. (1958) A neurophysiological test for psychiatric diagnosis: results in 750 patients. *Am J Psychiatry* 114:1002–10.

Shankel LW, Dimassimo DA, Whittier JR. (1960) Changes with age in electrical reactions in mental patients. *Psychiatr Q* 34:284–92.

Shapira B, Zohar J, Newman M, Drexler H, Belmaker RH. (1985) Potentiation of seizure length and clinical response to electroconvulsive therapy by caffeine pretreatment: a case report. *Convuls Ther* 1:58–60.

Shapira B, Lerer B, Gilboa D, Drexler H, Kugelmass S, Calev A. (1987) Facilitation of ECT by caffeine pretreatment. *Am J Psychiatry* 144:1199–1202.

Shapira B, Lerer B, Kindler S, Lichtenberg P, Gropp C, Coooper T, Calev A. (1992) Enhanced serotonergic responsivity following electroconvulsive therapy in patients with major depression. *Br J Psychiatry* 160: 223–29.

Shapira B, Lidsky D, Gorfine M, Lerer B. (1996) Electroconvulsive therapy and resistant depression: clinical implications of seizure threshold. *J Clin Psychiatry* 57:32–8.

Shapiro MF, Goldberg HH. (1957) Electroconvulsive therapy in patients with structural diseases of the central nervous system. *Am J Med Sci 233*: 186–95.

Shepley WH, McGregor JS. (1939) Electrically induced convulsions in treatment of mental disorders. *Br Med J* 2:1269–71.

Shettar MS, Grunhaus L, Pande AC, Tandon RC, Knonfol ZA, Haskett RF. (1989) Protective effects of intramuscular glycopyrrolate on cardiac conduction during ECT. *Convuls Ther* 5:349–52.

Shimamura AP, Squire LR. (1987) A neuropsychological study of fact memory and source amnesia. *J Exp Psychol [Learn Mem Cog]* 13:464–73.

Siekert RG, Williams SC, Windle WF. (1950) Histologic study of the brains of monkeys after experimental electroshock. *Arch Neurol Psychiatry* 63:79–86.

Silverskiöld P, Gustafson L, Risberg J, Ingmar R. (1986) Acute and late effects of electroconvulsive therapy: clinical outcome, regional cerebral blood flow, and electroencephalogram. *Ann N Y Acad Sci 462*: 236–48.

Siris SG, Glassman AH, Stetner F. (1982) ECT and psychotropic medication in the treatment of depression and schizophrenia. In: R Abrams, WB Essman, eds. *Electroconvulsive Therapy: Biological Foundations and Clinical Applications*. New York: Spectrum Publications. pp. 91–112.

Skrabanek P, Balfe A, Webb M, Maguire J, Powell D. (1981) Electroconvulsive therapy increases plasma growth hormone, prolactin, luteinizing hormone and follicle-stimulating hormone but not thyrotropin or substance P. *Psychoneuroendocrinology* 6:261–67.

Slade AP, Checkley SA. (1980) A neuroendocrine study of the mechanism of action of ECT. *Br J Psychiatry* 137:217–21.

Slawson P. (1985) Psychiatric malpractice: the electroconvulsive therapy experience. *Convuls Ther* 1:195–203.

Slawson P. (1989) Psychiatric malpractice and ECT: a review of national loss experience. *Convuls Ther* 5:126–30.

Slawson P. (1991) Psychiatric malpractice and ECT: a review of 1,700 claims. *Convuls Ther* 7:255–61.

Slawson PF, Guggenheim FG. (1984) Psychiatric malpractice: a review of the national loss experience. *Am J Psychiatry* 141:979–81.

Small IF. (1974) Inhalant convulsive therapy. In: M Fink, S Kety, J McGaugh, TA Williams, eds. *Psychobiology of Convulsive Therapy*. Washington DC: V.H. Winston and Sons. pp. 65–77.

Small IF, Small JG, Milstein V, Moore JE. (1972) Neuropsychological observations with psychosis and somatic treatment. Neuropsychological examinations of psychiatric patients. *J Nerv Ment Dis* 155:6–13.

Small IF, Small JG, Milstein V, Sharpley P. (1973) Interhemispheric relationships with somatic therapy. *Diseases of the Nervous System 34*: 170–7.

Small IF, Milstein V, Small JG. (1981) Relationship between clinical and cognitive change with bilateral and unilateral ECT. *Biol Psychiatry 16*: 793–4.

Small JG. (1985) Efficacy of ECT in schizophrenia, mania and other disorders. II: mania and other disorders. *Convuls Ther* 1:271–6.

Small JG, Small IF, Perez HC, Sharpley P. (1970) Electroencephalographic and neurophysiological studies of electrically induced seizures. *J Nerv Ment Dis* 150:479–89.

Small JG, Kellams JJ, Milstein V, Small IF. (1980) Complications with electroconvulsive treatment combined with lithium. *Biol Psychiatry 15*: 103–12.

Small JG, Small IF, Milstein V, Kellams JJ, Klapper MH. (1985) Manic symptoms: an indication for bilateral ECT. *Biol Psychiatry 20*: 125–34.

Small JG, Klapper MH, Kellams JJ, Miller MJ, Milstein V, Sharpley PH, Small IF. (1988) ECT compared with lithium in the management of manic states. *Arch Gen Psychiatry* 45:727–32.

Smith JE, Williams K, Burkett S, Glue P, Nutt DJ. (1990) Oxytocin and vasopressin responses to ECT. *Psychiatry Res 32*:201–2.

Smith S. (1956) The use of electroplexy (ECT) in psychiatric syndromes complicating pregnancy. *J Ment Sci* 102:796–800.

Snow SS, Wells CE. (1981) Case studies in neuropsychiatry: diagnosis and treatment of coexistent dementia and depression. *J Clin Psychiatry 42*: 439–41.

Sobel DE. (1960) Fetal damage due to ECT, insulin coma, chlorpromazine or reserpine. *Arch Gen Psychiatry 2*:606–11.

Sobin C, Sackeim HA, Prudic J, Devanand DP, Moody BJ, McElheiney MC. (1995) Predictors of retrograde amnesia following ECT. *Am J Psychiatry 152*:995–1001.

Sobin C, Prudic J, Devanand DP, Nobler MS, Sackheim HA. (1997) Who responds to electroconvulsive therapy?

Solan WJ, Khan A, Avery D, Cohen S. (1988) Psychotic and nonpsychotic depression: comparison of response to ECT. *J Clin Psychiatry 49*: 97–9.

Sommer BR, Satlin A, Friedman MS. (1989) Glycopyrrolate versus atropine in post-ECT amnesia in the elderly. *J Geriatr Psychiatry Neurol 2*: 18–21.

Sørensen PS, Bolwig TG, Lauritsen B, Bengtson O. (1981) Electroconvulsive therapy: a comparison of seizure duration as monitored with electroencephalograph and electromyograph. *Acta Psychiatry Scand 64*:193–8.

Sørensen PS, Hammer M, Bolwig T. (1982) Vasopressin release during electro-convulsive therapy. *Psychoneuroendocrinology 7*:303–8.

Sperling MR, Wilson CL. (1986) The effects of limbic and extralimbic electrical stimulations upon prolactin secretions in humans. *Brain Res 371*: 293–7.

Sperling MR, Pritchard PB, III, Engel J, Jr, Daniel C, Sagel J. (1986) Prolactin in partial epilepsy: an indicator of limbic seizures. *Ann Neurol 20*: 716–22.

Sperling MR, Melmed S, McAllister T, Price TR. (1989) Lack of effect of naloxone on prolactin and seizures in electroconvulsive therapy. *Epilepsia 30*:31–44.

Spiker DG, Dealy RS, Hanin I, Weiss JC, Kupfer DJ. (1986) Treating delusional depression with amitriptyline. *J Clin Psychiatry 47*:243–5

Squire LR. (1982) Neuropsychological effects of ECT. In: R Abrams, WB Essman, eds. *Electroconvulsive Therapy: Biological Foundations and Clinical Applications*. New York: Spectrum Publications. pp. 169–86.

Squire LR. (1986) Memory functions as affected by electroconvulsive therapy. *Ann N Y Acad Sci 462*:307–14.

Squire LR, Chace PM. (1975) Memory functions six to nine months after electroconvulsive therapy. *Arch Gen Psychiatry 32*:1557–64.

Squire LR, Miller PL. (1974) Diminution of anterograde amnesia following electroconvulsive therapy. *Br J Psychiatry 125*:490–5.

Squire LR, Slater PC. (1978) Bilateral and unilateral ECT: effects on verbal and nonverbal memory. *Am J Psychiatry 135*:1316–20.

Squire LR, Slater PC. (1983) Electroconvulsive therapy and complaints of memory dysfunction: a prospective three-year follow-up study. *Br J Psychiatry 142*:1–8.

Squire LR, Zouzounis JA. (1986) ECT and memory: brief pulse versus sine wave. *Am J Psychiatry 143*:596–601.

Squire LR, Slater PC, Chace PM. (1975) Retrograde amnesia: temporal gradient in very long-term memory following electroconvulsive therapy. *Science 187*:77–9.

Squire LR, Slater PC, Chace PM. (1976) Anterograde amnesia following electroconvulsive therapy: no evidence for state-dependent learning. *Behavioral Biology 17*:31–41.

Squire LR, Wetzel CD, Slater PC. (1979) Memory complaint after electroconvulsive therapy: assessment with a new self-rating instrument. *Biol Psychiatry 14*:791–801.

Squire LR, Slater PC, Miller PL. (1981) Retrograde amnesia and bilateral electroconvulsive therapy. Long-term follow-up. *Arch Gen Psychiatry 38*:89–95.

Squire LR, Shimamura AP, Graf P. (1985) Independence of recognition memory and priming effects: a neuropsychological analysis. *J Exp Psychol [Gen] 11*:37–44.

Srinivasaraghavan, Abrams. (1996) Court-ordered electroconvulsive therapy: The Illinois experience. Proc. 11th World Congress on Medical Law, Vol. 2, pp. 405–15.

Stack CG, Abernethy MH, Thacker M. (1988) Atracurium for ECT in plasma cholinesterase deficiency. *Br J Anaesth 60*:244–5.

Staton RD, Hass PJ, Brumback RA. (1981) Electroencephalographic recording during bitemporal and unilateral non-dominant hemisphere (Lancaster position) electroconvulsive therapy. *J Clin Psychiatry 42*:264–9.

Staton RD, Enderle JD, Gerst JW. (1981) The electroencephalographic pattern during electroconvulsive therapy: V. Observations on the origin of phase III delta energy and the mechanism of action of ECT. *Clin Electroencephalogr 19*:176–98.

Stenfors C, Theodorsson E, Mathe AA. (1989) Effect of repeated electroconvulsive treatment on regional concentrations of tachykinins, neurotensin, vasoactive intestinal peptide, neuropeptide Y, and galanin in rat brain. *J Neurosci Res 24*:445–50.

Stengel E. (1951) Intensive ECT. *J Ment Sci 97*:139.

Stevenson GH, Geoghegan JJ. (1951) Prophylactic electroshock. *Am J Psychiatry 107*:743–8.

Stieper DR, Williams M, Duncan CP. (1951) Changes in impersonal and personal memory following electroconvulsive therapy. *J Clin Psychol 7*:361–6.

Stoker MJ, Spencer CM, Hamilton M. (1981) Blood-pressure elevation during ECT and associated cognitive deficit. In: RL Palmer, ed. *Electroconvulsive Therapy: An Appraisal.* Oxford: Oxford University Press. pp. 106–12.

Stone AA. (1977) Recent mental health litigation: A critical perspective. *Am J Psychiatry 134*:273–9.

Stoudemire A, Knos G, Gladson M, Markwalter H, Sung YF, Morris R, Cooper R. (1990) Labetalol in the control of cardiovascular responses to electroconvulsive therapy in high-risk depressed medical patients. *J Clin Psychiatry 51*:508–512.

Strain JJ, Bidder TG. (1971) Transient cerebral complication associated with multiple monitored electroconvulsive therapy. *Diseases of the Nervous System 32*:95–100.

Strain JJ, Brunschwig L, Duffy JP, Agle DP, Rosenbaum AL, Bidder TG. (1968) Comparison of therapeutic effects and memory changes with bilateral and unilateral ECT. *Am J Psychiatry 125*:294–304.

Strömgren LS. (1973) Unilateral versus bilateral electroconvulsive therapy. Investigations into the therapeutic effect in endogenous depression. *Acta Psychiatr Scand Suppl 240*:8–65.

Strömgren LS. (1975) Therapeutic results in brief-interval unilateral ECT. *Acta Psychiatr Scand 52*:246–55.

Strömgren LS. (1984) Is bilateral ECT ever indicated? *Acta Psychiatr Scand 69*:484–90.

Strömgren LS. (1987) Optimum frequency of electroconvulsive therapy. *Convuls Ther 3*:75.

Strömgren LS. (1988) Electroconvulsive therapy in Aarhaus, Denmark, in 1984: its application in nondepressive disorders. *Convuls Ther 4*: 306–13.

Strömgren LS. (1990) Frequency of ECT treatments. *Convuls Ther 5*: 317–8.

Strömgren LS, Juul-Jensen P. (1975) EEG in unilateral and bilateral electroconvulsive therapy. *Acta Psychiatr Scand 51*:340–60.

Strömgren LS, Christensen AL, Fromholt P. (1976) The effects of unilateral brief-interval ECT on memory. *Acta Psychiatr Scand 54*:336–46.

Strömgren LS, Dahl J, Fjeldborg N, Thomsen A. (1980) Factors influencing seizure duration and number of seizures applied in unilateral electroconvulsive therapy. Anaesthetics and benzodiazepines. *Acta Psychiatr Scand 62*:158–65.

Summers WK, Robins E, Reich T. (1979) The natural history of acute organic mental syndrome after bilateral electroconvulsive therapy. *Biol Psychiatry 14*:905–12.

Summerskill J, Seeman W, Meals DW. (1952) An evaluation of post-electroshock confusion with the Reiter apparatus. *Am J Psychiatry 108*: 835–8.

Sutherland EM, Oliver JE, Knight DR. (1969) E.E.G., memory and confusion in dominant, non-dominant and bi-temporal E.C.T. *Br J Psychiatry 115*:1059–64.

Swartz CM. (1985) The time course of post-ECT prolactin levels. *Convuls Ther 1*:81–8.

Swartz CM. (1989a) Safety and ECT stimulus electrodes: I. Heat liberation at the electrode-skin interface. *Convuls Ther 5*:171–5.

Swartz CM. (1989b) Safety and ECT stimulus electrodes: II. Clinical procedures. *Convuls Ther 5*:176–9.

Swartz CM. (1990) Electroconvulsive therapy, emergence agitation and succinylcholine dose. *J Nerv Ment Dis* 178:455–7.

Swartz CM. (1991a) Quantity of prolactin released by ECT seizure [letter]. *Convuls Ther* 7:63.

Swartz CM. (1991b) Electroconvulsive therapy-induced prolactin release as an epiphenomenon. *Convuls Ther* 7:85–91.

Swartz CM. (1992) Review: Propofol anesthesia in ECT. *Convuls Ther* 8: 262–6.

Swartz CM. (1993a) Editorial: Beyond seizure duration as a measure of treatment quality. *Convuls Ther* 9:1–7.

Swartz CM. (1993b) Clinical and laboratory predictors of ECT response. In: CE Coffey, ed. *The Clinical Science of Electroconvulsive Therapy.* Washington DC: American Psychiatric Press. pp. 53–72.

Swartz CM. (1994a) Asymmetric bilateral right frontotemporal left frontal stimulus electrode placement for electroconvulsive therapy. *Neuropsychobiology* 29:174–8.

Swartz CM. (1994b) Electroconvulsive therapy (ECT) stimulus charge rate and its efficacy. *Ann Clin Psychiatry* 6:205–6.

Swartz CM. (1995) Setting the ECT stimulus. *Psych Times*, June, pp. 33–4.

Swartz CM. (1996) Case report: Disconnection of electroencephalographic, motoric, and cardiac evidence of ECT seizure. *Convuls Ther* 12: 25–30.

Swartz C, Abrams R. (1984) Prolactin levels after bilateral and unilateral ECT. *Br J Psychiatry* 144:643–5.

Swartz CM, Abrams R. (1986) An auditory representation of ECT-induced seizures. *Convuls Ther* 2:125–8.

Swartz CM, Abrams R. (1991a) Electroconvulsive therapy apparatus and method for monitoring patient seizures. *U.S. Patent Application* 07/698,304.

Swartz CM, Abrams R. (1991b) *The ECT Cognitive Monitor.* In: R Abrams, CM Swartz, eds. *The Technique of ECT: Documentation and Forms.* Lake Bluff, IL: Somatics Inc. p. 65.

Swartz CM, Abrams R. (1993) Electroconvulsive therapy apparatus and method for automatic monitoring of patient seizures. U.S. patent 5,269,302.

Swartz CM, Chen JJ. (1985) ECT-induced cortisol release: Changes with depressive state. *Convuls Ther* 1:15–21.

Swartz CM, Inglis AE. (1990) Blood pressure reduction with ECT response. *J Clin Psychiatry* 51:414–6.

Swartz CM, Inglis AE. (1990) Blood pressure reduction with ECT response. *J Clin Psychiatry* 51:414–16.

Swartz CM, Larson G. (1986) Generalization of the effects of unilateral and bilateral ECT. *Am J Psychiatry* 143:1040–41.

Swartz CM, Larson G. (1987) A reply to Brumback [letter]. *Convuls Ther* 3: 153–4.

Swartz CM, Larson G. (1989) ECT stimulus duration and its efficacy. *Ann Clin Psychiatry 1*:147–52.

Swartz CM, Lewis RK. (1991) Theophylline reversal of electroconvulsive therapy (ECT) seizure inhibition. *Psychosomatics 32*:47–51.

Swartz CM, Mehta R. (1986) Double electroconvulsive therapy for resistant depression. *Convuls Ther 2*:55–7.

Swartz CM, Saheba NC. (1989) Comparison of atropine with glycopyrrolate for use in ECT. *Convuls Ther 5*:56–60.

Swartz CM, Saheba N. (1990) Dose effect on dexamethasone suppression testing with electroconvulsive therapy. *Ann Clin Psychiatry 2*:183–8.

Swartz CM, Breen K, Wahby VS. (1989) Pharmacologic provocation and dexamethasone suppression test sensitivity. *Neuropsychobiology 22*: 11–13.

Swartz CM, Abrams R, Rasmussen K, Pavel J, Zorumski CF, Srinivasaraghavan J. (1994a) Computer automated versus visually determined electroencephalographic and electromyographic seizure duration. *Convuls Ther 10*:165–70.

Swartz CM, Abrams R, Lane RD, DuBois MA, Srinivasaraghavan J. (1994b) Heart rate differences between right and left unilateral ECT. *J Neurol Neurosurg Psychiatry 57*:97–9.

Swartz CM, Manly DT. (1997) Stimulus efficiency by pulsewidth and frequency. Presented at the Annual Scientific Meeting of the Association for Convulsive Therapy, May, 1997.

Swift MR, LaDu BN. (1966) A rapid screening test for atypical cholinesterase. *Lancet 1*:513–74.

Szirmai I, Boldizsar F, Fischer J. (1975) Correlation between blood gases, glycolytic enzymes and EEG during electroconvulsive treatment in relaxation. *Acta Psychiatr Scand 51*:171–81.

Tancer ME, Evans DL. (1989) Electroconvulsive therapy in geriatric patients undergoing anticoagulation therapy. *Convuls Ther 5*:102–9.

Tancer ME, Pedersen CA, Evans DL. (1987) ECT and anticoagulation. *Convuls Ther 3*:222–7.

Tancer ME, Golden RN, Ekstrom RD, Evans DL. (1989) Use of electroconvulsive therapy at a university hospital: 1970 and 1980–81. *Hosp Community Psychiatry 40*:64–8.

Tandon R, Grunhaus L, Haskett RF, Krugler T, Greden JF. (1988) Relative efficacy of unilateral and bilateral electroconvulsive therapy in melancholia. *Convuls Ther 4*:153–9.

Taubøll E, Gjerstad L, Stokke KT, Lundervold A, Telle B. (1987) Effects of electroconvulsive therapy (ECT) on thyroid function parameters. *Psychoneuroendocrinology 12*:349–54.

Taylor JR, Kuhlengel BG, Dean RS. (1985) ECT, blood pressure changes and neuropsychological deficit. *Br J Psychiatry 147*:36–8.

Taylor MA. (1982) Indications for electroconvulsive therapy. In: R Abrams, WB Essman, eds. *Electroconvulsive Therapy: Biological Foundations and Clinical Applications.* New York: Spectrum Publications. pp. 7–40.

Taylor MA, Abrams R. (1975) Acute mania: Clinical and genetic study of responders and non-responders to treatments. *Arch Gen Psychiatry 32*: 863–5.

Taylor MA, Abrams R. (1978) The prevalence of schizophrenia: A reassessment using modern diagnostic criteria. *Am J Psychiatry 135*:945–8.

Taylor MA, Abrams R. (1985) Short-term cognitive effects of unilateral and bilateral ECT. *Br J Psychiatry 146*:308–11.

Taylor MA, Gaztanaga P, Abrams R. (1974) Manic-depressive illness and acute schizophrenia: a clinical, family history, and treatment-response study. *Am J Psychiatry 131*:678–82.

Taylor P, Fleminger JJ. (1980) ECT for schizophrenia. *Lancet 1*:1380–2.

Taylor PJ, von Witt RJ, Fry AH. (1981) Serum creatine phosphokinase activity in psychiatric patients receiving electroconvulsive therapy. *J Clin Psychiatry 42*:103–5.

Taylor RM, Pacella PO. (1948) The significance of abnormal electroencephalograms prior to electroconvulsive therapy. *J Nerv Ment Dis 107*: 220–7.

Tchou PJ, Piasecki E, Gutmann M, Jazayeri M, Axtell K, Akhtar M. (1989) Psychological support and psychiatric management of patients with automatic implantable cardioverter defibrillators. *Int J Psychiatry Med 19*:393–407.

Tewfik GI, Wells BG. (1957) The use of Arfonad for the alleviation of cardiovascular stress following electro-convulsive therapy. *J Ment Sci 10*: 636–44.

Thenon J. (1956) Electrochoque monolateral. *Acta Neuropsiquiatria Argentina 2*:292–6.

Thiagarajan AB, Gleiter CH, Nutt DN. (1988) Electroconvulsive shock does not increase plasma insulin in rats. *Convuls Ther 4*:292–6.

Thienhaus OJ, Margletta S, Bennett JA. (1990) A study of the clinical efficacy of maintenance ECT. *J Clin Psychiatry 51*:141–4.

Thomas J, Reddy B. (1982) The treatment of mania. A retrospective evaluation of the effects of ECT, chlorpromazine, and lithium. *J Affect Disord 4*: 85–92.

Thompson JW, Weiner RD, Myers CP. (1994) Use of ECT in the United States in 1975, 1980, and 1986. *Am J Psychiatry 151*:1657–61.

Thorell JI, Adielsson G. (1973) Antidepressive effects of electroconvulsive therapy and thyrotrophin-releasing hormone. *Lancet 2*:43.

Thornton JE, Mulsant BH, Dealy R, Reynolds CF. (1990) A retrospective study of maintenance electroconvulsive therapy in a university-based psychiatric practice. *Convuls Ther 6*:121–9.

Thorogood M, Cown P, Mann J, Murphy M, Vessey M. (1992) Fatal myocardial infarction and use of psychotropic drugs in young women. *Lancet 340*:1067–70.

Thorpe JG. (1959) Learning ability during a course of 20 electroshock treatments. *J Ment Sci 105*:1017–21.

Troup PJ, Small JG, Milstein V, Small IF, Zipes DP. (1978) Effect of electroconvulsive therapy on cardiac rhythm, conduction and repolarization. *PACE 1*:171–7.

Tsuang MT, Tidball JS, Geller D. (1979) ECT in a depressed patient with shunt in place for normal pressure hydrocephalus. *Am J Psychiatry 136*:1205–6.

Turner TH, Ur E, Grossman A. (1987) Naloxone has no effect on hormonal responses to ECT in man. *Psychiatry Res 22*:207–12.

Ulett GA, Smith K, Gleser GC. (1956) Evaluation of convulsive and subconvulsive shock therapies utilizing a control group. *Am J Psychiatry 112*: 795–802.

Ulett GA, Das K, Hornung F, Davis D, Johnson M. (1962) Changes in the photically-driven EEG following electroconvulsive therapy. *Journal of Neuropsychiatry 3*:186–9.

Umlauf CW, Gunter RC, Tunnicliffe WW. (1951) Impedance of the human head as observed during electro-shock treatment. *Confinia Neurologica 11*:129–38.

Ungerleider JT. (1960) Acute myocardial infarction and electroconvulsive therapy. *Diseases of the Nervous System 21*:149–53.

Usubiaga JE, Gustafson W, Moya F, Goldstein B. (1967) The effect of intravenous lignocaine on cardiac arrhythmias during electroconvulsive therapy. *Br J Anaesth 39*:867–75.

Valentine M, Keddie KM, Dunne D. (1968) A comparison of techniques in electro-convulsive therapy. *Br J Psychiatry 114*:989–96.

Varma NK, Lee SI. (1992) Nonconvulsive status epilepticus following electroconvulsive therapy [letter]. *Neurology 42*:263–4.

Varma SL, Lal N, Trivedi JK, Anand M. (1988) Post-dexamethasone plasma cortisol levels in depressive patients receiving electro-convulsive therapy. *Indian J Med Res 87*:86–91.

Vetulani J. (1984) Changes in responsiveness of central aminergic structures after chronic ECS. In: B Lerer, RD Weiner, RH Belmaker, eds. *ECT: Basic Mechanisms.* London: John Libbey. pp. 33–45.

Vetulani J. (1986) Relationship between receptor and behavioral changes in the course of chronic treatment with antidepressants and ECT. In: C Shagass, R Josiassen, WH Bridger, KJ Weiss, D Stoff, GM Simpson eds. *Biological Psychiatry 1985.* New York: Elsevier. pp. 162–4.

Villalonga A, Bernardo M, Gomar C, Fita G, Escobar R, Pacheco M. (1993) Cardiovascular response and anesthetic recovery in electroconvulsive therapy with propofol or thiopental. *Convuls Ther 9*:108–11.

Villalonga A, Planella T, Castillo J, Hernandez C, Cabrer C, Manalich M, Towas A, Nalda MA. (1989) Nitroglicerina en nebulizador en la profilaxis de la hipertension inducida por la terapia electroconvulsiva. *Rev Esp Anestesiol Reanim 36*:264–6.

Viparelli U, Viparelli G. (1992) ECT and grand mal epilepsy. *Convuls Ther* 8:39–42.

Viparelli U, Di Lorenzo R, Capasso G, Manieri L, Sciorio G, Viparelli G. (1976) Trattamento con e.shock di inserma psicotica gia operata di commissurotomia mitralica. *Ospedale Psichiatrico* 8:1–10.

Vitkun SA, Boccio RV, Poppers PJ. (1990) Anesthetic management of a patient with neuroleptic malignant syndrome. *J Clin Anesth* 2:188–191.

Volavka J, Feldstein S, Abrams R, Fink M. (1972) EEG and clinical change after bilateral and unilateral electroconvulsive therapy. *Electroencephalogr Clin Neurophysiol* 32:631–9.

Volkow ND, Bellar S, Mullani N, Jould L, Dewey S. (1988) Effects of electroconvulsive therapy on brain glucose metabolism: a preliminary study. *Convuls Ther* 4:199–205.

Walker R, Swartz CM. (1994) Electroconvulsive therapy during high-risk pregnancy. *Gen Hosp Psychiatry* 16:348–53.

Ward C, Stern GM, Pratt RT, McKenna P. (1980) Electroconvulsive therapy in Parkinsonian patients with the ''on-off'' syndrome. *J Neural Transm* 49:133–5.

Warmflash VL, Stricks L, Sackeim HA, Decina P, Nelley P, Malitz S. (1987) Reliability and validity of measures of seizure duration. *Convuls Ther* 3:18–25.

Warnecke L. (1975) A case of manic-depressive illness in childhood. *Can Psychiatr Assoc J* 20:195–200.

Warren AC, Holroyd S, Folstein MF. (1989) Major depression in Down's syndrome. *Br J Psychiatry* 155:202–5.

Watterson D. (1945) The effect of age, head resistance, and other physical factors on the stimulus threshold of electrically induced convulsions. *J Neurol Neurosurg Psychiatry* 8:121–5.

Weatherly J, Villien LM. (1958) Treatment of a case of psychotic depression complicated by aortic homograph replacement. *Am J Psychiatry* 114:1120–1.

Weaver LA, Jr, Williams RW. (1982) The electroconvulsive therapy stimulus. In: R Abrams, WB Essman, eds. *Electroconvulsive Therapy: Biological Foundations and Clinical Applications*. New York: Spectrum Publications. pp. 129–56.

Weaver LA Jr, Ives J, Williams R. (1982) Studies in brief-pulse electroconvulsive therapy: the voltage threshold, interpulse interval, and pulse polarity parameters. *Biol Psychiatry* 171:131–43.

Weaver L, Williams R, Rush S. (1976) Current density in bilateral and unilateral ECT. *Biol Psychiatry* 11:303–12.

Webb MC, Coffey CE, Saunders WR, Cress MM, Weiner RD, Sibert TR. (1990) Cardiovascular response to unilateral electroconvulsive therapy. *Biol Psychiatry* 28:758–766.

Wechsler D. (1945) A standardized memory scale for clinical use. *J Psychol* 19:87–95.

Weckowicz TE, Yonge KA, Cropley AJ, Muir W. (1971) Objective therapy predictors in depression: a multivariate approach. *J Clin Psychol 27*: 4–29.

Weeks D, Freeman CP, Kendell RE. (1980) ECT: III: Enduring cognitive deficits? *Br J Psychiatry 137*:26–37.

Weil-Malherbe H. (1955) The effect of convulsive therapy on plasma adrenaline and noradrenaline. *J Ment Sci 101*:156–62.

Weinberger DR, Torrey EF, Neophytides AN, Wyatt RJ. (1979) Structural abnormalities in the cerebral cortex of chronic schizophrenic patients. *Arch Gen Psychiatry 36*:935–6.

Weiner N. (1985) Drugs that inhibit adrenergic nerves and block adrenergic receptors. In: AG Gilman, LS Goodman, eds. *The Pharmacologic Basis of Therapeutics*, 7th ed. New York: Macmillan. pp. 178–210.

Weiner R. (1980) Review of Breggin P. *Electroshock: Its Brain Disabling Effects. Am J Psychiatry 137*:1144.

Weiner RD. (1979) The psychiatric use of electrically induced seizures. *Am J Psychiatry 136*:1507–17.

Weiner RD. (1980a) ECT and seizure threshold: Effects of stimulus wave form and electrode placement. *Biol Psychiatry 15*:225–41.

Weiner RD. (1980b) The persistence of electroconvulsive therapy-induced changes in the electroencephalogram. *J Nerv Ment Dis 168*:224–8.

Weiner RD. (1981) ECT-induced status epilepticus and further ECT: a case report. *Am J Psychiatry 138:*1237–8.

Weiner RD. (1982) Electroencephalographic correlates of ECT. *Psychopharmacol Bull 18*:78–81.

Weiner RD. (1983a) EEG related to electroconvulsive therapy. In: JR Hughes, WP Wilson, eds. *EEG and Evoked Potentials in Psychiatry and Behavioral Neurology*. Boston: Butterworths, pp. 101–27.

Weiner RD. (1983b) ECT in the physically ill. *Journal of Psychiatric Treatment Evaluation 5*:457–62.

Weiner RD. (1984) Does electroconvulsive therapy cause brain damage? *Behavioral and Brain Sciences 7*:1–53.

Weiner RD. (1988) The first ECT devices. *Convuls Ther 4*:50–61.

Weiner RD, Coffey CE. (1986) Differential ability of ECT devices to produce seizures [letter]. *Convuls Ther 2*:134–5.

Weiner RD, Coffey CE. (1988) Constant current vs constant voltage ECT devices [letter]. *Br J Psychiatry 152*:292–3.

Weiner RD, Coffey CE. (1989) Comparison of brief-pulse and sine wave stimuli [letter]. *Convuls Ther 5*:184–5.

Weiner RD, Krystal AD. (1993) EEG monitoring of ECT seizures. In: CE Coffey, ed. *The Clinical Science of Electroconvulsive Therapy*. Washington DC: American Psychiatric Press. pp. 93–109.

Weiner RD, Henschen GM, Dellasega M, Baker JS. (1979) Propranolol treatment of an ECT-related ventricular arrythmia. *Am J Psychiatry 136*: 1594–5.

Weiner RD, Volow MR, Gianturco DT, Cavenar JO, Jr. (1980a) Seizures terminable and interminable with ECT. *Am J Psychiatry 137*: 1416–8.

Weiner RD, Whanger AD, Erwin CW, Wilson WP. (1980b) Prolonged confusional state and EEG seizure activity following concurrent ECT and lithium use. *Am J Psychiatry 137*:1452–3.

Weiner RD, Rogers HJ, Davidson JRT, Kahn EM. (1986a) Effects of electroconvulsive therapy upon brain electrical activity. *Ann N Y Acad Sci 462*:270–81.

Weiner RD, Rogers HJ, Davidson JRT, Squire LR. (1986b) Effects of stimulus parameters on cognitive side effects. *Ann N Y Acad Sci 462*: 315–25.

Weiner RD, Coffey CE, Krystal AD. (1991) The monitoring and management of electrically induced seizures. *Psychiatr Clin North Am 14*:845–69.

Weingartner H, Gold P, Ballenger JC, Smallberg SA, Summers R, Rubinow DR, Post RM, Goodwin FK. (1981) Effects of vasopressin on human memory functions. *Science 211*:601–3.

Weinger MB, Partridge BL, Hauger R, Mirow A. (1991) Prevention of the cardiovascular and neuroendocrine response to electroconvulsive therapy: I. Effectiveness of pretreatment regimens on hemodynamics. *Anesth Analg 73*:556–62.

Weinstein EA, Kahn RL, Bergman PS. (1959) The effect of electroconvulsive therapy on intractable pain. *Archives of Neurology and Psychiatry 81*: 37–42.

Weinstein MR, Fischer A. (1967) Electroconvulsive treatment of a patient with artificial mitral and aortic valves. *Am J Psychiatry 123*:882–4.

Weiss DM. (1955) Changes in blood pressure with electroshock therapy in a patient receiving chlorpromazine hydrochloride (Thorazine). *Am J Psychiatry 111*:617–9.

Weizman A, Gil-Ad I, Grupper D, Tyano S, Laron Z. (1987) The effect of acute and repeated electroconvulsive treatment on plasma betaendorphin, growth hormone, prolactin and cortisol secretion in depressed patients. *Psychopharmacology 93*:122–6.

Welch CA. (1982) The relative efficacy of unilateral nondominant and bilateral stimulation. *Psychopharmacol Bull 18*:68–70.

Welch CA, Drop LJ. (1989) Cardiovascular effects of ECT. *Convuls Ther 5*: 35–43.

Welch CA, Weiner RD, Weir D, Kahill JF, Rogers HJ, Davidson J, Miller RD, Mandell MR. (1982) Efficacy of ECT in the treatment of depression: waveform and electrode placement considerations. *Psychopharmacol Bull 18*:31–4.

Wells DG, Davies GG. (1987) Hemodynamic changes associated with electroconvulsive therapy. *Anesth Analg 66*:1193–5.

Wells DG, Zelcer J, Treadrae C. (1988) ECT-induced asystole from a subconvulsive shock. *Anesthesia Intensive Care 16*:368–71.

Wells DG, Davies GG, Rosewarne F. (1989) Attenuation of electroconvulsive therapy induced hypertension with sublingual nifedipine. *Anesthesia Intensive Care 17*:31-3.

West ED. (1981) Electric convulsion therapy in depression: a double-blind controlled trial. *Br Med J 282*:355-7.

Whalley LJ, Rosie R, Dick H, Levy G, Watts AG, Sheward WJ, et al. (1982) Immediate increases in plasma prolactin and neurophysin but not other hormones after electroconvulsive therapy. *Lancet 2*:1064-8.

Whalley LJ, Eagles JM, Bowler GM, Bennie JG, Dick HR, McGuire RJ, Fink G. (1987) Selective effects of ECT on hypothalamic-pituitary activity. *Psychol Med 17*:319-28.

White RK, Shea JJ, Jonas MA. (1968) Multiple monitored electroconvulsive treatment. *Am J Psychiatry 125*:622-6.

Widepalm K. (1987) Comparison of fronto-frontal and temporo-parietal unilateral non-dominant ECT. A retrograde memory study. *Acta Psychiatr Scand 75*:441-4.

Widerlöv E, Ekman R, Jensen L, Borglund L, Nyman K. (1989) Arginine vasopressin, but not corticotropin releasing factor, is a potent stimulator of adrenocorticotropic hormone following electroconvulsive treatment. *J Neural Trans 75*:101-9.

Wilcox KW. (1985) The pattern of cognitive reorientation following loss of consciousness. *Papers of the Michigan Academy of Science, Art and Letters 41*:357.

Willerson JT. (1982) Acute myocardial infarction. In: JB Wyngaarden, LH Smith, eds. *Textbook of Medicine*, 16th ed. Philadelphia: WB Saunders. pp. 247-5.

Williams KM, Iacono WG, Remick RA, Greenwood P. (1990) Dichotic perception and memory following electroconvulsive treatment for depression. *Br J Psychiatry 157*:366-72.

Williams M. (1966) Memory disorders associated with electroconvulsive therapy. In: CWM Whitty, OL Zangwill, eds. *Amnesia*. London: Butterworths. pp. 139-49.

Williams M. (1973) Errors in picture recognition after E.C.T. *Neuropsychologia 11*:429-36.

Wilson GF. (1985) Multiple-monitored ECT. *Convuls Ther 1*:144.

Wilson IC, Gottlieb G. (1967) Unilateral electroconvulsive shock therapy. *Diseases of the Nervous System 28*:541-5.

Wilson IC, Vernon JT, Guin T, Sandifer MG. (1963) A controlled study of treatments of depression. *J Neuropsychiatry 4*:331-7.

Wilson WP, Schieve JF, Durham NC, Scheinberg P. (1952) Effect of series of electric shock treatments on cerebral blood flow and metabolism. *Archives of Neurology Psychiatry 68*:651-4.

Windle WF, Groat RA, Fox CA. (1944) Experimental structural alterations in brain during and after concussion. *Surg Gynec Obstetr 79*:561-572.

Windle WF, Krieg WJS, Arieff AJ. (1945) Failure to detect structural changes in the brain after electrical shock. *Quart Bull Northwestern U Med Schl 19*:181–8.

Winkelman NW, Moore MT. (1944) Neurohistopathologic findings in experimental electric shock treatment. *J Neuropathol Exp Neurol 3*:199–209.

Winslade WJ, Liston EH, Ross JW, Weber KD. (1984) Medical, judicial, and statutory regulation of ECT in the United States. *Am J Psychiatry 141*: 1349–55.

Wise MG, Ward SC, Townsend-Parchman W, Gilstrap LC, III, Hauth JC. (1984) Case report of ECT during high-risk pregnancy. *Am J Psychiatry 141*:99–101.

Witztum J, Baker M, Woodruff RA, Jr, Pitts FN, Jr. (1970) Electrotherapy: the effects of methohexital on EKG. *Diseases of the Nervous System 31*:193–5.

Wolff GE. (1957) Results of four years active therapy for chronic mental patients and the value of an individual maintenance dose of ECT. *Am J Psychiatry 114*:453.

Wolford JA. (1957) Electroshock therapy and aortic aneurysm. *Am J Psychiatry 113*:656.

Woodruff RA, Pitts FM, Jr, McClure JN, Jr. (1968) The drug modification of ECT. *Arch Gen Psychiatry 18*:605–11.

Wyant GM, MacDonald WB. (1980) The role of atropine in electroconvulsive therapy. *Anaesthesia Intensive Care 8*:445–50.

Yalow RS, Varsano-Aharon N, Echemendia E, Berson SA. (1969) HGH and ACTH secretory responses to stress. *Horm Metab Res 1*:3–8.

Yassa R, Hoffman H, Canakis M. (1990) The effect of electroconvulsive therapy on tardive dyskinesia: A prospective study. *Convuls Ther 6*:194–8.

Yatham LN, Barry S, Dinan TG, Webb M. (1989) Which patients will respond to ECT? *Br J Psychiatry 154*:879–80.

Yesavage JA, Berens ES. (1980) Multiple monitored electroconvulsive therapy in the elderly. *J Am Geriatr Soc 28*:206–9.

Youmans CR, Jr, Bourianoff G, Allensworth DC, Martin WL, Derrick JR. (1969) Electroshock therapy and cardiac pacemakers. *Am J Surg 118*: 931–7.

Young RC, Alexopoulos GS, Shamoian CA. (1985) Dissociation of motor response from mood and cognition in a parkinsonian patient treated with ECT. *Biol Psychiatry 20*:566–9.

Yudofsky SC. (1979) Parkinson's disease, depression, and electroconvulsive therapy: a clinical and neurobiologic synthesis. *Compr Psychiatry 20*: 579–81.

Zamora EW, Kaelbling R. (1965) Memory and electroconvulsive therapy. *Am J Psychiatry 122*:546–54.

Zamrini EY, Meador KJ, Loring DW, Nichols FT, Lee GP, Figueroa RE et al. (1990) Unilateral cerebral inactivation produces differential left/right heart responses. *Neurology 40*:1408–11.

Zeidenberg P, Smith R, Greene L, Malitz S. (1976) Psychotic depression in a patient with progressive muscular dystrophy: treatment with multiple monitored electroconvulsive therapy. *Diseases of the Nervous System* 37:21–3.

Zhu W-X, Olson DE, Karon BL, Tajik AJ. (1992) *Ann Intern Med 117*: 914–15.

Zibrak JD, Jensen WA, Bloomingdale K. (1988) Aspiration pneumonitis following electroconvulsive therapy in patients with gastroparesis. *Biol Psychiatry 24*:812–14.

Zielinkski RJ, Roose SP, Devanand DP, Woodring S, Sackeim HA. (1993) Cardiovascular complications of ECT in depressed patients with cardiovascular disease. *Am J Psychiatry 150*:904–9.

Zimmerman M, Coryell W, Pfohl B. (1985) The treatment validity of DSM-III melancholic subtyping. *Psychiatr Res 16*:37–43.

Zimmerman M, Coryell W, Stangl D, Pfohl B. (1986) An American validation study of the Newcastle scale. III. Course during index hospitalization and six-month prospective follow-up. *Acta Psychiatr Scand 73*:412–5.

Zimmerman M, Pfohl B, Coryell W, Stangl D. (1987) The prognostic validity of DSM-III Axis IV in depressed patients. *Am J Psychiatry 144*:102–6.

Zinkin D, Birtchnell J. (1968) Unilateral electroconvulsive therapy: Its effects on memory and its therapeutic efficacy. *Br J Psychiatry 114*:973–88.

Zis A, McGarvey KA, Clark CM, Lam RW, Patrick L, Adams SA. (1993) Effect of stimulus energy on electroconvulsive therapy-induced prolactin release. *Convuls Ther 9*:23–7.

Zis AP, Manji HK, Remick RA, Grant BEK, Clark CM. (1989a) Effect of the 5-HT2 antagonist ketanserin on the ECT-induced prolactin release. *Biol Psychiatry 26*:102–6.

Zis AP, Remick RA, Clark CM, Grant BEK, Brown GM. (1989b) Blockade of the postictal prolactin surge by methysergide. *Arch Gen Psychiatry 46*:385–9.

Zis AP, Goumeniok AD, Clark CM, Grant BEK, Remick RA, Lam RW, Garland EJ. (1991) ECT-induced prolactin release: effect of sex, electrode placement and serotonin uptake inhibition. *Hum Psychopharmacology 6*:155–60.

Zis AP, McGarvey KA, Clark CM, Lam RW, Adams SA. (1992) The role of dopamine in seizure-induced prolactin release in humans. *Convuls Ther 8*:126–30.

Zorumski CF, Burke WJ, Rutherford JL, Reich T. (1986) ECT: Clinical variables, seizure duration, and outcome. *Convuls Ther 2*:109–19.

Zung WW, Rogers J, Krugman A. (1968) Effect of electroconvulsive therapy in memory in depressive disorders. *Recent Advances in Biological Psychiatry 10*:160–78.

Zwil AS, Bowring MA, Price TRP, Goetz KL, Greenbarg JB, Kane-Wagner G. (1990) Prospective electroconvulsive therapy in the presence of intracranial tumor. *Convuls Ther 6*:299–307.

Index